Research methods in pharmacy practice

Research Methods in Pharmacy Practice

Felicity Smith

BPharm, MA, PhD, MRPharmS

Reader in Pharmacy Practice
School of Pharmacy
University of London, UK

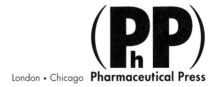

London • Chicago **Pharmaceutical Press**

Published by the Pharmaceutical Press
Publications division of the Royal Pharmaceutical Society of Great Britain

1 Lambeth High Street, London SE1 7JN, UK
100 South Atkinson Road, Suite 206, Grayslake, IL 60030-7820, USA

© Pharmaceutical Press 2002

First published 2002

Text design by Barker/Hilsdon, Lyme Regis, Dorset
Typeset by Type Study, Scarborough, North Yorkshire
Printed in Great Britain by TJ International, Padstow, Cornwall

ISBN 0 85369 481 8

A catalogue record for this book is available from the British Library

Contents

Preface

There are many books devoted to health services research methodology which provide practical guidance on planning and execution of research and/or address the theoretical bases of different approaches and methods. This book differs in two respects from existing texts: firstly, it is dedicated to research in pharmacy settings and the particular challenges that these settings present, and secondly, it focuses on the work of researchers, drawing on their experiences in attending to methodological problems to ensure a robust approach to meeting their research objectives.

This book comprises a review of published research undertaken in pharmacy practice and related settings, which is presented according to the methods employed. Earlier versions of most chapters were published in the *International Journal of Pharmacy Practice*. These original articles have been revised to include recent work, as well as the addition of new sections.

The material is designed to provide guidance for researchers in the preparation, planning and execution of their work. Researchers embarking on a project for the first time will find here a background to the application of different health services research methodologies in pharmacy that will assist them in selecting the approaches best suited to their objectives, and that will be workable in the context of their study setting. This book will aid established researchers, who may be new to the field of pharmacy or undertaking a project employing methods that are unfamiliar, in the identification of potential problems and pitfalls (which should be considered in planning the research) together with details of how they have been addressed by others. The strengths and weaknesses of different methods of health services research are well documented and readily identifiable from many generic research texts on health services. However, throughout the research literature in pharmacy practice there are many examples of innovative approaches that address practical methodological problems. Rather than 're-inventing the wheel', this book should provide researchers with tips and suggestions for addressing potential problems and ensuring feasible methodologies that are practicable and workable in *pharmacy* settings, and will enhance the quality and value of their own work.

Pharmacy practice research is sometimes described as a new discipline. While many factors support this argument (e.g. emergence of new journals, new centres and departments in academic institutions, interest in professional bodies), the preparatory work for this book revealed the vast extent and range of work that has been carried out. Recognition of this expertise was a major impetus for writing this book. It provided an opportunity to draw together past research experiences to enable researchers to benefit from, and build on, the accomplishments and expertise of their colleagues in their future work.

Felicity Smith
December 2001

Acknowledgements

This book could not have been written without the commitment of the pharmacy practice research community to high quality studies. The huge volume and wide range of published research undertaken by fellow pharmacy practice researchers has made the collection and analysis of material both a challenging and stimulating task. Most of the chapters in this book are based on a series of articles that appeared in the *International Journal of Pharmacy Practice*. I would like to thank Jo Lumb, former editor of the Journal, for her enthusiasm and careful reviewing of the original articles.

I am greatly indebted to George Smith for his detailed reading of the manuscript of this book and his constructive comments on both the content and the presentation. I would also like to acknowledge the support of colleagues past and present, in particular from the former Department of General Practice and Primary Care at St Bartholomew's Hospital Medical College and at the School of Pharmacy, University of London. Finally, I would like to thank my family and friends for their interest and encouragement throughout the preparation and writing of this book.

About the author

Felicity Smith is a registered pharmacist with experience of hospital and community pharmacy. After completing her MA in African Studies and her PhD, evaluating the contribution of community pharmacists to primary health care in London, at the Department of General Practice and Primary Care at St Bartholomew's Hospital Medical College in London, Dr Smith joined the academic staff of the School of Pharmacy, University of London. She is currently a Reader in its Centre for Practice and Policy.

Throughout her research career Felicity Smith has remained actively involved in research into many aspects of pharmacy services and drug use. She is experienced in the application of a wide range of health services research methodologies and tools in pharmacy settings. In 1998 she was awarded the first British Pharmaceutical Practice Research Award.

Introduction

Review of health services is an important feature of the agenda of governments across the world. Health care systems are subject to pressures of rising costs, increased use of high technology interventions, higher proportions of elderly people within the populations and rising public expectations. Public sector health services in many countries (in particular Britain and some other European countries) have seen major reforms, and pharmacy services are being reviewed in the light of new policy directions in the delivery and provision of care. In terms of the provision and delivery of health care, issues discernible as priorities to the British Government include information regarding and the assessment of current services, service provision appropriate to the needs and expectations of clients, equality of access to care, evidence-based decision-making in health care, professional accountability and systems for ensuring high standards of care, openness regarding standards and cost-effectiveness to ensure the best use of resources. In both industrialised and developing countries pharmacy has been recognised as possessing unrealised potential in contributing to the health care needs of their populations.

In the context of evolving health policy priorities, the implications for pharmacy services are continually being addressed, both in terms of ensuring existing services meet current needs and in the realisation of potential contributions of the profession to the achievement of wider goals of health policy. Individuals and bodies responsible for the development of health and pharmacy policy and its implementation require information about the needs of their populations, current service provision, the extent to which services meet the population's needs, the feasibility of new developments and the associated costs.

The immediate goals of health services research are to provide background data and experimental evidence from which policy makers can make informed decisions. To perform this role effectively attention must be paid to ensuring the quality of the work, demonstrating that any conclusions can be supported. The principles of rigour in research may be relatively straightforward, for example: appropriate study design, reliability of data collection processes, validity of instruments, clear analytical procedures, and interpretation of the findings in the light of the paradigms and methods employed. However, the relative simplicity of these can mask the difficulties that are encountered in health care and pharmacy practice settings; researchers may be operating among people who are in poor health and possibly preoccupied with subjective experiences and/or practitioners who have many other overriding and immediate priorities.

Although sometimes described as a new discipline, there is a huge body of published research in health services and pharmacy practice. It is a research field that attracts researchers and practitioners from many disciplines. Academics from disciplines including sociology, anthropology, psychology, economics, history and statistics have identified and addressed pertinent questions relevant to health, pharmacy and drug use. In applying their approaches and methods they have drawn on the perspectives of practitioners; at the same time they have stimulated health services and pharmacy practice researchers to incorporate different approaches and methods in their own research.

Health services research methods are commonly distinguished as quantitative or qualitative. Much of the early research draws principally on quantitative approaches. However, qualitative techniques are now well established and their value in addressing important issues in the provision and delivery of health care is acknowledged. Health services research, including pharmacy practice, is eclectic. In planning their work researchers are guided by their research objectives, adopting and adapting methods from many disciplines, that will, most importantly, be effective in meeting their objectives.

The eclectic nature of the pharmacy practice research was taken into account in the preparatory work for this book. Its purpose is to provide guidance for researchers in pharmacy settings in the identification of the major issues (including potential problems and pitfalls) that different methodologies present, and to indicate ways in which these have been, and can be, addressed. Thus, in the selection of published research papers for this review, the aim was to enable the major issues important to the application of different methodological approaches in pharmacy settings to be identified and discussed. Extensive hand-searches of published papers were undertaken covering the main English language journals of the research field. Studies in non-pharmacy but related settings which addressed methodological issues relevant to pharmacy issues and/or provided alternative perspectives on problems faced by pharmacy practice researchers were also included. Conference abstracts were excluded as they would not contain the level of methodological detail required, and many studies presented would subsequently appear as full papers.

While the generic strengths and weaknesses of different methods are well documented in many texts, the focus of this book is on their application by pharmacy practice researchers. By drawing on the experience of previous research for the different approaches that have been employed, it has been possible to identify the potential problems that may arise and describe ways in which they can be addressed. Thus, this book differs from extant research texts on health services in that it draws on the research experience and expertise of established researchers and is dedicated to the particular challenges of pharmacy settings.

Each chapter is devoted to the application of particular research methods and techniques. Chapters 1 and 2 focus on the application of survey methodology in pharmacy practice. Survey research accounts for a greater proportion of pharmacy practice research than any other approach. Issues important to the success of survey research include the identification of suitable sampling frames and adoption of appropriate sampling procedures, achievement of good response rates and management of non-response, the development of survey instruments, and ensuring validity, reliability and generalisability of data.

The wide application of survey methods means that there is great experience and expertise in their use in pharmacy settings and thus many examples to draw on. Surveys have been employed in many settings and applied to a wide range of topic areas, from the documentation of activities to the measurement of views and attitudes. The availability of computer statistical software packages has led to widespread application of sophisticated analytical procedures. The application of survey methods to the development of theoretical perspectives is discussed in Chapter 3.

Qualitative research, which is perhaps less familiar to researchers from traditional science disciplines, is reviewed in Chapter 4. This work typically involves small samples, non-probability sampling procedures, and the collection of detailed data which frequently comprises subjective opinions of individuals who may be describing their views or reporting their experiences. But in qualitative work, it remains important to maintain a scientific approach and demonstrate that attention has been paid to the important principles of qualitative inquiry throughout the planning and conduct of the research, for example, informed sampling procedures, validity of data collection and objectivity in analytical procedures. The development of health services that are sensitive to the needs of consumers is an important focus of health policy. Focus groups, discussed in Chapter 5, have been widely used to identify and explore issues from the perspective of different population groups. They provide a technique in which priorities of participants can be identified and insights gained into their reasoning and argument. Group techniques have also been used in the establishment of consensus.

Observation studies are the subject of Chapter 6. The majority of these studies involved non-participant observation (i.e. an independent observer); however, there are some examples of research by participant observers. Observation has the advantages that the researcher has control over the quality and completeness of data, and that data relates to actual events rather than depending on people's self-reports, which may be marred by poor estimates, memory effects and doubtful diligence in adherence to study procedures. However, the major drawback is the 'Hawthorne' effect, in which people being observed, knowingly or unknowingly, modify their behaviour when being observed.

Triangulation (Chapter 7), which is the combination of different methods or approaches in a single study, is common in health services research. There is some controversy regarding the mixing of methods which purists argue emanate from different scientific disciplines with their own ontologies and epistemologies. The theoretical rationale of triangulation has been addressed on the different levels of approaches, methods and data. However, the decisions of health services and pharmacy practice researchers regarding the selection of methods are based on which methods will be most effective in meeting their study objectives. All methods have their own strengths and weaknesses; combining methods enables investigation from different perspectives as well as providing a means of validation of findings.

The final two chapters focus on the evaluation of both existing and innovative pharmacy services. These studies are numerous, demonstrating the commitment of many pharmacists to extending the services they offer and to a genuine interest in the assessment of their value. Chapter 8 discusses the application of different study designs and frameworks. The choice of design will depend on the study objectives and must be workable in the context of the delivery of services, but it will also determine the extent to which outcomes can be attributed to antecedent care. A wide range of methods has been employed in the evaluation of services. Although discussed in earlier chapters their application to service evaluation is briefly considered in Chapter 9. The evaluation of health care interventions requires the identification of outcome measures relevant to the expected outcomes. For a successful and fair evaluation these measures must be sensitive to anticipated change and be reliable. Chapter 9 also reviews the development and selection of measures which have been employed in the evaluation of pharmacy services. In the context of changing health care policies and priorities, pharmacy services are continually evolving. Researchers have an important role in the development of the profession by documenting current practices, identifying needs and assessing the extent to which pharmacy services meet these needs, evaluating the feasibility and effectiveness of existing and extended services to ensure that the potential contribution of the professional to health care in the 21st century is realised.

In the preparatory work for this book, the wide range and large volume of research in pharmacy rapidly became apparent. There is a committed body of researchers who demonstrate a contemporary awareness of health policy, changing priorities and expectations of professionals and the public, and the potential contribution of pharmacy to health care. Their research output provides an invaluable aid in informing and guiding future services. Thus, the pharmacy profession can benefit from an ongoing commentary from researchers on both existing activities and potential developments. The extensive literature testifies to researchers' readiness to adopt and apply new techniques, their resourcefulness and commitment to solving problems and their foresight in identifying important issues for the future of pharmacy. I hope that this book will be an aid to future researchers, who in their work will build on the experience and expertise of their colleagues.

1

Survey research: design, samples and response

Social survey methodology is the most widely used approach by pharmacy practice researchers, accounting for a higher proportion of published papers than any other. Many texts have addressed the general strengths and problems of conducting social surveys.[1-5] Survey techniques have encompassed a wide range of research objectives in a variety of populations in pharmacy and related settings. There is a vast literature representing a wealth of experience of the application of survey techniques by pharmacy practice researchers. The large number of studies enables identification of the strengths and difficulties of survey research that are particular to pharmacy settings. Even the briefest of reviews of this literature would demonstrate researchers' awareness of the need for sound scientific methodology. Their commitment to this endeavour is apparent from the range of techniques and approaches, often innovative, that were devised to address problems presented by survey research. The general problems of survey research are well documented. Based on the experience of pharmacy practice researchers, manifested in their published work, Chapters 1 and 2 of this book provide a review of the particular considerations that survey research in pharmacy settings present, explore the ways in which difficulties have been addressed, and the levels of success.

Throughout the planning and conduct of a survey, researchers have to contemplate the advantages and disadvantages of different approaches and make choices: for instance, balancing resources against sample size, sampling procedures and generalisability; choosing the number of mailings and achieving adequate response rates; selecting procedures for the conduct of the study and maintaining validity of findings.

Social surveys are often viewed as a relatively quick and cheap method of obtaining information from a large number of respondents. However, the time required and the costs are easily underestimated. Aside from steps in planning the research to ensure methodological rigour, including preliminary fieldwork and piloting, the administrative tasks alone of conducting a large-scale survey are appreciable. Preparation of letters, questionnaires, envelopes for despatch and return, reminders and follow-up of non-responders require diligent record keeping and are time-consuming tasks. In order to achieve acceptable response rates, repeat mailings a few weeks apart are usually conducted; thus the process of data collection may well span several months. The costs of a postal survey are generally lower than for data collected by interview, especially if the population is widespread. However, costs of postage for despatch and return of questionnaires, repeat mailings, telephone follow-up, stationery, printing, and administrative support are not insignificant.

In this first chapter, issues relating to research objectives and design, populations and samples, response rates and management of non-response are reviewed. The following chapter focuses on the development of survey instruments, and the issues of validity, reliability and generalisability.

Research objectives

Survey research is viewed as a quantitative approach, data being collected from a sample of sufficient size to enable generalisations to be made to a wider population. Researchers aim to quantify their populations in terms of predetermined characteristics, to identify frequencies of events, to establish the proportion of respondents who hold particular views and/or to describe association between variables.

Survey instruments generally are structured questionnaires, commonly designed for self-completion and often distributed by post. They can be useful for gathering factual information. The reliability and validity of the data depends on respondents being both able and willing to provide the information requested. For example, people may have difficulty in providing information that requires them to remember timing of events or they may be unwilling to provide sensitive information (e.g. that relating to business or personal issues). Self-completion questionnaires, as opposed to those administered by an interviewer, usually provide no opportunity for researchers to follow-up responses to clarify ambiguous replies or, in the case of unexpected responses, to gather more detail. Thus, in deciding to collect data by questionnaire, researchers must consider the extent to which this method will produce data of the reliability and validity required to meet the study objectives.

From the range of subjects of study and specific objectives of survey research in pharmacy, it is apparent that the profession has extensive documentation of current activities, and of the views of professionals and the public on both existing services and new developments. Not surprisingly, as pharmacy practice research is frequently undertaken by pharmacists and/or within pharmacy related organisations, the vast majority of surveys focus on issues that are important to the profession and its development, often with the explicit aim of informing change and facilitating progress; for example, 'Sports care and the pharmacist: an opportunity not to be missed'.[6] In recent years researchers have provided valuable and detailed information on the major debates and developments within pharmacy. Thus, examples of studies include surveys on workforce issues,[7–11] views and implementation of specific service initiatives and policy decisions,[12–20] the application of practice guidelines,[21–24] a wide range of aspects of consumer perspectives of pharmacy services[25–30] and perspectives of other professional groups on pharmacy related issues.[31–36]

Survey techniques have been applied to identify the views, beliefs and attitudes of pharmacists, the public and other professional groups on pharmacy-related issues. Beliefs and attitudes are often seen as important determinants of practice and indicators of the feasibility of change. However, the complexities of attitudes as constructs present difficulties for researchers in ensuring the validity and reliability of instruments (see Chapter 2).

There are many examples of surveys in which a theoretical framework (e.g. sociological or psychological) provides a basis for the research. Theories to explain or predict people's health beliefs or behaviour, which have been operationalised as a survey instrument (e.g. theories of health beliefs and their associated measures) have also been incorporated into survey research by pharmacy researchers. Through survey work, researchers have endeavoured to apply, test and/or contribute to the development of health-related theories relevant to aspects of pharmacy services and drug use (see Chapter 3).

Study design

Most of the surveys that have been undertaken are descriptive studies in that they aim to portray the characteristics, activities and/or opinions of a population. The vast majority of studies are also cross-sectional in that the population is approached on a single occasion. In a cross-sectional survey, retrospective data are sometimes collected, in that respondents are asked to recall events. In a study of prescribing and dispensing for drug misusers in primary care in Scotland, information was requested on the prescriptions held in the pharmacy at the time of the survey.[37] This was a cross-sectional study in that the data related to one point in time. The reliability of the information would not have been hampered by the effect of memory.

If sample sizes are adequate, survey data enable the exploration of associations between the responses of population subgroups on variables within the data set. Such comparisons in cross-sectional surveys are common. Any associations are generally reported descriptively, although researchers may hypothesise regarding the direction of associations (e.g. possible causal relationships) which may warrant further investigation.

Some studies are specifically designed (through sampling and analytical procedures) to compare the opinions or practices of two or more population groups. These have included studies of the views of different professional groups,[31,32,34,38–48] comparisons of pharmacists and their clients,[47,49] or studies spanning international[50–52] or regional boundaries.[44] Researchers have also designed studies to establish differences between pharmacy populations, for example comparison of career paths and aspirations of white and ethnic minority pharmacists.[53]

Experimental studies designed to test a hypothesis, although a less common feature of survey research, have been undertaken.[54–57] A study to investigate the influence of health locus of control and perceived susceptibility to illness on the use of self-care protocols divided participants into two groups prior to data collection, one which received self-care protocols and one which did not.[54] In a study comparing the acceptability and degree of understandability of drug information leaflets, differences between groups were assessed using a structured questionnaire.[57]

Use of non-prescription medications by patients with congestive heart failure was compared with that of a matched control group. Participants in the study were requested to identify and recruit individuals to act as 'controls' who were 'loosely matched' to participants in terms of economic status and education.[56]

Longitudinal (or cohort) studies, in which a sample is followed-up over a period of time, are less common. Longitudinal studies enable researchers to obtain data on the course of events (i.e. descriptive data), providing more reliable information on the timing of events and the temporal relationships between variables. Thus, longitudinal studies are generally more powerful than cross-sectional studies in providing information on possible causal relationships. In a study of schoolchildren in Luo, Kenya, to observe associations between single symptoms and specific measures taken to deal with them, data were gathered in weekly interviews with the children for a period of 30 weeks. In each interview the child was asked about illness episodes, events, and actions in the previous week. Thus, children had to recall over a seven-day period, but the researchers obtained descriptive data of sequences of events over a period of many weeks.[58]

Longitudinal studies, appropriate for many research questions, are often less attractive to researchers (and funders) because of the time-lag to conclusions. Studies that involve follow-up of individuals over a period of time require at least this specified period for the data collection. Problems of follow-up and attrition are also greater for these studies. Tracing individuals who have moved, which can be essential for reliable, generalisable data, can be expensive and time-consuming, and may not be successful. Longitudinal studies in the pharmacy literature include the follow-up of a cohort of pharmacy students into their early careers,[59] and a study of mefloquine and chloroquine/proguanil users after return from their travels to assess adherence and associated factors.[60] Longitudinal data on symptoms and illness behaviour have also been obtained through diaries which were maintained by study participants over a period of four weeks.[61]

To investigate changes in practice or views over time, data have been collected in a series of cross-sectional studies. These differ from longitudinal studies in that the initial and subsequent questionnaires are not necessarily completed by the same individuals. Repeat cross-sectional studies have been used to investigate use of patient medication records at two points in time,[62–64] changes in medical practitioners' views on pharmacists giving advice to clients,[65,66] services to intravenous drug users,[67] and to study product use before and after switching from prescription-only to non-prescription status.[68,69]

Populations and settings

There are examples of surveys among pharmacists from all branches of the profession. The greatest number involve community pharmacists, but others include pharmacists in various hospital specialities,[70–73] health authorities,[21,74–78] and industrial personnel.[79,80] Survey research has also been conducted among general medical practitioners, for example on interprofessional issues[33,34,40–45,47,48,65,66,81–85]; studies among other professional groups have been undertaken, although there are less of them.[6,21,31,32,75,76,86–89] In addressing the public's perspectives, samples ranged from those that were population-based (representative of the population as a whole) to surveys of specific patient or client groups, one of the most unusual being employees of Danish slaughterhouses.[90]

Sampling procedures

Identification of, and access to, the population of interest is one of the first considerations of any researcher. A random sample is desirable as this allows the application of probability statistics and generalisation to the population from which the sample is drawn.

A random sample is defined as one into which every member of the population has an equal chance of being selected. The selection of a random sample from a population requires a sampling frame, which comprises a list of all members of the population. From this list a random sample can be selected using random numbers or, provided the researcher can be confident that there is no ordering of entries or patterns within the sampling frame, a systematic procedure such as the selection of every tenth person on the list[23,91] can be employed.

Successful random sampling requires a complete and up-to-date sampling frame. Computerised pharmacy records, which are almost universally maintained in the Netherlands, were used to identify the characteristics of users of benzodiazepines.[92] In a survey of pharmacies and herbal medicines in the USA, 6% of questionnaires were returned 'undeliverable', possibly indicating an incomplete sampling frame or one that was not regularly updated.[93]

Cluster sampling and stratified sampling are alternative sampling procedures that still may maintain features of randomness, such that probability statistics can be applied. Cluster sampling involves the division of the population into clusters (for instance, dividing a large geographical area into smaller ones), from which a number of clusters is then selected at random, individuals being, in their turn, randomly selected from within these clusters. Cluster sampling may be conducted in one[13] two[94,95] or more stages, and is sometimes combined with stratification[26] (see below). To investigate the characteristics of pharmacy's clientele, researchers commissioned a survey by the Office for National Statistics (ONS) which undertakes the decennial census of the British population. This survey, which formed part of one of the ONS omnibus surveys, included a random sample of the British population drawn from a sampling frame based on the Postcode Address File, which includes all private household addresses. Sampling was conducted in two stages. A random sample of 100 postal sectors was drawn (i.e. the respondents were selected from within 100 clusters) which were then stratified by region. Interviews were then conducted with selected members of the public in private households.[26]

In a survey of consumer perspectives of pharmacy services in which data were collected by telephone, a multistage sampling procedure was adopted: a random sample of telephone exchanges, selection of households from telephone directories within these exchanges, followed by selection of individuals within each household.[94]

Stratified sampling has been employed by researchers wishing to compare population groups.[96–102] Researchers investigating the relationship between occupational inheritance and business orientation in pharmacy required samples of pharmacists with or without a familial background in pharmacy.[102] They conducted a screening questionnaire, on the basis of which they grouped the respondents into strata of those with and those without familial backgrounds in pharmacy, and then randomly sampled 200 pharmacists from each of the strata. By adopting a stratification procedure they were assured that the numbers in each group were adequate to undertake a statistical comparison. In a study of consumer satisfaction and loyalty to community pharmacies in which different levels of drug information were provided, researchers stratified pharmacies into high, medium and low providers. High providers were pharmacies that had implemented work-flow changes to accommodate a sit-down consultation style; pharmacies currently in the process of implementing work-flow changes were defined as medium providers, and low providers were those pharmacies that were operating in the traditional way.[103] Again, by stratifying the sample the researchers could ensure sufficient numbers of pharmacies in each group for comparisons to be made.

In a survey of the patterns of utilisation of pharmacies, data were collected in three private pharmacies in three 'contrasting' areas of the Gaza Strip, Palestine. Whilst this approach may illuminate possible diversity between pharmacies in different locations, it was unclear how these were selected and to what extent they were representative.[104]

Quota and convenience samples are not randomly selected and care should be taken before making any claims regarding the generalisability of results. Quota samples that depend on the selection of specific numbers of individuals in different age groups, and proportions of male and female respondents, are commonly used in market research. They have also been used to select individuals in public places to achieve a degree of representativeness when random sampling is not possible.

Convenience samples, the selection of the most readily accessible or willing individuals as participants, for which no claims to representativeness can generally be made, may be useful to obtain information rapidly and cheaply on an otherwise inaccessible population. In these cases, generalisation to a wider population is not appropriate, although findings may provide useful data, especially in the early or exploratory stages of survey research. However, convenience sampling when a random procedure could be employed diminishes the generalisability, and hence the value, of the research.

Convenience samples have been employed to select pharmacists in situations when a high degree of practitioner involvement is required, such as assistance with data collection.[105–108] In such cases, co-operation may be difficult to achieve from individuals who do not share an interest in the topic being studied. The data collected by 'volunteer' samples may or may not be representative of a wider population. However, potential biases as a result of self-selection of participants may be unrelated to variables under study and thus the generalisability of the findings may not be greatly compromised. Membership lists of special interest organisations provide readily accessible sampling frames, but they are self-selecting, and the extent to which members are representative of a wider population must be addressed.[54,73,86,109,110]

There are also examples of opportunistic samples, which share features of convenience samples in terms of the selection procedure, but may also be representative of the population of interest. Examples include conference delegates.[111,112] Specialist conferences in particular may attract a high proportion of the population of interest (e.g. a study of English prescribing advisors[111]) and thus provide representative results. To study the use of non-prescription complementary remedies by arthritis sufferers, researchers used as a sampling frame a list of individuals who contacted their university department following an incorrect report in a magazine that the department was recruiting patients for a trial of complementary therapy. Although representativeness with respect to a wider population was unclear, researchers did not wish to lose the opportunity to undertake some research among this population; they conducted a postal survey of use of complementary therapies.[113]

Sampling pharmacists

Community pharmacists

In Britain, many researchers have used the Register of Premises[114] maintained by the Royal Pharmaceutical Society of Great Britain, which provides a complete list of all registered pharmacies by postal district.

Similar lists maintained by professional associations have been used as sampling frames in other countries.[51,55,96,99,115–118] A common alternative is the lists maintained by health authorities of pharmacists who are contracted to provide services.[119–121]

In using these lists the unit of sampling becomes the pharmacy (via the contractor) rather than the pharmacist. In locations in which the vast majority of pharmacies employ a single regular pharmacist, the sample may be broadly representative of the population of pharmacists. However, with more complex employment patterns, the extent to which respondents truly reflect manager, proprietor, locum or second pharmacists will be unclear. Pharmacists in pharmacies with more than one pharmacist have a smaller chance of being recruited into the sample. The problem may be more important when investigating the views and practices of individual pharmacists than for information relating to service provision from the pharmacy.

A decision has to be made regarding to whom to address the questionnaire. This may depend on the objectives of the study; for example, pharmacy managers may be in a position to provide the most reliable information regarding the practice and activities of the pharmacy. Researchers have sometimes reported directing the postal questionnaire to 'the pharmacist-in-charge',[122,123] but in these cases second (third, fourth, etc.) pharmacists and locum pharmacists are excluded.[124] Locum pharmacists may leave correspondence for the managing pharmacist, thus excluding themselves from the data set. In a survey of community pharmacists' attitudes to research, questionnaires were addressed to 'the pharmacist working in the pharmacy today'.[125] This may result in a sample more representative of all practising community pharmacists.

Researchers in Australia investigating pharmacists' preferences for cough suppressants[126–127] directed the questionnaire to 'the pharmacist dealing with most non-prescription product recommendations'. As a result of this targeting they recognised that they were unable to investigate non-responders as a comparison group did not exist.

Another approach has been to forward more than one questionnaire to each address[128] or to 'larger' pharmacies[17] in the hope of obtaining responses from a higher proportion, and therefore more representative sample, of pharmacists. However, because the sample size is undefined, response rates cannot be determined and the researcher is unable to assess either representativeness of the sample or non-response bias.

One study of community pharmacists in Britain used Royal Pharmaceutical Society local branch registers, from which the researchers excluded from the mailing those pharmacists known to be employed in other sectors of the profession. Some forms were returned by individuals who indicated that they were not working as community pharmacists, the remaining respondents forming a sample of community pharmacists of varying occupational status.[18] A list of all pharmacists in Michigan in which community pharmacists were not identified was combined with practice site codes. This enabled the elimination of some practitioners but still did not allow identification of all community pharmacists; ultimately, all pharmacists possibly eligible were mailed and only those who were community pharmacists were asked to complete the questionnaire, the others being asked to indicate their ineligibility.[100]

In a study of Dutch and Swedish community pharmacists including those in a combined hospital–community setting, to obtain a sample of Dutch pharmacists,[52] pharmacy address lists had to be combined with practice site codes of pharmacists extracted from professional registers. In contrast, in Sweden, all pharmacies were part of the National Corporation of Swedish Pharmacies, which maintained a staff record.[52,129]

Lists maintained by health authorities and professional associations are generally believed to be up-to-date and reliable. Other sources such as telephone directories[130] have been used in the past. These may be less dependable, because directories may be incomplete, there is a time-lag in their compilation and publication, and pharmacies may have multiple lines, etc. A list provided by the Washington State Board, USA included the names and addresses of over 2000 pharmacists but whether this was a comprehensive listing of all pharmacists was unclear.[131]

Lists maintained by other organisations and used as sampling frames may represent subpopulations of pharmacists, for example the National Pharmaceutical Association in Britain,[23,91] pharmacies of a large multiple chain in the UK,[132] and those employed by a single (although large) company in the USA.[133] This confers an advantage of accessible sampling frames and possibly increased response rates following internal distribution. However, this must be offset by the restricted generalisability. In the case of studies conducted among members of a large organisation, the validity of the responses may also be questionable if respondents are in any doubt about the independence of the study or if it requests respondents to comment on issues for which there is a company policy.

Surveys in which pharmacists have been asked to collect data during the course of their work have sometimes necessarily involved self-selecting samples of pharmacist volunteers because of the level of involvement required. Participants have been recruited through professional journals, professional meetings or mass mailings.[105–108,111–113]

Other pharmacists

Lists of hospital pharmacists in Britain are not so easily available. To obtain samples of hospital pharmacists, researchers have generally used lists of hospitals[134,135] as sampling frames,[22,70,72,136] and from these selected hospital pharmacies followed by pharmacists. Some studies have focused on subgroups of hospital pharmacists, for example dispensary managers,[70] or those associated with drug and therapeutics committees or formularies,[71,72] or members of special interest organisations.[54,73,86,109,110]

Screening questionnaires have also been used to identify pharmacists with particular practices or interests.[16,102,137] The success of this approach to obtain a sampling frame depends on comprehensive distribution of, and good response rates to, the screening questionnaire.

To survey the views of pharmacists working with general practices on prescribing issues, for whom no sampling frame was readily available, potential participants were identified from the respondents to a previous advertisement in a professional journal which had provided a contact address for pharmacists working with general medical practitioners who were interested in forming a national association. This sample was supplemented by contacting health authority personnel to whom such pharmacists may be known.[138]

Sampling frames for pharmacy students will generally be readily available, especially if the study is restricted to one school of pharmacy.[53,59,139,140] A world-wide study of schools of pharmacy used an address list of all schools known to FIP (International Pharmacy Federation); the authors acknowledged that the completeness of the list was unknown.[50]

Sampling other professional groups

Sources of sampling frames for studies among general practitioners (GPs) and physicians vary between countries, often depending on the health care system. Medical practitioners may be salaried workers, health service contractors or private practitioners. Sampling frames may be accessible through health authorities, professional organisations and/or commercial lists. Health authority lists are most commonly used as sampling frames for general medical practitioners in

Britain.[31,33,40,41,65,66,83–85] These lists include all GPs contracted to the National Health Service and they allow researchers to sample by individual practitioner[41,66,84] or by practice,[65,85] depending on their study objectives. Other practitioners in community health settings have also been accessed through these routes.[31,89] Practitioners in secondary care in Britain are generally employees of, and therefore accessed through, the hospital or trust.[32] Elsewhere, studies involving random samples have been conducted among municipal GPs and others having financial agreements with the municipality in Oslo,[82] GPs in New Zealand,[81] and physicians in the Netherlands, Sweden and Finland.[34,45,141] Staff in residential or nursing homes in both Norway and Britain have been contacted through local or district authorities.[87,142]

In a survey intended to establish the views of health authority general managers on future pharmaceutical services, many of the questionnaires were re-directed by the targeted respondents to their pharmacy staff. Although the goals of the organisation may be reflected by either group, professional perspectives and personal opinions may differ.[76] Perhaps in this study, the health authority managers had not understood that their own views were being sought by the researchers, believing their pharmacy staff to be the most appropriate respondents. In another study of this population a similar problem was not reported.[21]

A survey of members of special interest organisations was conducted to investigate the attitudes of a range of health care professionals towards patient counselling on drug–nutrient interactions.[86] Although some interesting information might have been obtained, the membership (as for pharmacist special interest groups) will have been self-selecting and not necessarily representative of individuals outside the organisation.

Sampling for population-based surveys

A number of different approaches have been used to obtain samples representative of the total population. The ideal sampling frame is a list of all members of the population. However, where these exist they often present limitations.

In Britain, researchers have used electoral registers as sampling frames for defined geographical areas.[47,97,98,101,143–147] These lists include a high proportion of the population. They are less reliable in areas with populations of high mobility, in particular inner city areas. The comprehensiveness and representativeness may also be affected by their political and financial applications. For example, following the introduction of the short-lived 'poll tax' in Britain in the 1990s it was found that many individuals, often concentrated in particular population subgroups and geographical areas, were less likely to register. Similar considerations have led researchers to question the reliability of the decennial census in Britain.[148] Local population registers have been used as sampling frames for a population-based study by pharmacy practice researchers in Finland.[95] Population registers for areas of Sweden were successfully used as a sampling frame to recruit a random sample of people in a survey on deregulation of, and access to, non-prescription drugs.[149]

Electoral registers have also been used to sample for a study of ethnic minority consumers of community pharmacy services. The sample was selected by name from the registers of purposively selected locations; that is, those who would be expected to meet researchers' needs, in this case those including higher proportions of people in ethnic minority groups. The 'name' method was considered satisfactory for Asian groups. It was less successful for black Caribbeans, 23% of those selected being white, and as a result a booster sample was required to obtain sufficient numbers.[97,98]

Five hundred ethnic minority pharmacists and 500 non-ethnic minority pharmacists were identified by surname to determine whether career profiles and ambitions of UK pharmacists differed among ethnic groups and gender subpopulations. Authors recognised that this method of identification might fail to identify pharmacists of Afro-Caribbean origin, but believed that there were relatively few pharmacists in that group.[150] The response rates were also low, thus the participating ethnic minority pharmacists might not include a fair representation of the different groups in pharmacy employment.

To ensure a comprehensive sampling frame, a study of elderly people in their own homes combined electoral registers with lists held by health authorities for the same areas.[30]

The Postcode Address File has been used as a sampling frame to investigate characteristics of pharmacies' clientele.[26] This includes all private household addresses, but not the names of individual residents. For this reason, researchers conducting a postal survey opted to use electoral registers, believing that personalising the mailing would improve response rates.[144] The Postcode Address File is used in many large-scale social surveys in which data are collected by home interviews. In these cases researchers visit each selected household and follow procedures (e.g. Kish grids[1]) for random selection of individuals from within them.[151] Weightings may also be applied to adjust for different sized households: people in large households would otherwise have a smaller chance of being included in the sample.

Data on child illness and treatment behaviour in Guatemala came from a wider survey of family health which was based on a sample of households in rural communities. One hundred households from each of six communities were contacted and an adult member from each provided information on all household residents. The resulting household roster was used to identify all female residents aged 18–35 years who were eligible to participate in a detailed individual interview.[152]

Researchers collecting survey data by telephone have used telephone directories to sample their participants.[65,151,153] In the past this method was criticised for bias as people without a telephone would be excluded, although one group of researchers reported that 98% of US households had telephones.[153] Ex-directory numbers and households with multiple lines also lead to selection bias.

Selection of an individual within a household once a telephone number has been included can also present problems. For example, in conducting telephone surveys, it may be difficult to ensure that individuals living in residential homes or other institutions, those with disabilities, or those who speak a different language from the researcher are fairly represented.

Researchers investigating patient role orientation to pharmacy consultation randomly selected households through telephone directories and from within each household asked the 'person within the household who most often purchased prescriptions' to respond.[94] By targeting these individuals within a household, interesting data may be obtained, but it is unclear to what extent those interviewed may be representative of a wider population. To investigate consumer awareness, purchases and information sources for non-prescription drugs, random digit dialling was employed for the selection of people for a telephone interview in the State of Georgia, USA.[154] The authors reported that they used a two-stage procedure which included stratification of the household sample in terms of age and sex to ensure representativeness with respect to these variables. Following the selection of numbers from Australian electronic telephone directories, 'Kish' grids[1] were employed as a means of randomly selecting a single respondent from each contacted household.[151]

General medical practice databases have also been used to draw population based samples.[143,155] The proportion of individuals registered with a general medical practitioner in Britain is estimated to be around 98%, although there is variation between different areas and population groups. Thus a sample drawn from patients registered with local medical practices should provide a broadly representative sample of the people in an area. Use of these sources can present ethical problems regarding the confidentiality of information.

Few countries have a general medical practitioner system similar to the UK. In the USA, health maintenance organisation policy holders have been used as a sampling frame.[54] Because of non-uniformity of health care coverage in the USA, these lists will not be representative of the population as a whole, although they may provide useful information on particular population groups.

Recruitment of respondents by researchers stationed in public places has been used in a number of studies to obtain general population samples,[89,156–158] in particular, shopping areas. Attention has been paid to include shopping centres that are used by a wide cross-section of the population as well as to undertake visits at different times of day and days of the week. Although the sample may include diverse groups, the sample will be restricted to users of the shopping centre, the most frequent shoppers having a greater chance of being included in the sample. The extent to which respondents are representative of the total population may be questionable.

Selection of individuals for interview in these settings can also present a problem. Using dice to determine if each passing shopper should be approached[157] will maintain randomness, although it may be less practicable at busy times. Approaching every tenth person when busy and every fifth at quieter times has also been adopted as a workable procedure.[156] In this case, people who shop at quieter times have a greater chance of being included in the sample. Shopping centres can also be difficult settings in which to elicit co-operation and conduct interviews, as people are preoccupied and the settings afford little privacy. Potentially low response rates may mean the sample is less representative of the total general population than a more scientific sample of shoppers would be, if this were feasible.

Mailing lists that are obtained through commercial firms have been used as a source of consumers.[25,159–161] One list in New York included 151 million consumers in over 78 million households. However, despite the large numbers the representativeness of the sample to the total population is not known.[159]

Door-to-door canvassing of residential buildings in which researchers conducted screening interviews was undertaken to identify users of non-prescription analgesics.[162] Although a time and labour intensive procedure, it indicates the importance that researchers attach to achieving their objectives among a widespread and relatively inaccessible population.

To obtain the views of the public on an extended role for community pharmacy, an alternative to a population-based sample was employed.[163] This involved the selection of four population groups each of which would represent diverse experiences, priorities and views. Different sampling strategies were devised for each group: active elderly people (using age–sex registers of two general practices as the sampling frame), mothers of children under 5 years (from records of a health visitor), carers of people with disabilities (through a carers' newsletter) and people in full-time employment (from Brighton Polytechnic as an employer of a large number of people of diverse background).

Sampling patient and user groups

In many countries, pharmacies are virtually the sole suppliers of medication. Many studies have used community pharmacies as sampling points for pharmacy clients and specific patient groups.[27,48,69,101,108,164–175] Although they may be good sampling points for recruiting users of pharmacy services, data from infrequent or non-users of pharmacies, which may be important for some studies, will be excluded.

In studies involving pharmacy clientele, many researchers have depended on the pharmacists or pharmacy staff to select potential respondents and/or to distribute questionnaires for return either to the pharmacy or with a freepost envelope direct to the researchers. Although eligibility criteria may be clearly stated by the researchers, the actual selection is out of their control. The extent to which protocols are observed may vary for logistical reasons (e.g. between quiet and busy times), as a result of lack of awareness of the importance of adhering to documented selection procedures, or because staff feel more comfortable approaching certain clients (e.g. those they know or do not know, or those considered to be less likely to refuse). Many authors, aware of the sampling bias that may result, acknowledged the importance of ensuring that recruitment procedures are understood by pharmacy staff, that they are workable within the pharmacy setting at busy and quiet times and that they are acceptable to clients. In a study of clients purchasing specific non-prescription products for dyspepsia, pharmacy staff were requested to maintain a record of the number of customers who refused to participate. This enabled the calculation of a refusal rate (40%).[175] In general, the lack of control over recruitment and only limited knowledge of the extent to which they are followed may present problems for researchers who wish to ascertain the extent to which the respondents are representative of the population. Pharmacy clients may also be reluctant to provide honest opinions or experiences if they are concerned how this may reflect on a pharmacist with whom they have a relationship.

In a study of consumers' views of health promotion by pharmacists, data were collected in interviews with clients in the pharmacy. Researchers recognised that once the interviewer was engaged in an interview, others entering the pharmacy would not be approached and would therefore be excluded from participation. This would result in over-representation of people coming in at quieter times. Although this could have been addressed by employing more than one interviewer on the study, it was not possible within the resources of the study.[27] Alternative sampling strategies, such as planning more visits at busier times or interviewing every fifth client, may lead to a more representative sample, but may also compromise the total number of interviews obtained.

Community pharmacy prescription databases have successfully been used to identify patient groups. These have included hypertensive patients,[169] people using hypnotics,[108] and prescription users of non-steroidal anti-inflammatory drugs.[171] In the second of these pharmacy-based studies, a network of 318 community pharmacies in Spain was set up. Participating pharmacy owners interviewed patients coming to the pharmacy for one of the study drugs. A total of 5324 of the 6683 individuals approached were interviewed. Such a study may not be workable in all situations; for example, a lone pharmacist in a busy pharmacy. However, a good response rate was obtained in this case. In the third of these studies, users were invited by pharmacy staff to participate, and once recruited took part in a telephone interview. In another study of patients with osteoarthritis who were prescribed non-steroidal anti-inflammatory drugs, a hospital computer database was used as a sampling frame.[176] A range of hospitals and private surgeries have been successfully used by other researchers to survey self-medication practices of hypertensive patients.[177]

Patient groups have also been identified and selected through medical practices and other health professionals.[46,155,176,178–181] Once again, unless the researcher is directly involved, adherence to study protocols cannot always be assured. Researchers depending on nursing staff to screen for incorrect inhaler use were aware that patients were chosen for the study only when the nursing staff had time.[180] In an interview survey of patients' perspectives of the importance of drug information, ward staff selected patients they perceived as capable of participating.[56]

Patients have been recruited from hospital wards to study aspects of the primary–secondary care interface. Researchers[182–184] reported that for what appeared to be a 'captive' population, recruitment was unexpectedly time-consuming as a result of absences from the ward, ward activity or sleep.

Special interest organisations have also been used as sources of specific patient groups.[110] A postal survey on pharmacy services for breast-feeding mothers included GPs, pharmacists and mothers. The mothers were recruited through a database held by a voluntary organisation, the National Childbirth Trust, UK, which although open to all mothers is, as the authors acknowledge, biased towards people in higher socio-economic groups, educational level and possibly more likely to breast-feed.[185] The sample for a study of use of complementary remedies by people with arthritis was identified following a magazine advertisement.[113] Although self-selecting, such samples may provide a useful source of study participants who are able to contribute data for many studies.

To obtain a sample for a control group in a study of the use of non-prescription medications by patients with congestive heart failure, researchers recruited a matched control group through the study participants. Each participant in the study was requested to give a questionnaire to a friend, neighbour or relative of similar age (within five years) and the same gender who did not reside with him or her and who was not seeing a physician for any heart condition. Questionnaires from the control group were supplied with a stamped addressed envelope for return direct to the investigators. However, the response rates were lower than anticipated, such that patients in the latter part of the study were asked to recruit two others. It is unclear why this method was not as successful as expected; it may be that participants were uncomfortable in approaching family members and friends and/or that 'controls' were less motivated to complete and return the questionnaires.[56]

To investigate adverse events associated with the use of antimalarials, a postal and telephone survey of travellers selected from lists of people who had contacted a health line and been advised to use one of the drugs of interest was conducted.[186] Although not necessarily representative of users of antimalarial drugs, these records provided a source of a large sample of travellers who would otherwise be difficult to identify. To study adherence to medication for malaria prophylaxis, participants were recruited through tour representatives who distributed and collected questionnaires on the final day of their clients' holidays. These clients were also asked for their telephone numbers so they could be contacted regarding their consumption of malaria tablets after their return home.[60]

Other sources of study participants have included schools that were used to investigate management by mothers of childhood fever,[187] and rugby clubs, amateur football clubs and ice skaters to investigate a potential role for pharmacists in sports care.[6] In the latter study the sample was not random but purposively selected to include players of differing ages and abilities in a range of sports.

Ethical issues in identification of samples

There are a number of ethical issues associated with the use of medical records or databases as sampling frames for research. Because a very high proportion of the population of the UK are registered with a general medical practitioner, their records may provide an effective sampling frame for the selection of a sample representative of a local population. They are also valuable for the identification of samples of patients with particular conditions or using specified drugs. Community pharmacies also increasingly maintain records of drugs used by individuals in a local area, based on the supplies they make. However, the data held on these systems are confidential. Researchers do not have the right to access records unless this is specifically granted by the individuals concerned. Thus, identification of samples, survey mailings and/or invitations to participate in research can in the first instance be made only by practitioners who have legitimate access. Researchers commonly work in collaboration with health professionals. For researchers who wish to undertake studies that are clearly independent of the health care establishment or professionals known to potential respondents, these databases may be unsuitable as sampling frames; however, finding alternatives can be problematic. Ethical problems regarding access also present a major disadvantage for researchers in that there may be very limited opportunities for the researcher to follow-up non-responders or assess non-response bias.

A further ethical issue raised by involving health professionals in recruitment of potential participants is ensuring that participants feel free to make a genuine choice regarding whether or not to take part. Although guidelines exist regarding recruitment procedures,[188] the decision of the potential participant could be influenced by their relationship with the practitioner and concerns about possible repercussions. Researchers, of course, for whom representative samples are important, will be keen to encourage participation.

Research in Britain that involves patients and/or resources of the National Health Service must be approved by the appropriate research ethics committees. Research among independent practitioners (including community pharmacists and general practitioners), members of the public or particular population subgroups including members of voluntary organisations, special interest groups that are not overseen by these committees should, of course, comply with accepted guidelines,[188] observing relevant priniciples and meeting similar standards.

Response rates and non-responders

Achieving a high response rate is a major consideration in the planning and execution of survey research. The problem is that the non-responders may differ in some way from the responders such that the data do not represent the population as a whole. The results cannot therefore be generalised to the total population from which the sample was drawn. Studies that have investigated responders and non-responders have found significant differences important to the findings of the study.[189-194] For example, a study into violent crime in community pharmacy found that non-responders were less likely to have been a victim of particular events, with the result that generalisations based solely on the replies of the responders would have been misleading.[191] It is necessary to check for non-response bias and to adjust the findings accordingly before attempting to generalise results to the research population.

Non-responders may include those who refused to participate, people unable to respond (e.g. through disability or inability to read the language of the questionnaire), and those unable to provide the required information. Missing data may also result from researchers omitting to gather information or poorly constructed questions. Response rates of 100% are rarely achieved. When they are,[139,195] these are often studies among 'captive populations', perhaps where people are either unaware that a study is being undertaken or where they feel obliged to participate.

Any sizeable proportion of non-responders introduces potential bias into the findings. This bias cannot be overcome by increasing the sample size.[196] In general, directing resources to achieve a high response is more beneficial, in terms of achieving accurate results, than increasing the sample size. Researchers planning a study should include ample time for the investigation and follow-up of non-responders and the assessment of the likely impact of non-response.

The efforts of pharmacy practice researchers to maximise their response rates demonstrate their awareness of the problems a low response rate presents and their commitment to ensuring high quality research. However, there are many studies in which response rates are not reported or are unclear.

An investigation of the management of oral disease in community pharmacies obtained a response rate of 32%. The authors acknowledged that the response rate was low but because of the quality of the data they did receive, they believed that valid observations could be made and no follow-up of non-responders was necessary.[197] However, without additional information, the data obtained could not be generalised to the two-thirds of pharmacies who did not respond. The high use of protocols (96%) found in a study of community pharmacists, without adjustment for non-response, could be misleading if generalised to a wider population of pharmacists without checking if practices were similar among non-responders.[14] In studies in which response rates are low and no investigation of non-responders is undertaken, the sample is effectively self-selecting and generalisation of findings beyond the sample is speculative.

Tactics used to maximise response rates

For postal questionnaires, the usual practice is to send the questionnaire with a covering letter and a pre-paid envelope for return. The contents of the covering letter are important, and are discussed by Moser and Kalton.[1] They are rarely discussed in published papers except to report that assurances of confidentiality were given.

Great efforts have been made by researchers to secure high response rates. The administrative burden of repeat mailings, reminder letters, telephone calls, careful timing of contacts, avoidance of holiday periods and attention to the content of the covering letter and presentation of questionnaires are all routine considerations for researchers.

Most researchers also send out reminders, generally two to four weeks after the first mailing. These are either postcard reminders, complete repeat mailings or a combination of the two. In the studies reviewed, the number of repeat mailings/reminders varied from none to four. Some researchers commented on these strategies in relation to response rates (see below). Telephone reminders were also used by some researchers, generally towards the end of the data collection when the number of calls required may be expected to be lower. Thus, the whole data collection may be expected to span a one-to-four month period (excluding any investigation of non-responders), although this will also vary with method of data collection, postal questionnaire, interview (telephone or face-to-face), and depending on the number of researchers, location of the study, size of the sample, and process and speed of recruitment.

In an effort to obtain good response rates, researchers have alerted potential respondents in advance to advise them of the study, sometimes by telephone.[12,87,151,198] They have also undertaken personal visits to pharmacies to remind respondents and/or to collect completed questionnaires.[199] They have also conducted telephone interviews with pharmacists to collect responses to pre-mailed questionnaires[200] or with consumers following their recruitment in pharmacies.[20,171,201]

Maximisation of response rates is an important consideration in the methodology. As part of the evaluation of a health promotion pro-gramme in community pharmacy, researchers wished to survey the views of consumers. A questionnaire was devised for self-completion by clients in the pharmacy. However, because pilot work revealed difficulties in obtaining co-operation, a researcher was employed to administer the questionnaire as a structured interview. Further pilot work showed this approach to be more successful.[27]

In a study of part-time community pharmacists, following initial mailing of questionnaires, reminders were sent after one month to non-responders, half of whom received an additional questionnaire with their reminder letter. The response rate from this group was three times that obtained from the group who received a letter only,[11] demonstrating that inclusion of a further questionnaire was worthwhile. An investigation of the effect of a contact by mail prior to a telephone survey obtained a response rate of 76% from those individuals who received a letter and 60% from those who did not.[151]

In a randomised trial of the impact of telephone and recorded delivery reminders on the response rate of patients to research question-naires, significantly more questionnaires were returned following recorded delivery than following telephone reminders. The latter was less expensive, taking account of the costs of time spent by an adminis-trator on each method and costs of calls and postage.[202]

In order to obtain high response rates a number of researchers omitted identification reference numbers from their questionnaires, in the hope that the anonymity that this afforded would encourage people to respond.[17,79,203] Many of these researchers acknowledged that this was at the expense of being able to target reminders to non-responders or investigate differences between responders and non-responders to assess bias. Also, the response rates obtained by these researchers did not suggest that this approach led to higher response rates. The ability to assess bias due to non-response greatly enhances the value of survey research.

Telephone surveys have generally achieved higher response rates. For some researchers this was the reason they opted to conduct the survey by telephone.[75] Researchers who switched part of the way through the data collection from postal to telephone administration of questionnaires achieved much improved response rates.[15,190] These researchers acknowledge that bias may have been introduced by a change in the method of data collection. To ensure a high response rate in a survey of users of non-steroidal anti-inflammatory drugs recruited in community pharmacies, researchers arranged telephone interviews for those people who had not been in a pharmacy (e.g. those for whom a third party collected their prescription) in an attempt to ensure the sample remained representative of all users of these drugs.[171]

Use of incentives

Payment to individuals for participation in research is increasingly a consideration for researchers. Payments may be reimbursement for time or other resources directly resulting from participation in a study, for example locum expenses or time spent collecting data, or nominal payments that serve as incentives to participate, rather than removing disincentives.

In most cases the objective of payments or gifts was to achieve better response rates. However, the true effect on response rates was untested in these studies and the actual impact on response rates was unclear, as overall the response rates achieved were not dissimilar from many other studies. As well as affecting the extent of non-response, incentives may also influence some individuals more than others, thus affecting the nature of non-response bias. Financial incentives, should they become the norm, will also have an impact for funding and ethical implications.

Incentives may be provided more often than they are reported in the literature. However, in a number of studies researchers reported that inducements were offered.[30,116,125,164,195,204–206] In some instances the amounts offered were unspecified, for example 'small honorarium for recruiting patients to a study'.[164] Other inducements included a book on pharmacy management,[116] and the offer of entry into a draw for a free day's locum on return of completed questionnaires,[204] and sachets of coffee and tea with first mailing and duplicate mailings to non-responders.[125]

Interviewees in a survey of consumer preferences among pharmacy needle exchange attendees were given a £5 (approximately 8 euros) voucher to spend in the pharmacy in which the interview took place. Researchers saw this as a way of compensating participants for their time and of thanking pharmacists for their co-operation. A high response rate (97%) was reported.[30]

The design of some studies has enabled researchers to assess the impact of incentives on the response rates by both pharmacists and pharmacy clients. In a study in which community pharmacists were asked to identify and recruit eligible clients from those purchasing one of a selected range of products, the pharmacies were divided into two groups. In 20 pharmacies the medicines were offered free of charge once customers agreed to participate in the study. In a second group, customers paid the normal retail price. Participants were required to complete and return a first questionnaire, following which they were sent a second. The response rate to the first questionnaire was higher among the customers who received the free medicines; however, there was no significant difference in the response rates between the two groups to the second questionnaire. The pharmacists were reported as divided regarding whether or not providing free medicines made recruitment easier.[205] In this study the researchers also investigated the effect of payments to pharmacists on their recruitment rates. The study was divided into two phases. In the first phase the pharmacists were offered no payment and in the second £50 (approximately 80 euros) per week to recruit five patients. Although there was an increase in the recruitment rates in the second phase the authors reported that there was no clear relationship vis-à-vis the incentives.[205]

In another pharmacy-based study in which respondents were recruited in five independent community pharmacies, clients purchasing non-prescription analgesics were allocated to one of four incentive groups: no incentive; £3 (approximately 5 euros) voucher with questionnaire; £3 voucher sent on receipt of questionnaire; and entry into prize draw on receipt of questionnaire. Researchers found no appreciable effect of these incentives on questionnaire returns.[206]

Response rates achieved

The wide variations in response rates are not easy to explain. Researchers sending the same questionnaire to pharmacists or medical practitioners in different regions may obtain very different response rates. A survey involving GPs in two different health regions obtained responses of 24% and 59%, respectively.[44] The response rates from pharmacists in different health authorities in and around London varied from 65 to 84%;[191] another study among pharmacists achieved a 65% response in London and the home counties and 85% in Wales.[64] Variation in response rates between countries is generally not more marked than differences within them.

External factors may have an important impact on response rates, although this is difficult to quantify. The response rate (15%) to a questionnaire survey of pharmacies in South Africa undertaken at the time of a postal strike contrasted with that among pharmacies in a small area local to the researchers where it was possible to hand deliver the questionnaires (100%).[207]

When repeat mailings were conducted and response rates at each stage reported, in general a larger proportion of replies was received following the initial mailing (between half and two-thirds) and usually within a shorter time.[64,124,208,209]

The findings regarding response rates reviewed here may not be representative in that studies that achieve higher response rates may be more likely to be submitted and accepted for publication. A survey of herbal medicines in pharmacies and pharmacists' perceptions of these products achieved a response rate of 26%. The authors described this level of response as 'common' in this population.[93] Response rates of published research, reviewed above, are generally considerably higher than this. However, these rates may not fairly represent researchers' experiences when both published and unpublished research are included.

Community pharmacists

The response rates achieved in published survey research among community pharmacists ranged from as low as 20% to over 90%. In approximately a third of cases the response rates were below 50%, and in a further third they were over 70%. Similar rates were obtained in studies among community pharmacies in many countries, although response rates among community pharmacists in the USA were generally lower. Surveys achieving the highest rates (over 80%) included those in which questionnaire distribution was internal to employees in a large store chain,[132] conducted by telephone[15,200] and involving special interest groups.[109] In general, higher response rates were also achieved by researchers who persisted with repeat mailings. Many researchers who achieved over 70% response performed at least three mailings. The most common practice was two reminders. Questionnaires unnumbered to assure confidentiality in the hope of achieving high response rates did not appear to do so and ruled out any possibility of investigating response bias. It is unclear whether advance warning of research affected the response rates.

Response rates among hospital pharmacists and pharmacy managers were generally higher than among community pharmacists, ranging from 75 to 92% in the studies reviewed. Among pharmacists working with general practices on prescribing issues, response rates varied with method of recruitment. A response rate of 71% was obtained among respondents identified through an advertisement in a professional journal; whereas 37% of pharmacists identified through health authority personnel responded.[138] A response rate of 71% was obtained among a national sample of pharmacists who had participated in a previous study on a related topic, but might reflect a more research friendly population from whom a relatively high response rate may be expected.[9]

Medical practitioners

Response rates among general medical practitioners were similar to those obtained among community pharmacists. In a review of response rates to surveys published in medical journals, a mean response rate of 60% was reported.[92] This was found to vary depending on the subject of study and technique used. Reminders, in writing with a copy of the instrument or by telephone, raised the rate by around 13%. Anonymity and financial incentives were not found to have an effect.[92]

Pharmacy clients

Surveys of pharmacy clients in which questionnaires were handed out at the time of purchase or with a prescription for later return obtained variable response rates ranging from 21 to 88%. In one study, variation in the response rate from different pharmacies ranged from 0 to 98%.[168] Possible reasons are not addressed by the authors. Variation may be a function of the relationship between pharmacists who agree to take part and their clients, differing clientele (e.g. regular or casual clients) or non-uniformity of selection procedures between pharmacies. In these studies it is not usually possible either to remind potential respondents or to follow-up non-responders. Community pharmacists interviewing their clients who were taking hypnotic drugs in Spain[108] achieved an 80% response rate. The sample of participating pharmacies was not random;

however, because of the large network of pharmacists involved, the results may be representative of Spanish users of hypnotics. The study may also have attracted pharmacists who believed that it would be workable in their pharmacy. The authors concluded that the response rate indicated that the method of research was acceptable to many clients.

General public

Response rates around 60% were reported following selection from electoral registers in the UK.[47,101,143–147] A study of members of different ethnic groups obtained response rates varying from 55% for Punjabi speakers to 86% for Gujerati speakers.[97,98] A 73% response was obtained following selection from population registers in Finland;[95] 68% was obtained in a Swedish study.[149] Researchers in the USA who used commercial mailing lists as sources of consumers[19,159,160,210] generally obtained lower response rates (between 15 and 40% in studies reviewed here).

Door-to-door screening interviews were conducted by researchers to identify elderly users of non-prescription analgesics. Screening interviews were successfully conducted with 85% of residents; 78% of residents identified as eligible agreed to a more in-depth interview and 86% of these allowed contact to be made with their physician.[162] Reliable data on response rates of surveys conducted in shopping centres may be difficult to maintain; thus, this information was often not reported.

Other groups

Studies of specific patient or population sub-groups often, but not always, achieved high response rates. Studies in which participants were recruited from 'captive populations' may be assured high rates.[29,59,139,194] A survey of the use of folic acid supplements, conducted with women in three maternity units after delivery of their babies, obtained a response rate of 95%.[29] It will be important to ethics committees that potential respondents in these studies are able to exercise a free choice regarding their participation.

Samples obtained through medical practices, clinics or other health personnel generally obtained high response rates (70–90%),[176,177,186,211] although there were exceptions. In a survey investigating gender differences in physical symptoms and illness behaviour, participants were asked to maintain daily diaries recording information regarding their relevant experiences. As all variables were operationalised as self-report scales, this meant that participants were required to respond to 115 questionnaire items each day. Eighty per cent of the sample which was identified from GP surgeries in the Netherlands completed the health diary for a period of four weeks.[61]

Variable response rates were achieved from samples drawn from membership lists of special interest organisations of patients or professionals[73,86,109,110,212] despite the expectation that these may be high. Studies involving mothers of children under 10 years old, contacted through schools[187] and workers in the Danish slaughterhouse and meat industry,[90] obtained response rates of 76% and 83%, respectively.

A response rate of 30% was obtained[113] in a study of the use of complementary remedies by arthritis sufferers who had supplied their contact details believing that they may be entering a trial of complementary therapies. Whilst this opportunistic sample may have been perceived as research-friendly, their perceptions regarding the nature of the research and the potential benefits to themselves may be important in influencing their decisions regarding participation.

Investigation of non-responders

There were many studies performed in which no investigation of the extent to which non-responders differed from the population as a whole was carried out. Efforts by researchers to determine important differences greatly enhance the generalisability of a study. For some methods of data collection (e.g. interviews in shopping centres) this would be very difficult. Where there is no discussion of potential response bias, it may appear that the researchers do not perceive the importance and relevance of this to their findings. Non-response has been found by a number of researchers to be associated with lack of interest or experience in the study area.[189–191]

When differences were investigated, the most common procedures were comparisons on the basis of demographic variables, geographical location and/or practice characteristics, the data for these being readily available. In the majority of cases, researchers were able to report that no significant differences were found, or to argue that any differences would be unlikely to have an impact on the study findings. However, the most important differences may be those for which data are not easily accessible. Researchers investigating GPs' opinions of drug problems compared responders and non-responders to the initial mailing on the basis of age, sex and practice characteristics and found no significant differences.[82] On the basis of this, they felt justified in not sending reminders. That no significant differences in these variables were found does not mean that important and confounding variation with other variables did not exist. A survey into the use of pharmacies and GPs for advice identified variation in response rates between different age and gender groups.[213] There may be variation between these age and gender groups in their use of services which should be taken into account in the results. There may also be other important differences between responders and non-respondents that are determinants of service use.

In a study of barriers and facilitators to pharmaceutical care, the analysis of non-response bias was based on selected variables collected through telephone interviews from a random sample of non-responders (a total of 30 interviews lasting 4–5 minutes each) in West Virginia, USA. This indicated that non-responders were more likely to be younger and have a less favourable attitude towards customers. The authors therefore urged caution in extrapolating the findings to all rural pharmacies in West Virginia.[214] Non-response bias was investigated in a lifestyle survey by telephoning 400 non-responders to collect information on a small number of important questions. Non-responders were found to differ significantly in their current smoking, hazardous alcohol consumption and lack of moderate or vigorous activity.[193] Characteristics of responders and non-responders were investigated in a study of infant feeding. Non-responders were found to be more similar to bottle-feeding responders than breast-feeding responders; they were also more likely to be smokers, from lower socio-economic groups and to bottle-feed.[215] A survey of the views of GPs on health service changes identified differences between responders and non-responders that would have implications for using research findings as a guide to informing policy making.[194]

Investigation of non-responders should include steps to establish differences in respect of variables central to the study, and not be restricted to those for which data are readily available. Non-responders to a survey of threats and violence at work were found to have been less likely to have experienced certain types of incident than community pharmacists who returned questionnaires. The data obtained in this follow-up of non-responders enabled adjustment of study findings.[191] Similar procedures followed in other studies have demonstrated the importance of conducting investigations of non-responders to assess the impact on the reliability and validity of the findings.[193,208,214,215]

In cases where follow-up of non-responders is not possible, the reasons for non-response may enable some comments to be made about the likely effects. A survey of carers in residential homes obtained a response rate of 75%. Investigation of the reasons for non-response revealed that these were largely due to vacant accommodation, holidays and rostering, which the authors felt would be unlikely to lead to systematic bias.[87]

Another approach that has been employed to assess non-response bias is to compare the replies of early and late responders.[93,100,129,192,216] The basis of this approach is the assumption that any differences between these groups may reflect more profound differences between responders and non-responders; that is, late responders may be similar to non-responders with respect to variables of interest. If no trend is evident between early and late respondents, then researchers assume non-responders may not differ significantly either. Although absence of demonstrable variation is not evidence that no significant differences exist, if a more detailed investigation of non-respondents is not possible this analysis may be a helpful indication of possible biases.

A survey of herbal medicines in pharmacies and pharmacists' perceptions of these products achieved a response rate of 26%. To estimate non-response bias, responses to eight variables were compared between early (first 10%) and late (final 10%) responders. The authors referred to this as a time trends extrapolation test which assumes that late responders are more likely to be similar to non-responders. The two groups were found to differ significantly on only one of the variables examined (staff position), which was not considered to be important to the interpretation of the results.[93]

This approach to the assessment of non-response bias was investigated by researchers who despatched questionnaires in four successive mailshots (initial mailing and three reminders) which was followed by a telephone call to a random sample of non-responders. Questionnaires returned following the first to third mailshots were compared with those from the fourth. All postal responders were then compared with the random sample of non-responders who were followed up by telephone. No significant differences were found between responders from mailshots 1–3 when compared with responders to mailshot 4, although some non-statistically significant trends were discernible. The extent to which differences existed in the respondents from the first three mailshots was not reported. However, statistically significant differences were identified in key variables between postal respondents and those telephoned. The researchers concluded that telephone follow-up of non-responders was required for the detection of non-response bias and corresponding correction of study findings.[192] This study questions the value of comparing early and late responders to draw inferences regarding non-response bias. It also confirms the findings of other researchers, who, when investigating non-responders, have identified significant response bias that affects the conclusion of the research.

Conclusion

Scientific sampling procedures, high response rates and assessment of the impact of non-response bias are important to the quality of survey research; in particular, the generalisability of the findings. The extent to which these can be achieved depends, in part, on the study population and the variables under study. In the survey work that has been undertaken in pharmacy, researchers have demonstrated an awareness of the potential problems, and have explored their implications and how they can be addressed in pharmacy settings.

References

1. Moser C A, Kalton G. *Survey Methods in Social Investigation*. Aldershot: Gower, 1989.
2. Robson C. *Real World Research*. Oxford: Blackwell, 1993.
3. De Vaus D A. *Surveys in Social Research*, 3rd edn. London: UCL Press, 1991.
4. *Pharmacy Practice Research Resource Centre Research Bulletins*. Manchester: PPRRC, 1992–1997.
5. Oppenheim A N. *Questionnaire Design, Interviewing and Attitude Measurement*, 2nd edn. London: Pinter Publishers, 1992.
6. Kayne S, Reeves A. Sports care and the pharmacist: an opportunity not to be missed. *Pharm J* 1994; 253: 66–7.
7. Blenkinsopp A, Boardman H, Jesson J, Wilson K. A pharmacy workforce survey in the West Midlands: 1. Current work profiles and patterns. *Pharm J* 1999; 263: 909–13.
8. Boardman H, Blenkinsopp A, Jesson J, Wilson K. A pharmacy workforce survey in the West Midlands: 2. Changes made and planned for the future. *Pharm J* 2000; 264: 105–8.
9. Gaither C A. An investigation of pharmacists' role stress and the work/ non-work interface. *J Soc Admin Pharm* 1998; 15: 92–103.
10. Ibrahim M I M, Wertheimer A I. Management leadership styles and effectiveness of community pharmacists: a descriptive analysis. *J Soc Admin Pharm* 1998; 15: 57–62.
11. Symonds B S. Work-coping and home-coping: achieving a balance in part-time community pharmacy. *Int J Pharm Pract* 2000; 8: 10–19.
12. Powis M G, Rogers P J, Wood S M. United Kingdom pharmacists' views on recent POM to P switched medicines. *J Soc Admin Pharm* 1996; 13: 188–97.
13. Erwin J, Britten N, Jones R. Pharmacists and deregulation: the case of H2 antagonists. *J Soc Admin Pharm* 1996; 13: 150–8.

14. Cantrill J A, Weiss M C, Kishida M, Nicolson M. Pharmacists' perceptions and experiences of pharmacy protocols: a step in the right direction? *Int J Pharm Pract* 1997; 5: 26–32.

15. John D N, Evans S W. South-east Wales community pharmacists' views on the new medicines sales protocols. *Pharm J* 1996; 256: 626–8.

16. Rogers P J, Fletcher G, Rees J E. Reasons for community pharmacists establishing patient medication records. *Int J Pharm Pract* 1993; 2: 44–8.

17. Krska J. Attitudes to audit among community pharmacists in Grampian. *Pharm J* 1994; 253: 97–9.

18. Oborne C A, Dodds L J. Seamless pharmaceutical care: the needs of community pharmacists. *Pharm J* 1994; 253: 502–6.

19. Shefcheck S L, Thomas J. Consumers' perceptions of access to medications and attitudes towards regulatory options. *J Soc Admin Pharm* 1998; 15: 149–63.

20. Raynor D K, Knapp P. Do patients see, read and retain the new mandatory medicines information leaflets? *Pharm J* 2000; 264: 268–70.

21. Hunt A J, Sheppard C, Lupton C, Brown D. Family health services authorities and community pharmacists at the purchaser–provider interface. *Int J Pharm Pract* 1995; 3: 200–8.

22. O'Brien K, Sibbald B, Cantrill J A. Hospital outpatient dispensing policy in the North-West Regional Health Authority. *Pharm J* 1996; 257: 902–5.

23. Thomas K A, Brown D, Hunt A, Jones I F. Community pharmacists and the NHS contract: 1. Attitudes to remuneration and terms of service. *Pharm J* 1996; 257: 854–8.

24. Marriott J F. BNF recommendations on substitution: are they followed in practice? *Pharm J* 1999; 263: 289–92.

25. Gore P R, Madhavan S. Consumers' preferences and willingness to pay for pharmacist counselling for non-prescription medicines. *J Clin Pharm Ther* 1994; 19: 17–25.

26. Tully M P, Temple B. The demographics of pharmacy's clientele: a descriptive study of the British general public. *Int J Pharm Pract* 1999; 7: 172–81.

27. Anderson C. Health promotion by community pharmacists: consumers' views. *Int J Pharm Pract* 1998; 6: 2–12.

28. Duggan C, Bates I. Development and evaluation of a survey tool to explore patients' perceptions of their prescribed drugs and their need for drug information. *Int J Pharm Pract* 2000; 8: 42–52.

29. McGovern E, Moss H, Grewal G, *et al.* Factors affecting the use of folic acid supplements in pregnant women in Glasgow. *Br J Gen Pract* 1997; 47: 635–7.

30. Clarke K, Sheridan J, Williamson S, Griffiths P. Consumer preferences among pharmacy needle exchange attendees. *Pharm J* 1998; 261: 64–6.

31. Read R W, Krska J. Potential roles of the pharmacist in chronic pain management: a multidisciplinary perspective in primary care. *Int J Pharm Pract* 1998; 6: 223–8.

32. Child D, Hirsch C, Berry M. Health care professionals' views on hospital pharmacist prescribing in the United Kingdom. *Int J Pharm Pract* 1998; 6: 159–69.

33. Bleiker P, Lewis A. Extending the role of community pharmacists: the views of GPs. *Int J Pharm Pract* 1998; 6: 140–4.

34. Tanskanen P, Jakala J, Airaksinen M, Enlund H. Physicians' views on co-operation with community pharmacists in Finland. *J Soc Admin Pharm* 1997; 14: 220–9.

35. Ranelli P L, Biss J. Physicians' perceptions of communication with, and responsibilities of, pharmacists. *J Am Pharm Assoc* 2000; 40: 625–30.

36. Ziebland S, Graham A, McPherson A. Concerns and cautions about prescribing and deregulating emergency contraception: a qualitative study of GPs using telephone interviews. *Fam Pract* 1998; 15: 449–56.

37. Matheson C, Bond C M, Hickey F. Prescribing and dispensing for drug misusers in primary care: current practice in Scotland. *Fam Pract* 1999; 16: 375–9.

38. Gaunt R, Whitfield M, Ghalamkari H, Millar M. General practitioner prescribing and community pharmacist recommendation for the sale of aciclovir topical cream. *Int J Pharm Pract* 1996; 4: 204–8.

39. Jepson M H, Strickland-Hodge B. Surveys of the frequency, purpose, influence and outcome of inter-professional contact between pharmacists and GPs in Britain. *J Soc Admin Pharm* 1995; 12: 18–32.

40. Holden J D, Wolfson D J. Comparison of attitudes of general medical practitioners and community pharmacists to prescribing matters. *Int J Pharm Pract* 1996; 4: 175–81.

41. Smith F. Referral of clients by community pharmacists: views of general medical practitioners. *Int J Pharm Pract* 1996; 4: 30–5.

42. Krska J, Kennedy E J. Responding to symptoms: comparing general practitioners' and pharmacists' advice. *Pharm J* 1996; 257: 322–4.

43. Dixon N H E, Hall J, Hassell K, Moorhouse G E. Domiciliary visiting: a review of compound analgesic use in the community. *J Soc Admin Pharm* 1995; 12: 144–53.

44. Sutters C A, Nathan A. The community pharmacist's extended role: GPs and pharmacists attitudes towards collaboration. *J Soc Admin Pharm* 1993; 10: 70–84.

45. Troein M, Rastam L, Selander S. Physicians' lack of confidence in pharmacists' competence as patient informants. *J Soc Admin Pharm* 1992; 9: 114–22.

46. Kilkenny M, Yeatman J, Stewart K, Marks R. Role of pharmacists and general practitioners in the management of dermatological conditions. *Int J Pharm Pract* 1997; 5: 11–15.

47. Jepson M H, Strickland-Hodge B. Attitudes to patient medication records and their optimization through patient registration. *Pharm J* 1994; 253: 384–8.

48. Hall J, Radley A S. A role for community pharmacists in the control of anticoagulant therapy. *Pharm J* 1994; 252: 230–2.

49. Hedvall M-B, Paltschik M. Perceived service quality in pharmacies: with empirical results from Sweden. *J Soc Admin Pharm* 1992; 8: 7–14.

50. Schaefer M, Leufkens H G M, Harris M F. The teaching of social pharmacy/pharmacy administration in colleges of pharmacy with special regard to the situation in Germany. *J Soc Admin Pharm* 1992; 9: 141–8.

51. Hagedorn M, Cantrill J, Nicolson M, Noyce P. Pharmaceutical care and the deregulation of medicines. A survey of British and German pharmacists. *J Soc Admin Pharm* 1996; 13: 1–7.

52. Blom A T H G, Kam A L, Bakker A, Claesson C. Patient counselling in community pharmacy: a comparative study between Dutch and Swedish pharmacists. *J Soc Admin Pharm* 1993; 10: 53–62.

53. Hassell K. White and ethnic minority pharmacists' professional practice patterns and reasons for choosing pharmacy. *Int J Pharm Pract* 1996; 4: 43–51.

54. Scott D M, Woodward J M B. The influence of locus of control and perceived susceptibility to illness on family managers' self-care chart use. *J Soc Admin Pharm* 1992; 9: 21–8.

55. Pendergast J F, Kimberlin C L, Berardo D H, McKenzie L C. Role orientation and community pharmacists' participation in a project to improve patient care. *Soc Sci Med* 1995; 40: 557–65.

56. Ackman M L, Campbell J B, Buzak K A, *et al.* Use of non-prescription medications by patients with congestive heart failure. *Ann Pharmacother* 1999; 33: 675–9.

57. Servizio di Informazione e di Educazione Sanitaria, Farmacie Comunali Italiane. What information for the patient? Large scale pilot study on experimental package inserts giving information on prescribed and over-the-counter drugs. *BMJ* 1990; 301: 1261–5.

58. Geissler P W, Nokes K, Prince R J, *et al.* Children and medicines: self treatment of common illnesses among Luo school children in Western Kenya. *Soc Sci Med* 2000; 50: 1771–83.

59. Hornosty R W, Muzzin L J, Brown G P. Faith in the ideal of clinical pharmacy among practising pharmacists seven years after graduation from pharmacy school. *J Soc Admin Pharm* 1992; 9: 87–96.

60. Abraham C, Clift S, Grabowski P. Cognitive predictors of adherence to malaria prophylaxis regimens on return from a malarious region: a prospective study. *Soc Sci Med* 1999; 48: 1641–54.

61. van Wijk C M T G, Huisman H, Kolk A M. Gender differences in physical symptoms and illness behaviour: a health diary study. *Soc Sci Med* 1999; 49: 1061–74.

62. Rodgers P J, Rees J E. Comparison of the use of PMRs in community pharmacy in 1991 and 1995: 1. PMR use and recording of product details. *Pharm J* 1996; 256: 161–6.

63. Rodgers P J, Rees J E. Comparison of the use of PMRs in community pharmacy in 1991 and 1995: 2. The recording of patients' details. *Pharm J* 1996; 256: 491–5.

64. Rodgers P J, Fletcher G, Rees J E. Patient medication records in community pharmacy. *Pharm J* 1992; 248: 193–6.

65. Erwin J, Britten N, Jones R. General practitioners' views on the over-the-counter sales by community pharmacists. *BMJ* 1996; 312; 617–18.

66. Spencer J A, Edwards C. Pharmacy beyond the dispensary: general practitioners' views. *BMJ* 1992; 304: 1670–72.

67. Sheridan J, Strang J, Barber N, Glanz A. Role of community pharmacies in relation to HIV prevention and drug misuse: findings from the 1995 national survey in England and Wales. *BMJ* 1996; 313: 272–4.

68. Lewis M A O, Chadwick B L. Management of recurrent herpes labialis in community pharmacies. *Pharm J* 1994; 253: 768–9.

69. Branstad J-O, Kamil I, Lilja J, Sjoblom M. When topical hydrocortisone

became an OTC drug in Sweden: a study of the users and their information sources. *Soc Sci Med* 1994; 39: 207–12.

70. Argyle M, Newman C. An assessment of pharmacy discharge procedures and hospital communications with general practitioners. *Pharm J* 1996; 256: 903–5.

71. Leach R H, Leach S J. Drug and therapeutics committees in the UK in 1992. *Pharm J* 1994; 253: 61–3.

72. Joshi M P, Williams A, Petrie J C. Hospital formularies in 1993: where, why and how? *Pharm J* 1994; 253: 63–5.

73. Smith S, Battle R. Use of information services by drug information pharmacists. *Pharm J* 1994; 253: 499–501.

74. Cotter S M, Barber N D, McKee M. Hospital clinical pharmacy services provided to primary care. *Int J Pharm Pract* 1994; 2: 215–21.

75. Anderson C. Community pharmacy health promotion activity in England: a survey of policy and practice. *Health Educ J* 1996; 55: 194–202.

76. Sheppard C P, Hunt A J, Lupton C A, Begley S. Community pharmacists in primary care: prospects for pharmacist–doctor collaboration. *J Soc Admin Pharm* 1995; 12: 181–9.

77. Schneider J S, Barber N D. Community pharmacist and general practitioner collaboration in England and Wales. *Pharm J* 1996; 256: 524–5.

78. Liddell H. Competency-based training for pre-registration trainers: what are the views of hospital trainers. *Pharm J* 1996; 256: 624–5.

79. Bradley B, McCusker E, Scott E, Li Wan Po A. Patient information leaflets on over-the-counter medicines: the manufacturer's perspective. *J Clin Pharm Ther* 1995; 20: 37–40.

80. Kong S X, Wertheimer A I, McGhan W F. Role stress, organisational commitment and turnover intention among pharmaceutical scientists: a multivariate analysis. *J Soc Admin Pharm* 1992; 9: 159–71.

81. Thomson A N, Craig B J, Barham P M. Attitudes of general practitioners in New Zealand to pharmaceutical representatives. *Br J Gen Pract* 1994; 44: 220–3.

82. Stromme H K, Botten G. Physicians' perceived drug-related problems and preventive strategies concerning old patients in general practice. *J Soc Admin Pharm* 1992; 9: 172–8.

83. Rodgers P J, Rees J E. General medical practitioners' attitudes towards the use of patient medication records. *Int J Pharm Pract* 1995; 3: 163–8.

84. Clark J C, Gerrett D. General medical practitioners' perceived use of drug information sources with special reference to drug information centres. *Int J Pharm Pract* 1994; 2: 247–52.

85. Voss S, Hardy N, Olds T, George S. The use of practice formularies by general practitioners in Southampton and south-west Hampshire. *Pharm J* 1997; 258: 38–9.

86. Teresi M E, Margan D E. Attitudes of health care professionals toward patient counselling on drug–nutrient interactions. *Ann Pharmacother* 1994; 28: 576–80.

87. Rivers P H. The impact of carers' attitudes on the safety of medication procedures in UK residential homes for the elderly. *J Soc Admin Pharm* 1995; 12: 132–43.

88. Newton S A, Black M. Nursing sisters' satisfaction with the pharmacy service – a survey. *Int J Pharm Pract* 1994; 2: 220–2.

89. Bhati M, Duxbury A J, Macfarlane T V, Downer M C. Analgesics recommended by dentists and pharmacists, and used by the general public for pain relief. *Int J Health Promotion Educ* 2000; 38: 95–103.

90. Kristensen T S. Use of medicine as a coping strategy among Danish slaughterhouse workers. *J Soc Admin Pharm* 1992; 8: 53–64.

91. Thomas K A, Brown D, Hunt A, Jones I F. Community pharmacists and the NHS contract: 2. Attitudes to its improvement, the extended role and the negotiation progress. *Pharm J* 1996; 257: 896–901.

92. Asch D A, Jedrziewski M K, Christakis N A. Response rates to mail surveys published in medical journals. *J Clin Epidemiol* 1997; 50: 1129–36.

93. Bouldin A S, Smith M C, Garner D D, *et al.* Pharmacy and herbal medicine in the US. *Soc Sci Med* 1999; 49: 279–89.

94. Schommer J C, Sullivan D L, Haugtvedt C L. Patients' role orientation for pharmacist consultation. *J Soc Admin Pharm* 1995; 12: 33–42.

95. Airaksinen M, Ahonen R, Enlund H. Customer feedback as a tool for improving pharmacy services. *Int J Pharm Pract* 1995; 3: 219–26.

96. Cockerill R W, Myers T, Worthington C, *et al.* Pharmacies and their role in the prevention of HIV/AIDS. *J Soc Admin Pharm* 1996; 13: 46–53.

97. Jesson J, Sadler S, Pocock R, Jepson M. Ethnic minority consumers of community pharmaceutical services. *Int J Pharm Pract* 1995; 3: 129–32.

98. Jesson J, Jepson M, Pocock R, *et al. Ethnic Minority Consumers of Community Pharmaceutical Services. A Report for the Department of Health.* Birmingham: Aston University/ MEL Research, 1994.

99. Paluck E C, Stratton T P, Eni G O. Pharmacists and health promotion: a study of thirteen variables. *J Soc Admin Pharm* 1996; 13: 89–98.

100. Farris K B, Kirking D M. Predicting community pharmacists' intention to try to prevent and correct drug therapy problems. *J Soc Admin Pharm* 1995; 12: 64–79.

101. Jesson J, Pocock R, Jepson M, Kendall H. Consumer readership and views on pharmacy health education literature: a market research survey. *J Soc Admin Pharm* 1994; 11: 29–36.

102. Carlson A M, Wertheimer A I. Occupational inheritance and business orientation in pharmacy. *J Soc Admin Pharm* 1992; 9: 42–8.

103. Whitehead P, Atkin P, Krass I, Benrimoj S I. Patient drug information and consumer choice of pharmacy. *Int J Pharm Pract* 1999; 7: 71–9.

104. Beckerleg S, Lewande-Hundt G, Eddema M, *et al.* Purchasing a quickfix from private pharmacies in the Gaza Strip. *Soc Sci Med* 1999; 49: 1489–500.

105. Cairns C, Marlow H, McCoig A, Hargreaves D. The Croydon community pharmacy accident survey. *Pharm J* 1996; 257: 817–9.

106. Greene R. Survey of prescription anomalies in community pharmacies: (1) Prescription monitoring. *Pharm J* 1995; 254: 476–81.

107. Greene R. Survey of prescription anomalies in community pharmacies: (2) Interventions and outcomes. *Pharm J* 1995; 254: 873–5.

108. Spanish group for the study of hypnotic drug utilization. Hypnotic drug use in Spain: a cross-sectional study based on a network of community pharmacies. *Ann Pharmacother* 1996; 30: 1092–100.

109. Boakes R M, Strickland-Hodge B, Jepson M H. Survey of use of the Pharmacy Information and News Service (PINS) among community pharmacists. *Int J Pharm Pract* 1991; 1: 98–101.
110. Gattera J A, Stewart K, Benrimoj S I, Williams G M. Usage of non-prescription medication by people with diabetes. *J Soc Admin Pharm* 1992; 9: 66–74.
111. Baines D L, Rafferty J P, McLeod H S T. A survey of English NHS prescribing advisors' roles, and their views on improving prescribing in the new NHS. *Pharm J* 2000; 264: 557–9.
112. Chang Z G, Kennedy D T, Holdford D A, Small R E. Pharmacists' knowledge and attitudes toward herbal medicine. *Ann Pharmacother* 2000; 34: 710–5.
113. Ernst E. Over-the-counter complementary remedies used for arthritis. *Pharm J* 1998; 260: 830–1.
114. *Annual Register of Pharmaceutical Chemists*. London: Royal Pharmaceutical Society of Great Britain.
115. Odedina F T, Segal R, Hepler C D, *et al*. Changing pharmacists' practice pattern. *J Soc Admin Pharm* 1996; 13: 74–88.
116. Laurier C, Poston J W. Perceived levels of patient counselling among Canadian pharmacists. *J Soc Admin Pharm* 1992; 9: 104–13.
117. Benjamin H, Motawi A, Smith F J. Community Pharmacists and primary health care in Egypt. *J Soc Admin Pharm* 1996; 12: 3–11.
118. Spencer M G, Smith A P. A multicentre study of dispensing errors in British hospitals. *Int J Pharm Pract* 1993; 2: 142–6.
119. Hughes C M, McFerran G. Pharmacy involvement in formulary development: community pharmacists' views. *Int J Pharm Pract* 1996; 4: 153–5.
120. Mottram D R, Jogia P, West P. Community pharmacists' attitudes to the extended role. *J Soc Admin Pharm* 1995; 12: 12–17.
121. Paxton R, Chapple P. Misuse of over-the-counter medicines: a survey in one county. *Pharm J* 1996; 256: 313–15.
122. Ortiz M, Walker W L, Thomas R. Development of a measure to assess community pharmacists' orientation towards patient counselling. *J Soc Admin Pharm* 1992; 9: 2–10.
123. Ortiz M, Walker W L, Thomas R. Job satisfaction dimensions of Australian community pharmacists. *J Soc Admin Pharm* 1992; 9: 149–58.
124. Brown J, Brown D. Pharmaceutical care at the primary–secondary interface in Portsmouth and south-east Hampshire. *Pharm J* 1997; 258: 280–4.
125. Rosenbloom K, Taylor K, Harding G. Community pharmacists' attitudes towards research. *Int J Pharm Pract* 2000; 8: 103–10.
126. Emmerton L, Benrimoj S. Factors influencing pharmacists' preferences for non-prescription cough suppressants. *J Soc Admin Pharm* 1994; 11: 78–85.
127. Emmerton L, Gow D J, Benrimoj S I. Dimensions of pharmacists' preferences for cough and cold products. *Int J Pharm Pract* 1994; 3: 27–32.
128. Liddell H. Attitudes of community pharmacists regarding involvement in practice research. *Pharm J* 1996; 256: 905–7.
129. Lindblad A K, Isacson D, Hyttsten A-C. Pharmacists' perceptions of the Swedish system for extemporaneous compounding. *J Soc Admin Pharm* 1996; 13: 139–49.
130. Hardy N, Hodgkins P, Luff A, *et al*. Counterprescribing for ophthalmic

conditions: a survey of community pharmacists. *Int J Pharm Pract* 1993; 2: 104–6.

131. Beal J F, Skaer T L, Day R D, Jinks M J. The comfort level of pharmacists who counsel contraceptive patients. *J Clin Pharm Ther* 1993; 18: 317–24.

132. Dickinson C, Howlett J A, Bulman J S. The community pharmacist: a dental health advisor. *Pharm J* 1994; 252: 262–4.

133. Olson D S, Lawson K A. Relationship between hospital pharmacists' job satisfaction and involvement in clinical activities. *Am J Health Syst Pharm* 1996; 53: 281–4.

134. *Chemist and Druggist Directory*. London: MG Information Services, 1995.

135. IHSM. *Health and Social Services Yearbook*. London: IHSM [annual].

136. Picton C L, Hewetson M L. Survey of pharmacy support for clinical trials. *Pharm J* 1995; 254: 126–7.

137. Murphy J E, Slack M K, Campbell S. National survey of hospital based pharmacokinetic services. *Am J Health Syst Pharm* 1996; 53: 2840–7.

138. Martin R M, Lunec S G, Rink E. UK postal survey of pharmacists working with general practices on prescribing issues: characteristics, roles and working arrangements. *Int J Pharm Pract* 1998; 6: 133–9.

139. Sheridan J, Barber N D. Pharmacy undergraduates' and preregistration pharmacists' attitudes towards drug misuse and HIV. *J Soc Admin Pharm* 1993; 10: 163–70.

140. Sheridan J, Bates I P, Webb D G, Barber N D. Educational intervention in pharmacy students' attitudes to HIV/AIDS and drug misuse. *Med Educ* 1994; 28: 492–500.

141. Ortiz M, Walker W L, Thomas R. Physicians – friend or foe? Comparisons between pharmacists' and physicians' perceptions of the pharmacist's role. *J Soc Admin Pharm* 1989; 6: 59–68.

142. Stromme H K, Botten G. Drug-related problems among old people living at home, as perceived by a sample of Norwegian home-care providers. *J Soc Admin Pharm* 1993; 10: 63–9.

143. Smith F J, Farquhar M, Bowling A P. Drugs prescribed for people aged 85 and over living in their own homes in an area of inner London. *Int J Pharm Pract* 1995; 3: 145–50.

144. Jepson M, Jesson J, Pocock R, Kendall H. *Consumer Expectations of Community Pharmaceutical Services. A Report for the Department of Health.* Birmingham: Aston University/MEL Research 1991.

145. Vallis J, Wyke S, Cunningham-Burley S. Users' views and expectations of community pharmacists in a Scottish commuter town. *Pharm J* 1997; 258: 457–60.

146. Forbes A J, Ross A J, Rees J A. Problems with medicines use: the Bolton project. *Int J Pharm Pract* 1991; 1: 34–7.

147. Rees J A, Forbes A J, Ross A J. Difficulties in the use of medicine packaging. *Int J Pharm Pract* 1992; 1: 160–3.

148. Majeed F A, Cook D G, Poloniecki J, Martin D. Using data from the 1991 census. *BMJ* 1995; 310: 1511–14.

149. Isacson D, Bingefors C. On prescription switches and access to over-the-counter drugs in Sweden. *J Soc Admin Pharm* 1999; 16: 13–25.

150. Platts A E, Tann J. A changing professional profile: ethnicity and gender issues

in pharmacy employment in the United Kingdom. *Int J Pharm Pract* 1999; 7: 29–39.

151. Smith W, Chey T, Jalaludin B, *et al*. Increasing response rates in telephone surveys: a randomised trial. *J Public Health Med* 1995; 17: 33–8.
152. Heuveline P, Goldman N. A description of child illness and treatment behaviour in Guatemala. *Soc Sci Med* 2000; 50: 345–64.
153. Brown C M, Segal R. The effects of health and treatment perceptions on the use of prescribed medications and home remedies among African American and White American hypertensives. *Soc Sci Med* 1996; 43: 903–17.
154. Kotzan J A, Carroll N V, Perri M, Fincham J E. The prescription to non-prescription switch: consumer awareness, purchases information sources and the pharmacist. *J Pharm Market Manag* 1987; 2: 43–61.
155. Richards S, Thornhill D, Roberts H, Harries U. How many people have hayfever and what do they do about it? *Br J Gen Pract* 1992; 42: 284–6.
156. Hargie O, Morrow N, Woodman C. Consumer perceptions of and attitudes to community pharmacy services. *Pharm J* 1992; 249: 688–91.
157. Charupatanapong N. Perceived likelihood of risks in self-medication practices. *J Soc Admin Pharm* 1994; 11: 18–28.
158. Bell H M, McElnay J C, Hughes C M. Societal perspectives on the role of the community pharmacist and community based pharmaceutical services. *J Soc Admin Pharm* 2000; 17: 119–28.
159. Gore P, Madhavan S. Credibility of the sources of information for non-prescription medicines. *J Soc Admin Pharm* 1993; 10: 109–22.
160. Carroll N V, Fincham J E. Elderly consumers' perceptions of the risks of using mail-order pharmacies. *J Soc Admin Pharm* 1993; 10: 123–9.
161. Gore M R, Thomas J. Non-prescription informational services in pharmacies and alternative stores: implications for a third class of drugs. *J Soc Admin Pharm* 1995; 12: 86–99.
162. Rantucci M, Segal H J. Hazardous non-prescription analgesic use by the elderly. *J Soc Admin Pharm* 1992; 8: 108–120.
163. Williamson V K, Winn S, Livingstone C R, Pugh A L G. Public views on an extended role for community pharmacy. *Int J Pharm Pract* 1992; 1: 223–9.
164. Livingstone C R, Pugh A L G, Winn S, Williamson V K. Developing community pharmacy services wanted by local people: information and advice about prescription medicines. *Int J Pharm Pract* 1996; 4: 94–102.
165. McElnay J C, McCallion R C. Non-prescription drug use by elderly patients. *Int J Pharm Pract* 1996; 4: 6–11.
166. Britten N, Gallagher K, Gallagher H. Patients' views of computerised pharmacy records. *Int J Pharm Pract* 1992; 1: 206–9.
167. Krska J, Kennedy E. Expectations and experiences of customers purchasing over-the-counter medicines in pharmacies in the north of Scotland. *Pharm J* 1996; 256: 354–6.
168. Whitaker P, Wilson R, Bargh J, *et al*. Use and misuse of purchased analgesics with age. *Pharm J* 1995; 254: 553–6.
169. Beto J A, Lisbecki R F, Meyer D A, *et al*. Use of pharmacy computer prescription database to access hypertensive patients for mailed survey research. *Ann Pharmacother* 1996; 30: 351–5.
170. Greco R, Lavack L, Rovers J. Assessment of the pharmacy service needs of

HIV-positive outpatients receiving zidovudine. *Ann Pharmacother* 1992; 26: 621–6.

171. Willison D J, Gaebel K A, Borden E K, *et al*. Experience in the development of a post-marketing surveillance network: the pharmacy medication monitoring program. *Ann Pharmacother* 1995; 29: 1208–13.

172. Payne K, Ryan-Woolley B M, Noyce P R. Role of consumer attributes in predicting the impact of medicines deregulation on National Health Service prescribing in the United Kingdom. *Int J Pharm Pract* 1998; 6: 150–8.

173. Grewar J, McDonald T M. Hayfever symptoms and over-the-counter remedies: a community pharmacy study. *Int J Pharm Pract* 1998; 6: 22–9.

174. Kayne S, Beattie N, Reeves A. Survey of buyers of over-the-counter homoeopathic medicines. *Pharm J* 1999; 263: 210–12.

175. Krska J, John D N, Hansford D, Kennedy E J. Drug utilisation evaluation of non-prescription H2-receptor antagonists and alginate-containing preparations for dyspepsia. *Br J Clin Pharmacol* 2000; 49: 363–8.

176. Long A, Wynne H A. Patient satisfaction with arthritis medication. *Int J Pharm Pract* 1996; 4: 52–4.

177. Chua S-S, Benrimoj S I, Stewart K, Williams G. Usage of non-prescription medications by hypertensive patients. *J Soc Admin Pharm* 1992; 8: 33–45.

178. Deshmukh A A, Sommerville H. Survey of the needs of patients in a private nursing home: a pharmacist's view. *Int J Pharm Pract* 1996; 4: 83–7.

179. Fairbrother J, Mottram D R, Williamson P M. The doctor–pharmacist interface, a preliminary evaluation of domiciliary visits by a community pharmacist. *J Soc Admin Pharm* 1993; 10: 85–91.

180. Elfellah M S, McDonald L, Thomson A, Smith A. Screening for incorrect inhaler use by regular users. *Pharm J* 1994; 253: 467–8.

181. Read R W, Krska J. Targeted medication review: patients in the community with chronic pain. *Int J Pharm Pract* 1998; 6: 216–22.

182. Duggan C, Bates I, Hough J. Discrepancies in prescribing: where do they occur? *Pharm J* 1996; 256: 65–7.

183. Cook H. Transfer of information between hospital and community pharmacy – a feasibility study. *Pharm J* 1995; 254: 736–7.

184. Francis S-A. Medication and quality of life: a study of people with a diagnosis of schizophrenia. [PhD thesis.] London: University of London, 1997.

185. Jones W, Brown D. The pharmacist's contribution to primary care support for lactating mothers requiring medication. *J Soc Admin Pharm* 2000; 17: 88–98.

186. Barrett P J, Emmins P D, Clarke P D, Bradley D J. Comparison of adverse events associated with use of mefloquine and combination of chloroquine and proguanil as antimalarial prophylaxis: postal and telephone survey of travellers. *BMJ* 1996; 313: 525–8.

187. Marchetti M, Minghetti P, Donzelli P. Treatment of children's fevers in Italy after the withdrawal of aspirin paediatric formulations from OTC products. *J Soc Admin Pharm* 1992; 8: 121–9.

188. Foster C, ed. *Manual for Research Ethics Committees*. London: Centre for Medical Law and Ethics, King's College London, 1997.

189. Templeton L, Deehan A, Taylor C, *et al*. Surveying general practitioners: does a low response rate matter. *Br J Gen Pract* 1997; 47: 91–4.

190. Sibbald B, Addington-Hall J, Brenneman D, Freeling P. Telephone versus

postal surveys of general practitioners: methodological considerations. *Br J Gen Pract* 1994; 44: 297–300.

191. Smith F J, Weidner D. Threatening and violent incidents in community pharmacies: 1. An investigation of the frequency of serious and minor incidents. *Int J Pharm Pract* 1996; 4: 136–44.

192. Sheridan J, Strang J. Late responders and non-responders to a postal survey questionnaire: analysis of potential further response and non-response bias. *Int J Pharm Pract* 1998; 6: 170–5.

193. Hill A, Roberts J, Ewings P, Gunnell D. Non-response bias in a life-style survey. *J Public Health Med* 1997; 19: 203–7.

194. Armstrong D, Ashworth M. When questionnaire response rates do matter: a survey of general practitioners and their views of NHS changes. *Br J Gen Pract* 2000; 50: 479–80.

195. Hawksworth G, Wright D J, Chrystyn H. A detailed analysis of the day-to-day unwanted products returned to community pharmacies for disposal. *J Soc Admin Pharm* 1996; 3: 215–22.

196. Cochran W G. *Sampling Techniques*. New York: John Wiley and Sons, 1977.

197. Stromme H K, Botten G. Support and service for the drug treatment of old people living at home: a study of a sample of Norwegian home-care providers. *J Soc Admin Pharm* 1993; 10: 130–7.

198. Generali J A, Danish M A, Rosenbaum S E. Knowledge of and attitudes about adverse drug reaction reporting among Rhode Island pharmacists. *Ann Pharmacother* 1995; 29: 365–9.

199. Sadik F, Reeder C E, Saket M, *et al.* Job satisfaction among Jordanian pharmacists. *J Soc Admin Pharm* 1992; 8: 46–51.

200. Leemans L, Laekeman G. Computer-assisted drug delivery in community pharmacies: pharmaco-epidemiological and scientific consequences. *J Soc Admin Pharm* 1994; 131–8.

201. Taylor J. Reasons consumers do not ask for advice on non-prescription medicines in pharmacies. *Int J Pharm Pract* 1994; 2: 209–14.

202. Tai S S, Nazareth I, Haines A, Jowett C. A randomised trial of the impact of telephone and recorded delivery reminders on the response rate to research questionnaires. *J Public Health Med* 1997; 19: 219–21.

203. Willett V J, Cooper C L. Stress and job satisfaction in community pharmacy: a pilot study. *Pharm J* 1996; 256: 94–8.

204. Rees L. The provision of disease prevention services from community pharmacies. [PhD thesis.] London: University of London, 1994.

205. Kennedy E, Krska J, John D, Hansford D. Effect of incentives on recruitment and response rates in a community-based pharmacy practice based study. *Int J Pharm Pract* 1999; 7: 80–5.

206. Grewar J, Matthews J, McMahon A D, McDonald T M. Capturing data on over-the-counter medicines in community pharmacies: a methodological study. *Pharm J* 1997; 259: 736–9.

207. Truter I, van Niekerk W P. Pharmacists' perception of mission statements for retail pharmacies in South Africa. *J Soc Admin Pharm* 1999; 16: 53–60.

208. Maslen C L, Rees L, Redfern P H. Role of the community pharmacist in the care of patients with chronic schizophrenia in the community. *Int J Pharm Pract* 1996; 4: 187–95.

209. Mudhar M S, Wilson K A, Irwin W J. Perceptions of preregistration graduates about the UK pharmacy undergraduate course. *Int J Pharm Pract* 1996; 4: 59–64.
210. Worley M M, Schommer J C. Pharmacist-patient relationships: factors influencing quality and commitment. *J Soc Admin Pharm* 1999; 16: 1557–73.
211. Taylor F C, Ramsay M E, Tan G, *et al.* Evaluation of patients' knowledge about anticoagulant treatment. *Qual Health Care* 1994; 3: 79–85.
212. Madhavan S. Factors influencing pharmacists' preferences for the legal classification of Rx-to-OTC switched drug products. *J Clin Pharm Ther* 1993; 18: 281–90.
213. Barker J, Blanch P, Burrall K. The increasing use of pharmacies for advice and the downward trend for GP consultation. *Pharm J* 1999; 264: 138–40.
214. Venkataraman K, Madhavan S, Bone P. Barriers and facilitators to pharmaceutical care in rural community practice. *J Soc Admin Pharm* 1997; 14: 208–19.
215. Shepherd C K, Power K G, Carter H. Characteristics of responders and non-responders in an infant feeding study. *J Public Health Med* 1998; 20: 275–80.
216. Latif D A, Berger B A, Harris S G, *et al.* The relationship between community pharmacists' moral reasoning and components of clinical performance. *J Soc Admin Pharm* 1998; 15: 210–24.

2

Survey research: instruments, validity and reliability

This chapter focuses on the development of survey instruments and the approaches of researchers to ensuring the reliability and validity of survey research. The majority of surveys gather descriptive data, the aims of which may be to characterise a population (pharmacists, clients, or other groups), to describe particular services, events, attitudes, views or perceptions; and/or to establish relationships between variables. The survey questionnaire is the instrument of data collection. The questions included must be shown to provide accurate and reliable data on variables relevant to the topic of interest.

Reliability is concerned with the repeatability or reproducibility of measurements; for example, consistency in interpretation of questions by different individuals and the application of study procedures and/or reproducibility of measurements. Validity is concerned with the accuracy of data, rather than its reproducibility; that is, ensuring responses are a true reflection of the issues of interest. For example, are respondents able and willing to provide accurate information relevant to study objectives? Thus, whilst reliability is concerned with the precision and reproducibility of data, validity relates to the accuracy or the truth of measurements.

Accurate and reliable measurement of some variables will be relatively straightforward; others may be very difficult to 'operationalise'. This chapter discusses problems of validity and reliability that arise in survey research in pharmacy settings and ways in which they have been addressed.

Survey instruments

The survey instrument refers to the questions or questionnaire used to collect the data. It is important that the instrument gathers relevant information effectively and efficiently, and that the responses are a reliable and valid reflection of the issues being measured. The survey instrument should also be acceptable and attractive to potential respondents (e.g. reasonable in length and well presented).

Most pharmacy practice researchers undertaking survey research develop their own questionnaire or survey instrument, devising questions to meet their study objectives. In these cases, issues of acceptability, reliability and validity, of both individual questions and the instrument as a whole, have to be addressed from scratch.

Rather than develop their own instruments, researchers sometimes use questions, or series of questions, that have been devised and developed by others.[1-8] For example, in a population-based survey of deregulation and use of non-prescription drugs questions were based on those employed in the 'Swedish survey of living conditions'.[9] The advantage of this is that much of the time-consuming, detailed and often expensive work required to ensure validity and reliability will have already been undertaken. Employing measures that have been used by others also enables comparisons to be made between population groups.

In some instances, instruments developed and tested by others are adopted in their entirety.[2,4,6,8] More often, the application of an instrument in a new setting, among a different population group or to serve specific objectives, will require modifications and/or additions.[5,10-13] It cannot be assumed that following modification an instrument necessarily retains its validity. Similarly, an instrument developed within a particular population group will not automatically be transferable for use in another.

The reliability and validity of any survey instrument cannot be taken for granted. Failure to address these issues may lead others to doubt the value of the work. Some researchers report that questions comprising different measures were validated but provide no indication of how this was done. However, there are many cases in which researchers comprehensively reported the processes they employed in the development of their survey instruments, providing descriptions of their approaches and procedures.

In the development of questionnaires, many variables present problems for researchers in ensuring that questions are a valid and reliable reflection of phenomena of interest; that is, they are difficult to operationalise as part of a survey instrument.

Instruments to measure variables such as attitudes, health status and satisfaction with services, if they are an accurate reflection of the attribute of interest, may be structurally complex. These attributes will comprise many components which may vary in their importance among different populations and across settings. When investigating these issues it is often sensible to incorporate or adapt an existing measure where a suitable one exists. However, if a suitable one does not exist researchers will have to embark on developing their own.

Population descriptors such as ethnicity and socio-economic status are often included in survey research. Inequalities in health status and access to care are of concern to health care providers[14] and it is therefore important that relevant data are collected in research on pharmacy services and drug use. However, it is recognised that these variables are social/cultural constructs that are not easy to define and consequently difficult to operationalise in research. The shortcomings of existing measures and the development of new ones have been widely discussed.[15]

Some variables are subjective (in that they relate to an individual's feelings) rather than being determined by factors which can be 'objectively' measured. Examples include health status, quality of life and pain.

Other attributes are difficult to measure directly. In these cases, a 'proxy' measure may be employed. That is, information is gathered indirectly using variables for which a relationship with the attribute of interest can be demonstrated, for example, socio-economic status (for which occupation, education and/or housing tenure have been used). Some researchers view a categorisation of individuals as male and female as a proxy, in that in social (and pharmacy practice) surveys, researchers may be more interested in identifying and exploring the social, psychological or occupational significance of being female or male rather than biological differences.

Validity

The validity of an instrument is the extent to which it actually measures what it is designed to measure. In survey work, this refers to the extent to which the questions collect accurate data relevant to the study objectives. The validation process involves testing the instrument, in its entirety or by selecting individual questions, in the population for which it is to be used to ensure that the responses are a true reflection of the variables or attributes of interest. Only after this process has been successful is an instrument assigned validity.

Different types of validity are often distinguished and are summarised here. General issues relating to each are discussed in many texts.[16–18]

Types of validity

Face validity

Face validity is generally the first test of validity of an instrument, that is, *prima facie* (without further investigation), would the instrument be expected to collect accurate information as required to meet the study objectives? If a question or instrument does not possess face validity, then it is unlikely to be valid.

Checking for face validity aims to uncover obvious problems such as identification of questions for which it might be expected that respondents would be unable or reluctant to provide the information requested (e.g. on issues that may be considered confidential), questions that might be ambiguous or misinterpreted, or those that might not be an accurate reflection of the variable of interest.

Although only rarely mentioned in the studies reviewed[19,20] (e.g. a check on face validity was carried out by another member of the research team[20]), it is highly likely that in most instances some checking for face validity would have been undertaken. Most researchers in the process of developing a questionnaire will ask colleagues or others for comments and suggestions before going on to do more detailed and structured investigations on the validity.

In a study to compare pharmacists' and customers' perceptions of service quality, questions were assessed for face validity by a co-researcher.[20] This is a sensible first step to identify immediate problems. Individuals from the same research team, especially experienced researchers, may offer constructive advice to enhance the validity of an instrument. However, they are also likely to share similar perspectives on the topic and may therefore be 'blind' to some potential problems. Assessment of face validity may best be carried out among people from the population in which the study is to be conducted. It is to be expected that pharmacists would be less effective at assessing face validity of an instrument from the perspective of customers than that of pharmacists.

Criterion validity

Criterion validity refers to the extent to which the instrument or questions correlate with other measures of the same variable. Thus, to demonstrate criterion validity, the results are compared with established methods of collecting the same information. Examples include questions to assess mental health, such as anxiety or confusion, comparing the results with clinical measures. The General Health Questionnaire (GHQ28), which was used in a study of elderly people and their pre-scribed medication,[4] has been extensively used to screen for anxiety and depression among different population groups. Its criterion validity is based on the fact that a score of five to six on the GHQ28 correlates well with clinical diagnoses of anxiety and depression.[21] To validate the responses and assess reporting bias in a study of cigarette smoking based on self-reports, serum cotinine (a biochemical marker of exposure to tobacco smoke) was measured in a sample of respondents.[22] Individuals' reports of their medication use has been validated by comparing with pharmacy refill data records.[5]

Construct validity

Construct validity is concerned with whether or not a question, or a group of questions, corresponds to what is understood by a construct or concept. To achieve construct validity, the researcher must include questions that can easily be answered and which provide a classifi-cation that reflects the components and complexities of a theoretical construct. For example, to classify individuals on the basis of socio-economic group, the question arises as to how this concept is 'oper-ationalised' or how people of different socio-economic groups are identified and classified in a questionnaire. As a social construct, socio-economic status (social class) is widely recognised and there is some common understanding regarding its interpretation. For example, when describing this variable, features such as lifestyle, opportunities, income, wealth, outlook on life may be cited. However, it is complex, difficult to define and presents a problem for researchers who require questionnaire items which provide a valid reflection of this attribute. In Britain, classifi-cation into six socio-economic groups has been according to the Registrar General's classification which is based on occupation and employment status. However, despite modifications over the years (partly in response to society's continuous changes in structure), the validity of this method has been questioned. A revised approach has been devised,[23] which considers both validity and operational issues in research. The new classification is based on a conceptual model of employment relations theory. Validation procedures have included con-struct validity, and the assessment of continuity and congruence with existing systems of classification. To ensure ease of use for researchers and adaptability according to the objectives of the research, the new system is hierarchical, which enables the classification to be collapsed in different ways, as well as providing flexibility in the extent of data that are required.

Thus, occupation and employment status remain the basis for social classification in official statistics in the UK. It is argued that these variables are determinants of social class, providing a theoretical basis, whereas other variables, often well correlated, are consequences of it.[15] Use of the most valid measure is preferable, but this can result in considerable lengthening of questionnaires, which, depending on study objectives, may be counter-productive. Health service and pharmacy researchers have used other variables as indicators of socio-economic status, either alone or in combination; these include education and housing tenure. As 'proxy' variables, they also possess their own strengths and weaknesses.

Measures have also been devised and incorporated as a measure of the socio-economic status of populations, as distinct from that of the individual participants in a survey. For example, such measures were used to investigate inequalities in service provision or drug use between population groups[11,24–26] (see below).

There have been a number of studies investigating health issues and pharmacy services among different ethnic groups. For survey researchers investigating ethnicity, the question arises of how different ethnic groups are to be distinguished in a questionnaire.[27] Possible classifications may be according to place of birth, nationality, skin colour, language group, self-perceived identity, parental origins, etc. or a combination of these variables, all of which may lead to different classifications of the same individual. Choice of measure may depend on the objectives of the research; for example, language may be important regarding the provision of information on health services and drugs, self-perceived cultural identity may be a determinant of certain health practices, whereas genetic traits are important predisposing factors for some diseases (e.g. sickle cell disease). Studies in pharmacy practice have variously used facial appearance from photographs,[28] selection by name from electoral registers or clinic records[13,29,30] or asked people to classify themselves.[11,31] Each method has its own advantages and disadvantages. Information on religion, language, country and region of origin and length of residence in the location of the research study was collected to explore the differences between ethnic groups. Data were collected in interviews, respondents being matched with interviewers for language and ethnicity.[32]

In any research, the categories selected will be influenced by the location of the study and objectives of the research. If a primary objective is to compare findings with those of other studies, then classification must be conducted on the same basis. Health services researchers in the UK often adopt the relevant questions from the most recent decennial census.

Smaje,[27] in addressing the problems of operationalising ethnicity in research, provides an example of classification by religion as either Protestant or Catholic. He points out that this classification has very different social or cultural significance in Northern Ireland from elsewhere in the UK or the world. By citing this example, Smaje[27] demonstrates how the meanings attached to ethnicity may be more important than the classification itself, and that ethnicity may be seen as a social or cultural construct. Thus, each classification will have its own meaning.

In investigating many cultural issues, an individual's self-perceived identity is generally considered the most pertinent classification and is most commonly employed. This approach requires researchers to make a decision about how many categories to include, and which ones. Individuals within any category may share experiences and background, but these will not necessarily be universal to all individuals in that category, and differences among these individuals will be not be identifiable in the analysis. In Britain, the ethnic minority population is around 5%, which means that, in much research, 95% of the population falls into a single category. This clearly includes people from a range of cultural backgrounds who would distinguish themselves from others within the 95%.

Concern has been expressed that in medical research the 'white' group is not generally subdivided, despite well-documented differences in mortality and morbidity between subgroups.[33] The health of ethnic minority groups is a focus of the British Government's aim to address social exclusion, although it has been argued that a suitable and comprehensive information database does not exist.[34] Parker[35] argues that when researching ethnicity and health, racism should be included as a variable. She notes that by dividing minority groups but not the majority, ethnicity becomes an explanatory variable for black, but not for white people. Parker claims that this denies the fact that there are frequently more similarities than differences between ethnic minority groups, in particular, that what is different for black people compared to white people is the experience of racism. In research, white people are often described by appearance, whilst black people are divided into ethnic categories. She argues that this procedure implies that white people are not distinguished by culture and that black people do not share the experience of racism.[35]

Construct validity is also important in the development of measures of health status, quality of life and other theoretical constructs such as satisfaction. In recent years, many new measures have emerged for the assessment of health status and quality of life and been incorporated by pharmacy practice researchers.[2,4,13,36] Researchers investigating job satisfaction developed a survey instrument based on theoretical constructs from the literature that distinguished 'facet-free' aspects (general satisfaction) and 'facet-specific' aspects (satisfaction with specified aspects of a job).[37] The development of a measure to assess pharmacists' orientation to patient counselling has also been described in terms of its reliability and processes of validation.[38]

Content validity

Content validity is concerned with the extent to which an instrument covers all the relevant issues. Omitting to gather data on issues that are of importance to a topic will result in an instrument that lacks content validity. Questionnaires that do not include the questions that provide the respondents with the opportunity to report on the issues they feel important, or a closed question that includes a range of responses but excludes any that respondents believe to be more appropriate, will not accurately reflect their views.

A range of techniques has been employed by researchers to ensure the content validity of survey instruments. This is generally undertaken as part of the preliminary fieldwork leading to the development of the instrument. The aim of this fieldwork is to uncover, from the perspective of the population of interest, the issues, considerations, experiences, practices and priorities that are important to them with regard to the objectives of the research. In this respect this preliminary fieldwork shares approaches and features of qualitative enquiry (see Chapter 4). Exploratory (in-depth) and/or semi-structured interviews have been used by many researchers to identify the issues (in both their depth and breadth) that are important to the population of interest which can then be included in a survey instrument.[39–54] These examples include in-depth interviews to uncover the dimensions of pharmacists' preferences for cough and cold products,[50] and to provide the basis for a tool to obtain customer comments with a view to improving pharmacy services.[46]

Field notes from early stages of a study may provide insights into relevant issues and also be a useful source of questions or items for the survey instrument.[49,55,56] A survey comparing perceptions and activities of patient counselling among Swedish and Dutch pharmacists derived their questionnaire items from data collected during Dutch pharmacists' postgraduate education courses.[57] Members of the public attending a diabetes seminar were involved in the refinement of a questionnaire for people with diabetes.[58]

Group discussions (e.g. focus groups) have also provided a means of identifying relevant issues, modifying and refining questionnaires and/or checking the interpretation of individual questions or items.[38,59-62] Group discussions may be more successful than one-to-one interviews in revealing the breadth and depth of relevant issues and concerns. Structured group interviews, such as those using the Nominal Group technique[63,64] and Delphi method[65,66] have also been used to generate a wide range of ideas and to reach a consensus regarding the important issues.

Many researchers highlight the importance of the published work of previous researchers in identifying relevant issues and/or as a source of questionnaire items.[20,28,62,65-67] To investigate aspects of pharmacy health promotion activity, a range of variables which were claimed in the literature to be of importance were used as a basis for the survey instrument.[68,69]

Exploratory interviews conducted in the early stages of research will often involve convenience samples. Ideally, they should be conducted among the population for whom the questionnaire is intended. For instance, interviews with hospital pharmacists to inform the development of a questionnaire intended for community pharmacists[48] could result in some issues of importance to the latter being missed.

There are many examples of questionnaires that focus on attitudes. Because of the complexity of attitudes, ensuring content validity of instruments (which requires that all the relevant components are identified) may present particular difficulties[17] (see below).

Problems and processes of validation

Validating self-reports

An important aspect of the validation process in social survey research is to ascertain if the questions are interpreted as intended and to assess the extent of response bias. It is well established that social surveys based on self-reporting may not provide accurate data on some variables. For example, it is recognised that survey questions on smoking behaviour based on self-reporting are likely to underestimate cigarette consumption and prevalence levels.[22] The biochemical marker, serum cotinine, has been used to validate survey data.[22] Authors reporting an investigation of perceived levels of patient counselling among Canadian pharmacists point out that responses may be influenced by social desirability bias, misperceptions or their own definitions of counselling.[70]

Self-reports have been validated by comparison of responses with data on the same variables collected from other sources. This is discussed in more detail in Chapter 7. Examples include claims of general medical practitioners on their use of drug information services, which were compared with the records of the information centres concerned.[71] A study investigating adherence among patients taking antihypertensives combined self-reports with medical record data, blood pressure control and prescription refills.[72] In a study of use of non-prescription analgesics to investigate hazards, data from respondents were combined with information from subsequent contact with their physicians.[73]

The importance of the method of survey data collection to the subsequent validity of data has been addressed in relation to surveys of the extent of patient counselling.[64] Here, self-completion questionnaires have been shown to over-estimate the frequency of this activity[74] while diaries have resulted in under-estimates.[75] Researchers switching from postal to telephone data collection suggest that this may have increased the tendency for participants to provide socially desirable responses.[76]

Self-reports and actions

To compare the advice of doctors and pharmacists in responding to symptoms, researchers presented respondents with scenarios and they were requested to comment on the action they would take.[77] Similarly, a study of pharmacists' approaches to harm minimisation initiatives associated with problem drug use relied on self-reports by pharmacists regarding their willingness to participate in needle exchange schemes and to supervise methadone consumption.[78] The validity issue that this presents is the extent to which the responses reflect actual behaviour of practitioners when faced with similar problems in the course of their practice. It may also be difficult for respondents to envisage the provision of an additional service, its associated problems and rewards, and thus to speculate easily on their likely involvement.

Researchers investigating management of hypertension by general medical practitioners compared reported behaviours obtained in self-completion questionnaires with the contents of patients' medical records, finding a 'variable' relationship between the two sources. They concluded that if researchers had no prior knowledge of the validity of self-reports then the questions should not be used.[79]

Validity and the research setting

The location of the survey may also affect the validity of responses. In questionnaires given out by pharmacists (especially if they are to be returned to that pharmacy), and in which comments pertaining to pharmacy services are requested, people may be reluctant to express themselves freely. Similarly, potential respondents may doubt the independence of any survey carried out in a health-care setting. Researchers need to consider the possible impact of these inhibitions on the validity of their findings and take steps to ensure these are not jeopardised. Inadequate privacy in any setting may inhibit true responses on sensitive issues.

Problems of validity also arise when the research is carried out by individuals who are seeking comments on their own services, for example, a study of nursing sisters' satisfaction with the pharmacy services undertaken by pharmacy staff,[80] and a survey of the value of a newsletter to its recipients.[81] Patients attending a musculo-skeletal clinic were interviewed on the day of their appointment about their use of complementary therapies and satisfaction with conventional medical treatment.[82] Unless they are successfully assured of independence and confidentiality of the research and anonymity in the findings, respondents may be reluctant to provide negative views, resulting in bias in responses, a problem which should be addressed both in the methodology and the interpretation of the findings.

Studies across populations

There are examples of both successful and less successful studies across international boundaries.[57,83,84] Questions and methods relevant to practices that work well in one population may lack face validity or be inappropriate in another.

Surveying 'social pharmacy' or 'pharmacy administration' components of undergraduate courses in different countries may present problems in that the terms may be used differently or not at all in some countries. Questions may not be viewed as relevant by all respondents or may not be interpreted as intended.[84] In applying a measure of health locus of control to a population in Thailand, researchers needed to ensure that it possesses the same validity as in the populations in which it was developed.[85] The validity of the structural model of the SF36 measure of health status among Maori and Pacific ethnic groups has also been challenged.[86]

In comparing practices in different settings, for example, the management of dermatological conditions in community pharmacy and general medical practice in the UK,[87] different considerations and variables will apply to each. Researchers investigating ethnic minority consumers and pharmaceutical services discussed the adaptation of questions to the needs and experiences of the ethnic minority communities.[73]

Quantification in questionnaires

Precise frequencies or predetermined categories

Many questionnaires include some questions that require estimation by the respondents. The questions can ask respondents to provide a precise figure or to select from a series of predetermined categories. If the researcher requires information, for example, on the age of respondents, this can be done by asking the respondents either to specify their age (or date of birth) or (as is common in social surveys) to assign themselves to a predetermined age range. The former method confers greater flexibility in that researchers can subsequently construct their own categories to suit their needs (e.g. to compare their sample with other surveys or official statistics that may have used a variety of classification systems). However, interviewees and interviewers may feel more comfortable with the latter approach, especially for questions on sensitive issues. If it is clear from the outset that only one set of categories will be needed in the analysis of data, this method may be preferred. Reliable and valid data on age are generally easy to obtain, unless data are being collected through a third party, but for other variables (e.g. frequency of requests for advice, or medicine sales) respondents may have difficulty providing a precise answer, but feel able to select a reply from a series of categories.

Numerical frequencies or subjective quantifiers

In studies requiring frequency data, researchers have used both numerical frequencies and subjective (imprecise) quantifiers. For example, respondents may be asked to describe the frequency with which they omit doses of their medication as 'often, sometimes, rarely or never' rather than providing an objective frequency such as 'more than once daily, less than once a week', etc. Selecting a response is subjective in that respondents will employ their own terms of reference, possibly comparing themselves to those around them, their expectations or previous experiences.

Depending on the questions employed, their place within a survey instrument and/or the objectives of the research, subjective quantifiers may be most appropriate. For example, in the measurement of health status, respondents are frequently asked to provide an estimate of their self-perceived health:

In general would you describe your health as:
- *Excellent*
- *Very Good*
- *Good*
- *Fair*
- *Poor*

This question is not an objective measure of an individual's health status (although it forms an important component of many measures and has predictive value in terms of present and future health status) but a measure of the individual's perception of it.

In a survey that included measures of pharmacists' perceptions of their safety when undertaking professional activities, researchers adapted a question from the British Crime Survey[11]:

How safe do you feel walking alone in the area of your pharmacy after dark?
- *Very safe*
- *Fairly safe*
- *A bit unsafe*
- *Very unsafe*
- *Don't know*

This question is not a measure of actual risks to an individual but a measure of their perception of their own safety. These perceptions may be what the researcher is interested in. For instance, irrespective of objective risks, if pharmacists feel unsafe in the area of their pharmacy this may influence their decisions of whether or not to offer particular services.

Questions employing subjective quantifiers cannot be readily translated into numerical frequencies. If two people were asked: 'How often do you forget to take your tablets?', a frequency of once a week may be viewed as 'occasionally' by one respondent but 'very often' by another.

In a study of hospital trainers of pre-registration pharmacists, respondents were asked to report their level of satisfaction as:

- *gravely concerned*
- *quite concerned*
- *no view*
- *quite confident*
- *totally confident*

This scale was not validated in terms of interpretation of the responses, or the extent to which the terms of reference of different respondents may coincide. It does provide an indication of the proportions of respondents who hold overall negative or positive views. However, the true differences, or meanings, reflected in the responses of, for example, *quite concerned* vis-à-vis *gravely concerned* are unclear.[88]

Thus, if the researcher wishes to provide some estimates of numerical frequencies of events, rather than an individual's perceptions of them, then questions using subjective quantifiers may not be the best approach.

Adopting and adapting measures in the literature

Many pharmacy practice researchers have adopted or adapted measures from the literature to serve their own research objectives. Examples of the incorporation of established health status and quality of life measures are increasingly common.[2,4,13] The well-established health belief model has been used as a theoretical framework against which to relate other variables (including the use of medicines).[5] The health locus of control has been employed in an experimental study to investigate the use of self-care protocols.[1] Researchers investigating job satisfaction used the job descriptive index and the occupational stress indicator to investigate stress among community pharmacists.[8,89] Instruments developed by many pharmacy practice researchers have been informed by the literature, either in terms of identifying a theoretical basis for the subsequent development of an instrument or as a source of questions to measure specific variables.[3,11,19,37,58,67,90,91] Compromises in survey instruments are sometimes made by researchers to keep the survey to a reasonable length, or to avoid questions that people may be unwilling to answer. For instance, incorporation of an entire health status measure could lengthen the questionnaire unacceptably. Unless the measurement of health status was of primary importance to the researcher, a briefer, possibly less robust, series of questions may be preferred.

In health services research there is an extensive literature on the assessment of satisfaction in terms of the development of instruments, their application to different services and the difficulties that both these issues present. With increasing emphasis on perspectives of consumers in the health service, the investigation of satisfaction with services has been the subject of numerous surveys,[66,67,69,80,88,92–95] many of which are components of studies evaluating pharmacy services. There are studies in which researchers have not acknowledged the complexities of developing instruments for this purpose, sometimes relying on just a single question, the reliability and validity of which would be questionable. Because measurement of satisfaction frequently forms a part of service evaluation, this research is reviewed in more detail in Chapter 9.

Reliability

The reliability of questions of a survey instrument (or individual questions within it) relates to the extent to which the findings are reproducible or internally consistent. That questions in a survey are reliable is not evidence that they are necessarily valid. For instance, respondents to a survey may consistently over- or under-estimate in the information they provide, for example the number of hours they work or the number of units of alcohol they consume. Consequently, the results although reproducible, may be consistently wrong. Thus, a survey instrument can be reliable but not valid. However, it cannot be valid if it is unreliable.

Factors that can result in poor reliability include ambiguity of question wording, inconsistent interpretation of questions by respondents, variation in the style of questioning by different interviewers, or inability of respondents to provide accurate information, leading to guesses or poor estimates.

Questionnaires are generally an efficient method for gathering factual data, but care must be taken to ensure that people are able to provide the information. For example, questions expecting people to recall events (e.g. recent use of drugs, last time they visited the doctor) may produce inaccurate data; information that is sensitive or too inaccessible may result in poor response rates or misleading data. Questions requiring respondents to recall events, or estimate their frequency, commonly present reliability problems. For instance, in surveying the frequency of cold sore symptoms and their management in community pharmacy, some assessment or evidence of the reliability of responses should be provided.[96] Two studies of non-prescription medication use among patients with diabetes[97] and hypertension[58] claimed that questions relating to the previous two weeks provided reliable information.

In a study of drug use by people with hypertension, recall sensitivity (reliability) was found to be higher for questions that asked about medications used for a specific condition than for more general questions.[98]

In surveys of violent crime, the period of the previous 12 months was adopted to enable comparison with other studies. For minor incidents this may be too long a period for reliable recall. However, as serious events may be rare and be remembered for a lifetime, data collected over a longer time period may be more reliable and further questions were included to collect this information.[11] In this study, additional questions were also included in the questionnaire to provide an internal check on the reliability of responses. Respondents were asked to report the number of events in the previous year and then asked how long ago the most recent event occurred. Whilst for any individual the total number of events in a given time period and the timing of the most recent could be variable, in analysis of the data set as a whole, an association between these variables would be expected.

Thus, researchers have demonstrated how issues of reliability should be considered during the development of the survey instrument. Questions that are not carefully formulated, for example that are ambiguous, double-barrelled, that contain double negatives or are poorly expressed, are more likely to lead to unreliable results.

The method of data collection may be important in facilitating reliable data; for instance, the use of diaries to record events rather than asking respondents to recall events retrospectively. However, events may be more likely to remain unrecorded at busy times, if events are so rare that regular use of the diary is not established, or so routine that actions go unnoticed. In a study in which pharmacists recorded details of accidents, researchers noted that at the start of the study the rate of reporting was much higher than later on.[99] Some checking would be required to establish whether this was a result of reporting fatigue, loss of interest on the part of the participants, or genuinely reflected a decrease in the number of accidents.

A first step in addressing the reliability of data is similar to the face-validity check, that is, to spot questions that might be expected to be inaccurately answered. The dependability of responses may also be assessed by comparison with similar data obtained from other sources. Pilot work is important in uncovering many of these problems. A procedure commonly adopted to check for consistency of interpretation and response is the test–retest procedure in which the instrument is administered to a sample of respondents on two separate occasions, generally a few weeks apart.[39,100,101]

In some publications, the full questionnaire, or an abridged version, was included, which allows interpretation of the findings in the context of the actual questions asked.[3,55,85,102–104]

Variation between interviewers

When multiple interviewers are involved in gathering data, it is important to ensure consistent administration of the questionnaire. In survey work, most questionnaires are highly structured and if procedures are standardised and directions are clear there should be limited scope for variation. Studies in which interviews are recorded on audiotape provide opportunities for some quality assurance, that is, checks that study procedures are followed. When relying on others, such as practising pharmacists or other health personnel, to collect data it is important to ensure that standardised procedures are acceptable, workable and followed in each setting. Researchers have reported involving just one interviewer to avoid problems of variation.[105] In larger projects this is not always feasible.

Internal consistency

To check for internal reliability of questions, researchers have used both the split-half method and Cronbach's alpha. In the split-half method, the data are divided into two halves; each half is analysed independently and the results compared.[38,55,100,106] Cronbach's alpha is a statistic (between 0 and 1) that reflects the correlations between questionnaire items which are intended to be part of the same measure.[6,19,31,46,51,66,103,107–110] Researchers employing this method generally consider a figure of not less than 0.7 as acceptable (see Chapter 3).

Measuring attitudes

In many surveys pharmacy practice researchers have included measures to describe respondents' views and attitudes. These include pharmacists' attitudes to patient counselling,[38,70] audit,[100] terms of service,[92,111] involvement in research,[53,112] deregulation of medicines,[113] herbal medicines and drug–nutrient interactions,[114–116] as well as surveys among other population groups towards pharmacy related issues.[104,116–118] The measurement of attitudes, including the processes of the development and testing of measures, is recognised as a complex task. In other surveys, researchers have aimed to provide descriptive information on views or perceptions of a population, a simpler approach being employed in the development of questions or instruments. Thus, in pharmacy practice research, methodology ranges from a description of views of different groups of people (with no explicit link to the representation of underlying attitudes) to the identification of these underlying attitudes and the development (or identification from the literature) of instruments for their measurement.

Attitudes generally comprise many components, some more important to the overall attribute than others. Instruments for their measurement will therefore necessarily be structurally complex. Furthermore, attitudes may not be stable over a period of time and may be influenced, sometimes quite markedly, by recent experience. Demonstrating that a series of questions is a reliable and valid measure of people's attitudes on an issue is problematic.

A text referred to by many authors as providing guidance in the development of instruments for the measurement of attitudes is Oppenheim's *Questionnaire Design, Interviewing and Attitude Measurement.*[17] Oppenheim recognises the theoretical expositions and complexities in the study of attitudes, but for the purposes of research suggests that an attitude is 'a state of readiness, a tendency to respond in a certain manner when confronted with certain stimuli'. He sees attitudes as 'dormant' until expressed in speech and behaviour. Thus their measurement focuses on providing stimuli (e.g. items in a questionnaire) which reflect the domains of an attitude and which evoke a response by individuals that illuminates the underlying attitude.

In the development of instruments the issues that have been addressed by pharmacy practice and health service researchers relate to the development and selection of questionnaire items, including a demonstration of their validity (in terms of being a true reflection of the attribute of interest) and reliability. Oppenheim[17] also identifies the complex nature of attitudes and the consequent considerations for researchers, both in terms of their content and intensity. He describes how people's opinions are indicative of their attitudes to particular issues which, in turn, may be reflective of an underlying system of values. Thus, a positive or negative view on one issue is often associated with either positive or negative views on another, reflecting this underlying set of attitudes or values.

In terms of the content, Oppenheim also questions the linearity of attitudes, which assumes that the issues which are important to people holding positive views may not be those which are determinants of negative views. Thus, positive views of medical practitioners regarding the potential contribution of clinical pharmacists to patient care may be based on favourable experiences, whilst negative views may not necessarily be a result of poor experiences but of beliefs about their knowledge base or professional outlook. Exposure to clinical pharmacists has been shown to have an effect on medical practitioners' attitudes.[119] Thus, in the development of measures, the content validity, in terms of including the issues that are relevant to the attribute, must be assured. Oppenheim[17] also identifies differences in intensity of attitudes. As well as including the relevant issues, reasoning and arguments of individuals who hold different views, to be discriminatory the instrument must also possess the sensitivity to distinguish people who hold these views with different strengths of feeling.

In some studies in pharmacy, instruments developed in previous research have been incorporated or adapted. For example, to compare attitudes and beliefs regarding self-care and personal responsibility, researchers applied two existing measures: the 'health locus of control' and Krantz health opinion study.[85] Other researchers have set out to devise their own measures.

To ensure content validity, the preliminary fieldwork leading to the development of the instrument must be comprehensive in identifying all the relevant issues and domains relating to the study objectives from the perspective of the population of interest. This has been conducted in a number of ways. Qualitative interviews and a review of the literature were used to develop a comprehensive list of possible influences for inclusion in a pilot questionnaire to uncover the dimensions of pharmacists' preferences for cough and cold preparations.[50] To investigate views of the public on pharmacy services,[46] community pharmacists' attitudes to research,[53] pharmacy students' attitudes to drug misuse and HIV[39] and the important issues determining physicians' interactions with and perceptions of pharmacists' responsibilities,[120] questionnaire items were derived following face-to-face interviews.

Group techniques are believed to be effective in generating a wide range of issues from the perspective of the population of interest, as individual group members may act as a stimulus to each other and enable the exploration of issues from different viewpoints (see Chapter 5). In a study of attitudes of pharmacists, medical practitioners and nurses to domiciliary and other pharmacy services, questionnaires were designed following semi-structured group discussion sessions involving 10–12 members of each profession to identify that profession's important issues and priorities.[61] To measure Pharmacy Board members' attitudes on freedom of choice of individuals in choosing a pharmacy, the Delphi technique was used to achieve a consensus regarding the important issues.[65] In a comparison of Swedish and Dutch pharmacists' beliefs and activities in patient counselling, items were derived from data that had been collected during Dutch postgraduate courses on patient education.[57] Changes in attitudes to clinical pharmacy services were evaluated in a longitudinal study of pharmacy students who were followed up seven years after graduation. Statements pertaining to clinical pharmacy and to the status of the profession were initially derived from field notes, informal discussions and written comments obtained during the early stages of the research.[49] To survey consumer perceptions and attitudes to community pharmacy services[12] and pharmacists' attitudes to injecting drug misusers,[90] questionnaire items were derived from instruments used in previous studies.

Once the domains and issues have been identified, researchers then have to generate an item pool; that is questionnaire items that reflect the sentiments to be investigated both in terms of content and intensity. The formulation of individual items for the 'item pool' and subsequent selection of items for inclusion in the final instrument require care to ensure clarity of expression, so that people can identify with statements and respond easily. In many studies, the preliminary fieldwork provided a source of actual questionnaire items, as well as identification of the relevant domains of the measures required for content validity. The words and expressions used by participants may be those which best capture an individual's feelings and concerns and with which others can identify. Thus in selection of items attention is paid to comprehensiveness (coverage of relevant issues including representation of different strengths of opinion), balance between positive and negative statements (especially if scaling procedures are to be employed), clarity of wording (avoidance of ambiguous or double-barrelled statements) and expression (with which respondents are able to identify). In a study of the impact of carers' attitudes on the safety of medicines procedures in residential homes, researchers reported that following pilot work they made improvements to the clarity of questionnaire items, discarding those which were non-discriminatory.[55] To investigate views of the public on pharmacy services, the researchers describe the inclusion of statements both worded favourably and unfavourably, to minimise bias.[46] In a survey of pharmacy trainees' perceptions of the need for cultural sensitivity in service provision, researchers reported attention to the wording of items, in particular for those to which a socially desirable response may be implicit.[31]

As with many surveys, researchers reported piloting the questionnaire with a small number of respondents prior to the distribution for the main study.[12,39,40,46,65] In a study of consumers' views of pharmacy services, instruments were assessed by asking a convenience sample to complete it; these individuals were then interviewed to establish whether or not questions had been interpreted as intended.[46] A similar procedure using a focus group was employed to check the interpretation of items in an instrument to assess pharmacy students' attitudes to HIV/AIDS and drug misuse. Participants were asked what they understood by each item, after which ambiguous items were amended or removed.[40]

Scales

To each item in a questionnaire where scales are used, respondents are usually requested to express their views within a range. The most frequently employed is a five-point Likert scale,[38,46,49,53,57,90,121,122] which commonly includes the points 'strongly agree, agree, neither agree nor disagree, disagree, strongly disagree'. Scales of differing numbers of points have also been employed: for example, a four-point scale in a survey of community pharmacists' and general practitioners' attitudes to extended roles and interprofessional collaboration.[123] A seven-point scale was employed in a survey of consumer perceptions of quality of pharmacy services.[20] Scales with a greater number of intervals may result in greater discriminatory power, respondents being dispersed across seven categories rather than the usual five. Too few intervals on a scale result in discernible differences between individuals in their views on an issue being lost to the researcher. Too many intervals will result in an unreliable scale as respondents have difficulty in selecting a category. This will be evidenced by poor reliability (e.g. on test–retest respondents are inconsistent in their responses). The researcher will wish to aim for maximum discriminatory power, whilst ensuring reliability of the instrument is maintained.

A decision has also to be made regarding an even or odd number of intervals. A scale with an even number of intervals has no middle point, and therefore does not allow the respondents to be non-committal, forcing them to express either a positive or negative view. However, if respondents are genuinely unable to locate themselves, such a scale may either be unreliable (e.g. on test–retest) or the researcher may be faced with a high proportion of missing responses.

The data from Likert scales are often presented descriptively, that is the responses to each questionnaire item are reported separately.

However, scaling procedures are sometimes employed in which items on the scale are scored and/or summed. In the scoring of individual items, scores of 1 to 5 and -2 to $+2$ have been used. Imposing a five-point scoring system assumes a linear scale, the differences between the points on each scale being the same. The validity of this assumption has been questioned, especially if the responses to different items are to be summed or combined in some way. As an alternative, in some cases researchers have grouped positive and negative responses together resulting in values of -1, 0 and $+1$.

If visual analogue scales are used in which respondents place themselves on a continuum or interval scale (rather than a scale that is anchored by a description at every point, representing a series of separate categories), assumptions of linearity in the scoring system may be deemed invalid.

Other scaling procedures

A Gutmann scale[17] comprises a hierarchical series of categories for which an individual selects the level which best represents their status or views. Each level corresponds to a score on the scale. A Guttman scale was devised to compare the views of hospital pharmacists and doctors regarding clinical activities of pharmacists. This involved the development of a series of scenarios organised into a hierarchy according to level of involvement. These were presented as part of a questionnaire and respondents were asked to indicate their agreement or disagreement to pharmacists performing these roles.[124] To identify views of hospital doctors, nurses and pharmacists on pharmacist-written prescriptions and pharmacist prescribing, respondents were asked to express their views regarding a number of scenarios describing potential activities of pharmacists.[125] In both studies researchers compared the responses of the different professional groups.

The techniques used in assessing the reliability of attitudinal measures are those employed widely in social surveys (see above). Thus, there are examples of split-half,[38,55] test–retest[40] and Cronbach's alpha.[31,38,46,108,109] Factor analysis (sometimes in combination with Cronbach's alpha) has been used to identify or confirm the underlying dimensions or constructs of attitudinal measures[31,46,52,53,58,91,108,126,127] (see Chapter 3).

Measures of attitudes have also formed part of studies to develop or test theoretical models. For example, in the assessment of a theoretical framework of factors influencing pharmacists' behaviour and provision of pharmaceutical care, an attitudinal measure was one component.[66] Community pharmacists' attitudes were examined as part of a theoretical construct to predict intention to intervene in drug related problems.[91] Five attitudinal attributes provided a basis for the construction of a causal model to predict pharmaceutical care behaviours. A sample of pharmacists received an attitude survey followed by a behavioural survey two weeks later.[127]

Characterising pharmacies, pharmacists and clientele

In recognition of the heterogeneity of pharmacy services, researchers commonly include variables to describe and distinguish pharmacies in their sample and/or to establish types of pharmacy that are associated with particular services or events. This characterisation of pharmacies and/or pharmacists also enables some assessment of the extent to which the sample is representative of a wider pharmacy or pharmacist population with respect to these variables (and thus consider the validity of generalisation of findings to other populations). These endeavours require that researchers include in their data set some variables that describe the pharmacies or pharmacists included in their study. In descriptive surveys, characterisation of pharmacies, pharmacists and other staff and clientele is common. Relevant variables and categories will depend on the structure and organisation of the pharmacy sector.

Thus researchers must gather information meaningful to the study objectives, both in terms of the variables on which data are collected and the values selected for each variable. Researchers must also ensure that any categorisation is an accurate reflection of important differences (i.e. is valid), and is reliable in that the information being sought is readily available, easily interpreted and consistently reported. The variables selected and their associated values will depend on the level of precision required to fulfil the study objectives, whilst maintaining a satisfactory level of reliability of reporting. The reliability of a classification system could be assessed by asking a number of researchers to categorise a series of cases, possibly on repeated occasions.

Commonly distinguished features of pharmacies include structural and organisational aspects of their services and characteristics of staff and clientele.

Patterns of ownership of pharmacies are among the most frequently used of variables. Variables relating to ownership will not be of universal relevance. The most appropriate categorisation will be determined by the structure and organisation of the pharmacy sector in the location of interest. In countries where all pharmacies are part of a single organisation, or where there are regulations governing the number of pharmacies which an individual or company may own, this variable would not be a useful descriptor. For example, in an area with universal corporate ownership, the most relevant variables of classification will differ from a location where there are diverse patterns of ownership.

In Britain, pharmacy businesses range from single proprietor to large organisations comprising tens or even hundreds of premises. Thus, in Britain, classifications have distinguished single independent pharmacies from those that are part of small or large multiples. Classification as just 'an independent' or 'a multiple' can be unclear. Classification of multiples/chains as small or large are also sometimes ill defined. Specifications which have been used include: independent, small multiple, national multiple; sole independent, independent chain, corporate chain[68]; independent, chain under 10 pharmacies, chain 10–20, chain over 20[128]; independent, small ownership (2–8), medium ownership (9–15), large ownership (16+).[53] Although divisions may be arbitrary, specification of these improves the precision of the categorisation and enables comparison to be made with other studies.

Premises and business features that have been used include measures of prescription throughput (e.g. the number of prescription items dispensed in a given time period) and sales of non-prescription medicine products. One study investigating consumers' views regarding information-giving in pharmacies classified pharmacies as high, medium and low providers based on the extent to which work-flow changes had been implemented to accommodate advice-giving.[129]

Other variables relating to individual premises are aspects of the layout of the pharmacy, for example, presence of a designated counselling area. In a study of 'the changing face of pharmacy', four pharmacy layouts were distinguished: traditional (pharmacist not visible), traditional with some modification, open, and raised open.[130]

In Britain, the size and style of pharmacies varies greatly, some pharmacies having only one or two members of staff, others being part of large department stores. The total number of staff employed in premises has been used as a proxy for the size of an establishment.[11]

Pharmacists and other staff. Information on staff that has been collected usually relates to their number, occupational status and/or qualifications. Pharmacists are commonly distinguished as owners, owner/managers,

managers, employee pharmacists and locum pharmacists. Information may also be requested on non-pharmacist dispensary staff, including pre-registration pharmacists, technicians and dispensers. Data on the number and qualifications of medicines counter staff may also be important to study objectives. The number of pharmacists and other staff groups employed may be expressed as the number of staff members, numbers of part-time and full-time staff, or in terms of full-time equivalents.

Other characterisations of pharmacists may be based on personal attributes: age, sex, and ethnicity; professional characteristics, for example years since qualification and seniority in terms of grade; qualifications including participation in postgraduate study; speciality (community, hospital, academic, industrial, other), and business versus professional orientation.

Location. Data on location are gathered in many studies. The variables regarding location should ideally reflect the range of locations in which pharmacies in the study population are situated and be pertinent to the study objectives.

Data on location in terms of town/city centre, suburban, urban or rural have been used in many studies. Other classifications of this variable have included: town/city-centre, other main shopping street, small group of local shops, an area without other shops[11]; residential area, secondary high street, main shopping area[130]; main shopping street, indoor shopping precinct, small group of local shops, in health centre, on a housing estate.[128] An additional category of 'health centre' pharmacy has sometimes been added. However, this could be compatible with many locations and, if included as an alternative response within this variable, it may result in data not being obtained for health centre pharmacies. These classifications can also present difficulties in terms of reliability. For example, a distinction between rural and small town or between urban and suburban may be difficult to define. In self-completion surveys respondents may perceive the location of their pharmacies differently. In some studies, information has been gathered on the proximity of a given pharmacy to others, for example, the number of other pharmacies within a 2 km radius, and proximity to local surgeries.

Local population and clientele. Pharmacies have also been distinguished in terms of characteristics of the local population or their clientele.

Data on the socio-economic status of local populations to enable the identification and investigation of inequalities has been important to policy makers and researchers. Hirschfield and Wolfson[131] examined the number of pharmacies per 10 000 residents in a region of England in relation to socio-economic characteristics, revealing a greater concentration of pharmacies in more deprived areas. The Townsend Deprivation Index was used as a socio-economic indicator in combination with an affluence indicator (the criteria being the proportion of households with two or more cars). The Townsend Deprivation Index is a composite score based on variables such as unemployment, overcrowding, households without a car, etc. Carstairs–Morris Deprivation Scores are based on similar variables and calculated from the decennial population census. They were used as indicators of socio-economic status in a pharmacy-based study of non-prescription ibuprofen use.[25] Jarman underprivileged area (UPA) scores were devised as an indicator of workload in general medical practice associated with socio-economic variation. Again they are composite scores based on a number of indicators of population deprivation. Jarman UPA scores were used to classify pharmacies in a study in south-east England of threats of violence and assaults against pharmacy staff.[11] The Cambridge Scale, devised as a continuous measure to relate mortality and morbidity ratios to material factors, has been compared both on theoretical and empirical grounds with the Registrar General's classification.[24] A study of neighbourhood characteristics and the use of benzodiazepines in the Netherlands investigated and found associations with the proportion of one parent families, the extent of social rented housing and the number of rooms per person.[26]

Other characteristics of pharmacy clientele on which data have been gathered include: relative proportions of regular and casual clients (an indicator of the extent to which an area is residential or non-residential), estimates of the proportion of people in different age groups (e.g. to identify high or low proportions of elderly people), estimates of the proportion of people in different ethnic groups (in the UK questions from the decennial census are sometimes used), and whether prescription clients come principally from one or more local surgeries. In self-completion surveys of pharmacists, responses to many of these questions will be based on pharmacists' impressions and estimates rather than precise information. The reliability of the data may be unclear.

There will generally be many inter-relationships among variables relating to characteristics of pharmacies, pharmacists and their clientele. For example, younger pharmacists may be more likely to work in particular types of pharmacy, casual clients may be more prominent in pharmacies in non-residential areas. Because of this confounding, some caution must be exercised when drawing conclusions regarding associations among variables.

Between countries there are major differences in the structure of pharmacy services and the practices of the pharmacy profession. However, there are also many similarities in professional developments and aspirations as well as in the pressures and constraints facing the professions in different countries. To optimise the relevance of research beyond national boundaries it may be useful to consider which variables may be effective when applied internationally, or to develop appropriate variables for this purpose.

Generalisability

The generalisability (sometimes referred to as external validity) is concerned with the extent to which the survey findings can be applied to individuals beyond the sample.

The most important issues that determine the generalisability of study findings are the sampling procedures, sample sizes and response rates. If probability sampling procedures (see Chapter 1) are employed, sample sizes are adequate and response rates good, then assuming the survey instrument has gathered valid data, probability statistics can be employed in generalising the findings to the population from which the sample was drawn (the sampling frame). However, for many studies, researchers may wish to address the issue of generalisability to populations beyond the sampling frame. There may be strong arguments for claiming that much wider generalisation is appropriate.

Sampling procedures and sampling frames

Sampling procedures should be random (representative) in that all individuals in a population have an equal chance of being included in the sample (see Chapter 1). Sampling frames (lists of all members of a population) which are incomplete or self-selecting limit the ability of the researcher to achieve a random or representative sample and thereby to generalise the findings.

Special interest groups,[58,81,116] samples of volunteers[77,132] or other self-selecting individuals may provide some advantages for researchers; for example, in a study among pharmacists from within a single organisation it may be easier to achieve a high response rate than from a more disparate population. However, the findings will only be generalisable to other pharmacists within the organisation.[7,133] Similarly, in a survey of industrial pharmacists which used the American Association of Pharmaceutical Scientists' directory of members as a sampling frame, the members were a self-selecting group and therefore may not be representative of industrial pharmacists as a whole.[134]

For population-based studies, researchers have used electoral registers,[4,9,13,45,62,117,135–138] telephone directories,[5,103] shopping malls[12,105] and commercial mailing lists,[9,139] all of which have their strengths and weaknesses (see Chapter 1). They may achieve sufficient representativeness such that the author feels justified in making wider claims for the findings. As long as the sampling procedures are clearly described, readers can also make their own assessments of generalisability. A survey of 'all key hospital pre-registration trainers', for which a sampling frame was not identified and procedures were unclear, leaves the reader with the task of considering who might or might not have been included and the consequent generalisability of the findings.[88]

Difficulties may arise when the researcher is dependent on others to recruit individuals into the sample. In a survey screening for incorrect inhaler use, researchers were dependent on nursing staff to recruit regular inhaler users and were aware that patients were chosen for the study only when the nursing staff had time. Nursing staff may also be concerned that if the research uncovers poor techniques it may reflect on them, which may affect their selection of patients.[140] Similarly, in studies in community pharmacy in which selection of individuals for inclusion in a questionnaire survey is left to pharmacy staff, researchers may have no way of ensuring that the specified procedures are closely followed.

Sample sizes

Observance of rules for calculating sample sizes in survey research is often difficult. The statistical approach to determining sample size is to perform a power calculation.[18] This depends on estimations of the differences between groups with respect to variables of interest and provides a measure of the likelihood that a difference between groups will be detected. In descriptive studies, the sample size must be sufficient to allow results to be extrapolated to the population with the required degree of accuracy; the smaller the sample, the wider the confidence intervals (and the less precise the estimate) will be when results are extrapolated from sample to population. If subgroup analysis of survey data is intended it is important that the sample size is adequate to ensure sufficient numbers in each subgroup so comparisons can be made. The expected response rate should also be taken into account (although a larger sample size will not reduce bias due to non-response). In the studies reviewed here, although the sampling strategies were often clear, derivation of the sample size was only rarely discussed.[58,59,103]

Poor response rates

A number of researchers have found that responders and non-responders differ in important ways, limiting the generalisability of findings unless the non-responders are followed-up and the results amended accordingly (see Chapter 1). If response rates are low, the respondents must be viewed as a self-selecting group. A survey of the management of oral disease in community pharmacies[141] achieved a response rate of 32%, and the authors 'felt that replies returned were of sufficient number and quality for valid observations to be made'; however, these only represented one-third of the pharmacist population. As they did not follow-up or investigate differences between responders and non-responders, it was not possible for any independent assessment of the likely representativeness of the sample to be made, limiting the generalisability of the findings.

In general, as long as appropriate sampling strategies are employed it is better to channel resources into obtaining higher response rates and investigating the characteristics that distinguish non-responders from responders than increasing the sample size.[142] Increasing the sample size will not rectify systematic bias due to differences between responders and non-responders.

Geographical localisation of the study

The vast majority of studies are undertaken within defined geographical areas. This is common in health services research. Resources will not often permit nationwide projects. Although findings from local studies cannot be assumed to be generalisable beyond their boundaries, a study that is carried out in a defined area does not necessarily limit the usefulness and wider relevance of the data and conclusions. The extent to which results obtained can be extrapolated to other areas is open to debate. If it is reasonable to claim that the findings from a localised study are more widely applicable, it may be unnecessary to commit resources to an expensive national or international study. However, in cases where particular locations or settings would be expected to differ, in order to make any claims of applicability of findings to other populations, these populations would have to be included in the sample.

Researchers investigating the attitudes of community pharmacists and general medical practitioners to pharmacists' extended roles and opportunities for collaboration selected two health authority areas in England on the basis of their dissimilarity in terms of geographical location and socio-economic population profile. The authors felt that if similar views existed within these two areas then they could be expected to represent the professional groups more widely.[123] Similar arguments may be applied to studies that recruit patients or clients from databases held by community pharmacies.[97,143–145] If a number of sites are used for sampling, then authors may argue that diversity in a wider population would be reflected by differences within the sample.

Similar arguments have been employed for localised studies. The authors of a study in one health authority area concluded that because it covered both rural and industrial areas the findings 'were relevant to most of Britain'.[146] In a survey of pharmacies in two English counties, because ownership patterns were similar to England and Wales as a whole, researchers believed the results would be more widely generalisable.[102] A comparison of pharmacists from different ethnic backgrounds focused on the graduates of one school of pharmacy. The author acknowledges that care should be taken in generalising results beyond the graduates of the school; conversely, there may be powerful arguments to support the validity of broad generalisations.[28]

In some cases there may be less scope for generalisations. For instance, there may be good reasons for believing that findings of a survey of violent crime in pharmacies in the London area would not be generalisable to all other areas.[11] In a study of the impact of patient counselling on drug purchasing behaviour involving one pharmacy and one consultant, it may, as the authors state, be expected that the findings could be researcher and/or pharmacy dependent.[147] A survey in one pharmacy in Thailand (associated with the university) involved 34 pharmacists who sometimes worked there. It may be expected in this case that these pharmacists may share characteristics that would distinguish them from colleagues elsewhere.[85]

Generalisation to other locations is not important in all research. The aim of some studies is to address a local issue or need. Local information may be important and interesting in itself. In a new research field it may be appropriate to restrict the study to a small area to facilitate a more detailed exploration of relevant issues and develop appropriate research tools before extending the study to a wider population.

Preliminary fieldwork and pilot studies

Preliminary fieldwork may include informal discussions of study objectives and procedures to inform their development. Developing and selecting instruments, ensuring their validity and reliability, may be an important part of the preliminary fieldwork, which ultimately leads to the development of a protocol. In many studies reviewed, extensive preliminary fieldwork preceded and informed the development and/or selection of research instruments ensuring their validity and reliability.

The purposes of a pilot study are two-fold: first, to ensure that it is workable in practice settings in terms of study procedures and data collection, acceptable to participants and others on whom the conduct of the study may impact; and second, to check that study procedures gather reliable and valid data effectively and efficiently. The pilot study mimics the main study on a small scale, employing all the methods and instruments planned for the main study.

In a study of health authorities to obtain information on employees and contractors, some respondents reported that they did not have access to the information requested.[148] As an important task of the pilot work is to ensure that the method is capable of gathering the information required for the study, many such potential problems should be uncovered at this stage. Only in rare cases did researchers report that a pilot study was not undertaken.[149] Authors commonly reported that following the pilot work some (often minor) modifications to the survey instrument were required.

One feature commonly reported was that pilot work was undertaken outside the designated study area.[42,71,118,121,150–152] While it is important that potential respondents are not biased in their responses as a result of early involvement in the study, in many cases this precaution may be unnecessary or avoidable, for example, if the sample for the main study is selected prior to the pilot study.

Analytical procedures in survey research

Statistical procedures

Survey research commonly generates large data sets, both in terms of the number of variables (questionnaire items) and the number of cases (respondents). Thus, computer statistical packages are generally employed. The most frequently cited was SPSS (Statistical Package for the Social Sciences). Other software packages included SAS, Minitab,

Epi-info, SNAP, EXCEL and STATVIEW. As the vast majority of surveys are descriptive studies, frequency data and summary statistics (e.g. means, medians, standard deviations) are widely used.

The choice of test depends on the objectives of the study. The structure of data and whether variables are nominal, ordinal or interval/ratio, will indicate whether non-parametric or parametric procedures are most appropriate. As is common in social surveys, data on many variables are nominal (categorical) or ordinal rather than interval/ratio. For such data it is appropriate to use non-parametric statistical procedures when exploring relationships between variables and undertaking comparisons between population subgroups. Thus, the most commonly reported procedures were chi-squared tests to compare counts between nominal variables, Mann–Whitney U-test for comparison of ordinal data between two independent groups, Kruskal–Wallis test when there were more than two groups being compared and Spearman's rank correlation as a measure of association between two variables on an ordinal scale. T-tests and analysis of variance were used for comparisons of two or more groups for which data was normally distributed on an interval/ratio scale.

Tests of statistical significance were common, but confidence intervals were less frequently reported. This may be in part an artefact of the statistics software packages which for many tests provide data on confidence intervals less readily than information on statistical significance. As is conventional in other survey and health services research, a $p < 0.05$ value was generally taken as conferring statistical significance. This provides a measure of the extent to which the observed relationship between variables in a data set could be expected to occur by chance (i.e. be apparent in the data set when there is no true underlying relationship between the variables). A $p = 0.05$ value indicates that there is a 5% (1 in 20) chance of this situation occurring. In many surveys, data are collected on a large number of variables, and many statistical tests may be performed to identify relationships between them. If a $p < 0.05$ value is used, then 1 in every 20 tests performed would be expected to lead to a spurious result. Thus, in investigating relationships between variables, researchers must be aware of the potential for misleading findings which could result in unfounded conclusions. To overcome this difficulty statisticians advise researchers to plan their analyses in advance (and thus avoid 'fishing expeditions') performing limited numbers of procedures as dictated by the study objectives.

Smaller p-values (e.g. $p < 0.01$) can also be used. However, there is then the possibility that genuine differences may be missed when sample sizes are small. In many studies researchers in reporting their findings commonly report the p-value for each test, thus enabling the reader to reflect on the likely importance of the findings.

If statistically significant relationships between variables are observed in the data set, researchers have to ensure that these are not a result of research process (e.g. response bias, recall bias in interviews, poor reliability or validity of measures, incomplete data sets and bias in missing data). In a study in which respondents were asked to recall their use of drugs, researchers found that data relating to drug use for specified indications were more reliable when compared with pharmacy records.[98] Thus, as a result of the recall bias, an inaccurate picture regarding overall drug use may be obtained. Similarly, in a study comparing adverse events in women taking and not taking oral contraceptives, the authors suggest that women who complain of leg pain who are taking oral contraceptives may be more likely to undergo further investigation that those not taking oral contraceptives. It was thought that this may contribute to the documentation of a higher rate of these adverse effects in the former group.[153] The development of causal models in which the values of one variable in a data set are explained in terms of the values of others requires that spurious associations are identified.

Relationships between variables may also be indirect, that is a consequence of the impact of a third variable (confounding variable). Multivariate techniques can be useful in identifying the collinearity within a data set. A study to describe the population characteristics of community pharmacy's clientele employed CHAID (chi-square automatic interaction detection), which enabled the identification of subgroups within each variable predictive of use of pharmacy services.[154]

There are many examples of the application of more sophisticated multivariate techniques in survey research. These were often used in the development and testing of explanatory models, which are discussed in Chapter 3.

Missing values

Missing values are common in survey data. They result from individuals being unable or unwilling to answer questions and/or interviewers or interviewees omitting questions. Questions for which there are many missing responses during the pilot work should raise the suspicion of the researcher. They may be questions that are ambiguous, considered too personal, those for which the information is not available, or for which a detailed response may be an arduous or unacceptable task. In an interview survey it may be a question that the interviewer feels uncomfortable asking. During the pilot work, the researchers should endeavour to identify such questions and modify the survey instrument accordingly. However, some missing data will usually be expected. The handling of missing values was rarely discussed in the studies reviewed. Common practice is to code missing data as missing and then to omit these cases from the analysis. In a study investigating a theoretical model of pharmacists' consultation patterns, which involved completion of two questionnaires, the analysis included only respondents who completed both questionnaires.[66] Exclusion of all cases with any missing data can result in much lost data, especially in multivariate procedures which require data on a large number of variables.

In a study in which researchers applied a range of multivariate procedures to develop a model to explain pharmacists' preferences for recommending specific products, missing values were replaced with sample means.[43] Other practices are sometimes followed and are discussed in various texts, for example, replacing missing data with estimates derived from other cases or variables.[155-156] The validity of any procedure must be verified.

Conclusion

The issues and problems of reliability and validity in survey research are many and complex. However, it is essential that potential problems are identified and addressed in all stages of the planning and execution of the research. The papers reviewed here demonstrate researchers' awareness of the wide range of problems that arise and their commitment to finding scientific approaches to address potential problems that are workable in pharmacy settings.

References

1. Scott D M, Woodward J M B. The influence of locus of control and perceived susceptibility to illness on family managers' selfcare chart use. *J Soc Admin Pharm* 1992; 9: 21–8.
2. Deshmukh A A, Sommerville H. Survey of the needs of patients in a private nursing home: a pharmacist's view. *Int J Pharm Pract* 1996; 4: 83–7.
3. Erwin J, Britten N, Jones R. Pharmacists and deregulation: the case of H2 antagonists. *J Soc Admin Pharm* 1996; 13: 150–8.
4. Smith F J, Farquhar M, Bowling A P. Drugs prescribed for people aged 85 and over, living in their own homes in an area of inner London. *Int J Pharm Pract* 1995; 3: 145–50.

5. Brown C M, Segal R. The effects of health and treatment perceptions on the use of prescribed medications and home remedies among African American and White American hypertensives. *Soc Sci Med* 1996; 43: 903–17.

6. Hartzema A G, Godbout N, Lee S D, Konrad R. Measuring health locus of control among caregivers in charge of medication administration in long-term care settings. *J Soc Admin Pharm* 1990; 7: 84–92.

7. Olson D S, Lawson K A. Relationship between hospital pharmacists' job satisfaction and involvement in clinical activities. *Am J Health Syst Pharm* 1996; 53: 281–4.

8. Willett V J, Cooper C L. Stress and job satisfaction in community pharmacy: a pilot study. *Pharm J* 1996; 256: 94–8.

9. Isacson D, Bingefors C. On prescription switches and access to over-the-counter drugs in Sweden. *J Soc Admin Pharm* 1999; 16: 13–25.

10. Carroll N V, Fincham J E. Elderly consumers' perceptions of the risks of using mail-order pharmacies. *J Soc Admin Pharm* 1993; 10: 123–9.

11. Smith F J, Weidner D. Threatening and violent incidents in community pharmacies: 1. An investigation of the frequency of serious and minor incidents. *Int J Pharm Pract* 1996; 4: 136–44.

12. Hargie O, Morrow N, Woodman C. Consumer perceptions of and attitudes to community pharmacy services. *Pharm J* 1992; 249: 688–91.

13. Jesson J, Sadler S, Pocock R, Jepson M. Ethnic minority consumers of community pharmaceutical services. *Int J Pharm Pract* 1995; 3: 129–32.

14. Secretary of State for Health. Saving lives: our healthier nation. Cm 4386. London: The Stationery Office, 1999.

15. Rose D, O'Reilly K, eds. *Constructing Classes: Towards a New Social Classification for the UK*. Swindon: Economic and Social Research Council and Office for National Statistics, 1997.

16. Streiner D L, Norman G R. *Health Measurement Scales: a Practical Guide to their Use and Development*. Oxford: Oxford University Press, 1991.

17. Oppenheim A N. *Questionnaire Design, Interviewing and Attitude Measurement*, 2nd edn. London: Pinter Publishers, 1992.

18. Bowling A. *Research Methods in Health*. Buckingham: Open University Press, 1997.

19. Gore P, Madhavan S. Credibility of the sources of information for non-prescription medicines. *J Soc Admin Pharm* 1993; 10: 109–22.

20. Hedvall M-B, Paltschik M. Perceived service quality in pharmacies: with empirical results from Sweden. *J Soc Admin Pharm* 1992; 8: 7–14.

21. Goldberg D P. *Manual of the General Health Questionnaire*. Windsor: NFER-Nelson, 1978.

22. *Health Survey for England 1993*. London: HM Stationery Office, 1995.

23. Rose D, O'Reilly K. *The ESRC Review of Government Social Classifications*. London: Office for National Statistics and Economic and Social Research Council, 1998.

24. Prandy K. Class stratification and inequalities in health: a comparison of the Registrar-General's Social Classes and the Cambridge Scale. *Sociol Health Illness* 1999; 21: 466–84.

25. Sinclair H K, Bond C M, Hannaford P C. Over-the-counter ibuprofen: how and why is it used? *Int J Pharm Pract* 2000; 8: 121–7.

26. Groenewegen P P, Leufkens H G, Spreeuwenberg P, Worm W. Neighbourhood characteristics and use of benzodiazepines in the Netherlands. *Soc Sci Med* 1999; 48: 1701–11.

27. Smaje C. *Health, Race and Ethnicity*. London: King's Fund Institute, 1995.

28. Hassell K. White and ethnic minority pharmacists' professional practice patterns and reasons for choosing pharmacy. *Int J Pharm Pract* 1996; 4: 43–51.

29. Platts A E, Tann J. A changing professional profile: ethnicity and gender issues in pharmacy employment in the United Kingdom. *Int J Pharm Pract* 1999; 7: 29–39.

30. Jessa F, Hampshire A J. Use of folic acid by pregnant British Pakistani women: a qualitative pilot study. *Health Educ J* 1999; 58: 138–45.

31. Agrawal M, Sause R. Serving multi-ethnic populations: measuring the cultural sensitivity of pharmacy interns in New York City. *Int J Pharm Pract* 1998; 6: 83–90.

32. Douglas J. Developing appropriate research methodologies with black and minority ethnic communities. Part 1: Reflections on the research process. *Health Educ J* 1998; 57: 329–38.

33. Aspinall P J. Describing the 'white' ethnic group and its composition in medical research. *Soc Sci Med* 1998; 47: 1797–808.

34. Aspinall P J. Ethnic groups and 'our healthier nation': whither the information base. *J Public Health Med* 1999; 21: 125–32.

35. Parker H. Beyond ethnic categories: why racism should be a variable in health services research. *J Health Serv Res Policy* 1997; 2: 256–9.

36. Francis S-A. Medication and quality of life: a study of people with a diagnosis of schizophrenia. [PhD thesis.] London: University of London, 1997.

37. Ortiz M, Walker W L, Thomas R. Job satisfaction dimensions of Australian community pharmacists. *J Soc Admin Pharm* 1992; 9: 149–58.

38. Ortiz M, Walker W L, Thomas R. Development of a measure to assess community pharmacists' orientation towards patient counselling. *J Soc Admin Pharm* 1992; 9: 2–10.

39. Sheridan J, Barber N D. Pharmacy undergraduates' and preregistration pharmacists' attitudes towards drug misuse and HIV. *J Soc Admin Pharm* 1993; 10: 163–70.

40. Sheridan J, Bates I P, Webb D G, Barber N D. Educational intervention in pharmacy students' attitudes to HIV/AIDS and drug misuse. *Med Educ* 1994; 28: 492–500.

41. Thomson A N, Craig B J, Barham P M. Attitudes of general practitioners in New Zealand to pharmaceutical representatives. *Br J Gen Pract* 1994; 44: 220–3.

42. Maslen C L, Rees L, Redfern P H. Role of the community pharmacist in the care of patients with chronic schizophrenia in the community. *Int J Pharm Pract* 1996; 4: 187–95.

43. Emmerton L, Benrimoj S. Factors influencing pharmacists' preferences for non-prescription cough suppressants. *J Soc Admin Pharm* 1994; 11: 78–85.

44. Oborne C A, Dodds L J. Seamless pharmaceutical care: the needs of community pharmacists. *Pharm J* 1994; 253: 502–6.

45. Vallis J, Wyke S, Cunningham-Burley S. Users' views and expectations of

community pharmacists in a Scottish commuter town. *Pharm J* 1997; 258: 457–60.

46. Airaksinen M, Ahonen R, Enlund H. Customer feedback as a tool for improving pharmacy services. *Int J Pharm Pract* 1995; 3: 219–26.

47. Britten N, Gallagher K, Gallagher H. Patients' views of computerised pharmacy records. *Int J Pharm Pract* 1992; 1: 206–9.

48. Brown J, Brown D. Pharmaceutical care at the primary–secondary interface in Portsmouth and south-east Hampshire. *Pharm J* 1997; 258: 280–4.

49. Hornosty R W, Muzzin L J, Brown G P. Faith in the ideal of clinical pharmacy among practising pharmacists seven years after graduation from pharmacy school. *J Soc Admin Pharm* 1992; 9: 87–96.

50. Emmerton L, Gow D J, Benrimoj S I. Dimensions of pharmacists' preferences for cough and cold products. *Int J Pharm Pract* 1994; 3: 27–32.

51. Roins S, Benrimoj S I, Carroll P R, Johnson L W. Factors used by pharmacists in the recommendation of active ingredient(s) and brand of non-prescription analgesics for simple, tension and migraine headaches. *Int J Pharm Pract* 1998; 6: 196–206.

52. Duggan C, Bates I. Development and evaluation of a survey tool to explore patients' perceptions of their prescribed drugs and their need for drug information. *Int J Pharm Pract* 2000; 8: 42–52.

53. Rosenbloom K, Taylor K, Harding G. Community pharmacists' attitudes towards research. *Int J Pharm Pract* 2000; 8: 103–10.

54. Aldrich S, Eccleston C. Making sense of everyday pain. *Soc Sci Med* 2000; 50: 1631–41.

55. Rivers P H. The impact of carers' attitudes on the safety of medication procedures in UK residential homes for the elderly. *J Soc Admin Pharm* 1995; 12: 132–43.

56. Smith F J. General medical practitioners and community pharmacists in London: views on the pharmacist's role and responsibilities relating to benzodiazepines. *J Interprofess Care* 1993; 7: 37–45.

57. Blom A T H G, Kam A L, Bakker A, Claesson C. Patient counselling in community pharmacy: a comparative study between Dutch and Swedish pharmacists. *J Soc Admin Pharm* 1993; 10: 53–62.

58. Gattera J A, Stewart K, Benrimoj S I, Williams G M. Usage of non-prescription medication by people with diabetes. *J Soc Admin Pharm* 1992; 9: 66–74.

59. Cockerill R W, Myers T, Worthington C, *et al.* Pharmacies and their role in the prevention of HIV/AIDS. *J Soc Admin Pharm* 1996; 13: 46–53.

60. Murphy J E, Slack M K, Campbell S. National survey of hospital based pharmacokinetic services. *Am J Health Syst Pharm* 1996; 53: 2840–7.

61. Begley S, Livingstone C, Williamson V, Hodges N. Attitudes of pharmacists, medical practitioners and nurses towards the development of domiciliary and other community pharmacy services. *Int J Pharm Pract* 1994; 2: 223–8.

62. Jesson J, Pocock R, Jepson M, Kendall H. Consumer readership and views on pharmacy health education literature: a market research survey. *J Soc Admin Pharm* 1994; 11: 29–36.

63. Cantrill J A, Sibbald B, Buetow S. The delphi and nominal group techniques in health services research. *Int J Pharm Pract* 1996; 4: 67–74.

64. Aslanpour Z, Smith F J. Oral counselling on dispensed medication: a survey

of its extent and associated factors in a random sample of community pharmacies. *Int J Pharm Pract* 1997; 5: 57–63.

65. Gupta S, Rappaport H M. Pharmacy board members' attitudes on freedom of choice. *J Soc Admin Pharm* 1996; 13: 65–73.

66. Odedina F T, Segal R, Hepler C D, *et al.* Changing pharmacists' practice pattern. *J Soc Admin Pharm* 1996; 13: 74–88.

67. Gore M R, Thomas J. Nonprescription informational services in pharmacies and alternative stores: implications for a third class of drugs. *J Soc Admin Pharm* 1995; 12: 86–99.

68. Paluck E C, Stratton T P, Eni G O. Pharmacists and health promotion: a study of thirteen variables. *J Soc Admin Pharm* 1996; 13: 89–98.

69. Mottram D R, Jogia P, West P. Community pharmacists' attitudes to the extended role. *J Soc Admin Pharm* 1995; 12: 12–17.

70. Laurier C, Poston J W. Perceived levels of patient counselling among Canadian pharmacists. *J Soc Admin Pharm* 1992; 9: 104–13.

71. Clark J C, Gerrett D. General medical practitioners' perceived use of drug information sources with special reference to drug information centres. *Int J Pharm Pract* 1994; 2: 247–52.

72. Gilbert A, Owen N, Sansom L, Innes J M. High levels of medication compliance and blood pressure control among hypertensive patients attending community pharmacies. *J Soc Admin Pharm* 1990; 7: 78–83.

73. Rantucci M, Segal H J. Hazardous non-prescription analgesic use by the elderly. *J Soc Admin Pharm* 1992; 8: 108–20.

74. Krska J, Kennedy E J, Milne S A, McKessack K J. Frequency of counselling on prescription medicines in community pharmacy. *Int J Pharm Pract* 1995; 3: 178–86.

75. Ortiz M, Walker W L, Thomas R. Comparison between methods of assessing patient counselling in Australian community pharmacies. *J Soc Admin Pharm* 1989; 6: 39–48.

76. Sibbald B, Addington-Hall J, Brenneman D, Freeling P. Telephone versus postal surveys of general practitioners: methodological considerations. *Br J Gen Pract* 1994; 44: 297–300.

77. Krska J, Kennedy E J. Responding to symptoms: comparing general practitioners' and pharmacists' advice. *Pharm J* 1996; 257: 322–4.

78. Jones P, van Teijlingen E R, Matheson C I, Govin S. Pharmacists' approach to harm minimisation initiatives associated with problem drug use: the Lothian survey. *Pharm J* 1998; 260: 324–6.

79. Eccles M, Ford G A, Duggan S, Steen N. Are postal questionnaire surveys of reported activity valid? An exploration using general practitioner management of hypertension in older people. *Br J Gen Pract* 1999; 49: 35–8.

80. Newton S A, Black M. Nursing sisters' satisfaction with the pharmacy service– a survey. *Int J Pharm Pract* 1994; 2: 220–2.

81. Ritchie D J, Manchester R F, Rich M W, *et al.* Acceptance of pharmacy based, physician edited hospital pharmacy and therapeutics committee newsletter. *Ann Pharmacother* 1992; 26: 886–9.

82. Chandola A, Young Y, McAlister J, Axford J S. Use of complementary therapies by patients attending musculo-skeletal clinics. *J R Soc Med* 1999; 92: 13–16.

83. Hagedorn M, Cantrill J, Nicolson M, Noyce P. Pharmaceutical care and the deregulation of medicines. A survey of British and German Pharmacists. *J Soc Admin Pharm* 1996; 13: 1–7.

84. Schaefer M, Leufkens H G M, Harris M F. The teaching of social pharmacy/pharmacy administration in colleges of pharmacy with special regard to the situation in Germany. *J Soc Admin Pharm* 1992; 9: 141–8.

85. Charupatanapong N, Chairojkanjana K, Tanapaisalkit A. Comparison of attitudes and beliefs about self-care and personal responsibility for health held by consumers and pharmacists in Thailand. *Int J Pharm Pract* 1996; 4: 103–8.

86. Scott K M, Sarfati D, Tobias M I, Haslett S J. A challenge to the cross-cultural validity of the SF-36 health survey: factor structure in Maori, Pacific and New Zealand European ethnic groups. *Soc Sci Med* 2000; 51: 1655–64.

87. Kilkenny M, Yeatman J, Stewart K, Marks R. Role of pharmacists and general practitioners in the management of dermatological conditions. *Int J Pharm Pract* 1997; 5: 11–5.

88. Liddell H. Competency-based training for pre-registration trainers: what are the views of hospital trainers? *Pharm J* 1996; 256: 624–5.

89. Sadik F, Reeder C E, Saket M, *et al.* Job satisfaction among Jordanian pharmacists. *J Soc Admin Pharm* 1992; 8: 46–51.

90. Harding G, Smith F J, Taylor K M G. Injecting drug misusers: pharmacists' attitudes. *J Soc Admin Pharm* 1992; 9: 35–41.

91. Farris K B, Kirking D M. Predicting community pharmacists' intention to try to prevent and correct drug therapy problems. *J Soc Admin Pharm* 1995; 12: 64–79.

92. Thomas K A, Brown D, Hunt A, Jones I F. Community pharmacists and the NHS contract: 1. Attitudes to remuneration and terms of service. *Pharm J* 1996; 257: 854–8.

93. Long A, Wynne H A. Patient satisfaction with arthritis medication. *Int J Pharm Pract* 1996; 4: 52–4.

94. Lustig A, Zusman P. Professional self-image among Israeli pharmacists: sectoral differences. *Ann Pharmacother* 1992; 26: 1296–9.

95. Vincent-Ballereau F, Schrive I, Rousseau F. Dispensing of HIV drugs in France. *J Soc Admin Pharm* 1996; 13: 30–40.

96. Lewis M A O, Chadwick B L. Management of recurrent herpes labialis in community pharmacies. *Pharm J* 1994; 253: 768–9.

97. Chua S-S, Benrimoj S I, Stewart K, Williams G. Usage of non-prescription medications by hypertensive patients. *J Soc Admin Pharm* 1992; 8: 33–45.

98. Klungel O H, de Boer A, Paes A H P, *et al.* Influence of question structure on the recall of self-reported drug use. *J Clin Epidemiol* 2000; 53: 273–7.

99. Cairns C, Marlow H, McCoig A, Hargreaves D. The Croydon community pharmacy accident survey. *Pharm J* 1996; 257: 817–19.

100. Krska J. Attitudes to audit among community pharmacists in Grampian. *Pharm J* 1994; 253: 97–9.

101. Beal J F, Skaer T L, Day R D, Jinks M J. The comfort level of pharmacists who counsel contraceptive patients. *J Clin Pharm Ther* 1993; 18: 317–24.

102. Powis M G, Rogers P J, Wood S M. United Kingdom pharmacists' views on recent POM to P switched medicines. *J Soc Admin Pharm* 1996; 13: 188–97.

103. Schommer J C, Sullivan D L, Haugtvedt C L. Patients' role orientation for pharmacist consultation. *J Soc Admin Pharm* 1995; 12: 33–42.

104. Troein M, Rastam L, Selander S. Physicians' lack of confidence in pharmacists' competence as patient informants. *J Soc Admin Pharm* 1992; 9: 114–22.

105. Charupatanapong N. Perceived likelihood of risks in self-medication practices. *J Soc Admin Pharm* 1994; 11: 18–28.

106. Ortiz M, Walker W-L, Thomas R. Community pharmacists' professional role orientation. *J Soc Admin Pharm* 1992; 9: 97–103.

107. Krass I. A comparison of clients' experiences of counselling for prescriptions and over-the-counter medications in two types of pharmacy. Validation of a research instrument. *J Soc Admin Pharm* 1996; 13: 206–14.

108. Shefcheck S L, Thomas J. Consumers' perceptions of access to medications and attitudes towards regulatory options. *J Soc Admin Pharm* 1998; 15: 149–163.

109. Gaither C A. An investigation of pharmacists' role stress and the work/non-work interface. *J Soc Admin Pharm* 1998; 15: 92–103.

110. Roins S, Benrimoj S I, Carroll P R, Johnson L W. Pharmacists' recommendations of the active ingredient(s) of non-prescription analgesics for a simple, tension and migraine headache. *J Soc Admin Pharm* 1998; 15: 262–74.

111. Thomas KA, Brown D, Hunt A, Jones I F. Community pharmacists and the NHS contract: 1. Attitudes to its improvement, the extended role and the negotiation process. *Pharm J* 1996; 257: 896–901.

112. Liddell H. Attitudes of community pharmacists regarding involvement in practice research. *Pharm J* 1996; 256: 905–7.

113. Bond C M, Sinclair H K, Winfield A J, Taylor R J. Community pharmacists' attitudes to their advice giving role and to the deregulation of medicines. *Int J Pharm Pract* 1993; 2: 26–30.

114. Chang Z G, Kennedy D T, Holdford D A, Small R E. Pharmacists' knowledge and attitudes toward herbal medicine. *Ann Pharmacother* 2000; 34: 710–15.

115. Bouldin A S, Smith M C, Garner D D, *et al*. Pharmacy and herbal medicine in the US. *Soc Sci Med* 1999; 49: 279–89.

116. Teresi M E, Margan D E. Attitudes of health care professionals toward patient counselling on drug–nutrient interactions. *Ann Pharmacother* 1994; 28: 576–80.

117. Jepson M H, Strickland-Hodge B. Attitudes to patient medication records and their optimization through patient registration. *Pharm J* 1994; 253: 384–8.

118. Rodgers P J, Rees J E. General medical practitioners' attitudes towards the use of patient medication records. *Int J Pharm Pract* 1995; 3: 163–8.

119. Ritchey F J, Raney M R. Effect of exposure on physicians' attitudes towards clinical pharmacists. *Am J Hosp Pharm* 1981; 38: 1459–63.

120. Ranelli P L, Biss J. Physicians' perceptions of communication with, and responsibilities of, pharmacists. *J Am Pharm Assoc* 2000; 40: 625–30.

121. Holden JD, Wolfson D J. Comparison of attitudes of general medical practitioners and community pharmacists to prescribing matters. *Int J Pharm Pract* 1996; 4: 175–81.

122. Rees L, Harding G, Taylor K M G. Supplying injecting equipment to drug misusers: a survey of community pharmacists' attitudes, beliefs and practices. *Int J Pharm Pract* 1997; 5: 167–75.

123. Sutters C A, Nathan A. The community pharmacist's extended role: GPs' and pharmacists' attitudes towards collaboration. *J Soc Admin Pharm* 1993; 10: 70–84.

124. Harris S K, Smith F J, Moss F. The pharmacist's contribution to medical audit: perceptions of doctors and pharmacists in the North West Thames Regional Health Authority. *J Soc Admin Pharm* 1993; 10: 36–41.

125. Child D, Hirsch C, Berry M. Health care professionals' views on hospital pharmacist prescribing in the United Kingdom. *Int J Pharm Pract* 1998; 6: 159–69.

126. Doucette W R, Jambulingam T. Pharmacy entrepreneurial orientation: antecedents and its effect on the provision of innovative pharmacy services. *J Soc Admin Pharm* 1999; 16: 26–37.

127. Farris K B, Schopflocher D P. Between intention and behaviour: an application of community pharmacists' assessment of pharmaceutical care. *Soc Sci Med* 1999; 49: 55–66.

128. Sheridan J, Strang J, Lovell S. National and local guidance on services for drug misusers: do they influence current practice? Results of a survey of community pharmacists in south-east England. *Int J Pharm Pract* 1999; 7: 100–6.

129. Whitehead P, Atkin P, Krass I, Benrimoj S I. Patient drug information and consumer choice of pharmacy. *Int J Pharm Pract* 1999; 7: 71–9.

130. Savage I. The changing face of pharmacy practice – evidence from 20 years of work sampling studies. *Int J Pharm Pract* 1999; 7: 209–19.

131. Hirschfield A, Wolfson D J, Swetman S. Location of community pharmacies: a rational approach using geographic information systems. *Int J Pharm Pract* 1994; 3: 42–52.

132. Gaunt R, Whitfield M, Ghalamkari H, Millar M. General practitioner prescribing and community pharmacist recommendation for the sale of aciclovir topical cream. *Int J Pharm Pract* 1996; 4: 204–8.

133. Dickinson C, Howlett J A, Bulman J S. The community pharmacist: a dental health advisor. *Pharm J* 1994; 252 :262–4.

134. Kong S X, Wertheimer A I, McGhan W F. Role stress, organisational commitment and turnover intention among pharmaceutical scientists: a multivariate analysis. *J Soc Admin Pharm* 1992; 9: 159–71.

135. Jesson J, Jepson M, Pocock R, *et al. Ethnic Minority Consumers of Community Pharmaceutical Services. A Report for the Department of Health.* Birmingham: Aston University/MEL Research, 1994.

136. Jepson M, Jesson J, Pocock R, Kendall H. *Consumer Expectations of Community Pharmaceutical Services. A Report for the Department of Health.* Birmingham: Aston University/MEL Research, 1991.

137. Forbes A J, Ross A J, Rees J A. Problems with medicines use: the Bolton project. *Int J Pharm Pract* 1991; 1: 34–7.

138. Rees J A, Forbes A J, Ross A J. Difficulties in the use of medicine packaging. *Int J Pharm Pract* 1992; 1: 160–3.

139. Gore P R, Madhavan S. Consumers' preferences and willingness to pay for pharmacist counselling for non-prescription medicines. *J Clin Pharm Ther* 1994; 19: 17–25.

140. Elfellah M S, McDonald L, Thomson A, Smith A. Screening for incorrect inhaler use by regular users. *Pharm J* 1994; 253: 467–8.

141. Chadwick B L, Lewis M A O. The management of oral disease in community pharmacies. *Pharm J* 1994; 253: 317–19 and 322.

142. Cochran W G. *Sampling Techniques*. New York: John Wiley and Sons, 1977.

143. Beto J A, Lisbecki R F, Meyer D A, *et al.* Use of pharmacy computer prescription database to access hypertensive patients for mailed survey research. *Ann Pharmacother* 1996; 30: 351–5.

144. Richards S, Thornhill D, Roberts H, Harries U. How many people have hayfever and what do they do about it? *Br J Gen Pract* 1992; 42: 284–6.

145. Spanish Group for the Study of Hypnotic Drug Utilization. Hypnotic drug use in Spain: a cross-sectional study based on a network of community pharmacies. *Ann Pharmacother* 1996; 30: 1092–100.

146. Paxton R, Chapple P. Misuse of over-the-counter medicines: a survey in one county. *Pharm J* 1996; 256: 313–15.

147. Nichol M B, McCombs J S, Boghossian T, Johnson K A. The impact of patient counselling on over-the-counter drug purchasing behaviour. *J Soc Admin Pharm* 1992; 9: 11–20.

148. Magirr P, Otterill R. Measuring the employee/contractor balance. *Pharm J* 1995; 254: 876–9.

149. Hughes C M, McFerran G. Pharmacy involvement in formulary development: community pharmacists' views. *Int J Pharm Pract* 1996; 4: 153–5.

150. Rodgers P J, Rees J E. Comparison of the use of PMRs in community pharmacy in 1991 and 1995: 1. PMR use and recording of product details. *Pharm J* 1996; 256: 161–6.

151. Rodgers P J, Rees J E. Comparison of the use of PMRs in community pharmacy in 1991 and 1995: 2. The recording of patients' details. *Pharm J* 1996; 256: 491–5.

152. Stromme H K, Botten G. Drug-related problems among old people living at home, as perceived by a sample of Norwegian home-care providers. *J Soc Admin Pharm* 1993; 10: 63–9.

153. Hannaford P C, Kay C R. The risk of serious illness among oral contraceptive users: evidence from the RCGPs oral contraceptive study. *Br J Gen Pract* 1998; 48: 1657–62.

154. Tully M P, Temple B. The demographics of pharmacy's clientele: a descriptive study of the British general public. *Int J Pharm Pract* 1999; 7: 172–81.

155. Robson C. *Real World Research*. Oxford: Blackwell, 1993.

156. Snedecor G W, Cochran W G. *Statistical Methods*, 7th edn. Iowa: Iowa State University Press, 1980.

3

Theoretical perspectives and models in survey research

The vast majority of survey research is descriptive, providing documentation of populations and events. Analytical procedures are also commonly employed to explore associations between variables in the data set. Although these descriptive analyses may lead the researcher to propose hypotheses regarding possible explanations for the relationships between variables, in many cases researchers have undertaken more sophisticated model building procedures with which to explain and/or predict phenomena, either in relation to existing concepts and theories, or in the proposition or development of new ones.

In the pharmacy practice literature there are many examples of the incorporation of theory (in particular sociological theory) into research. The incorporation and/or the development of theory has become an important component of the aims and objectives of many studies in pharmacy employing survey methods. In arguing the benefits of greater prominence of theory in pharmacy practice research, Norgaard et al.[1] present the following definition of theory:

> an account of the world which goes beyond what we can see and measure. It embraces a set of inter-related definitions and relationships that organises our concepts of, and understanding of, the empirical world in a systematic way.

Using examples of the application of theory in pharmacy practice research, Norgaard et al.[1] demonstrate how theory-based research can provide insights into human behaviour in its social context. In one study, in which research into gender related workforce issues were reviewed, the author reported a reliance on traditional employment categories; she argued that the lack of a theoretical base in much of the research limited the extent to which the work could contribute to relevant sociological debates.[2]

Theoretical frameworks and measures

Sociological approaches

A number of pharmacy researchers have drawn on sociological theory or frameworks to inform their work. Jones[3] provides an exposition and review of theories that have provided a basis for sociological research. For each of the different theories he identifies ontological (beliefs about the nature of the subject of study) and epistemological (the type of evidence base that is required for investigation of the subject of study) assumptions to determine the conceptual basis and methodological approach, respectively, of the research. He describes the dominance of positivism (which assumes that behaviour and events are a result of external stimuli that can be observed and measured) and empiricism (based on observation or experiment) in sociological research of both the nineteenth and twentieth centuries.[3] Although it is not usually explicitly stated, much pharmacy practice and related health services research is positivist in that the researcher's objectives frequently relate to the identification (and/or quantification) of external determinants of events and behaviours and/or the testing of hypotheses. In the execution of the work, researchers aim for 'objectivity' (independence from personal perspectives or value judgements) in their approach. To ensure reliability of measures they endeavour to follow a 'scientific' method in designing the research and in the analytical procedures (which is considered by some to threaten the validity, see Chapter 4). This contrasts with the interpretivists who see human behaviour as a product of how people interpret the world around them (their ontology) and thus in terms of epistemology, the perceptions and explanations (or interpretations of reality) by individuals become the focus of the research.

Phenomenology assumes that humans (unlike matter) have consciousness; they experience and understand the world in terms of meanings, and actively construct an individual social reality.[4] Thus the research process is concerned with identifying and interpreting these meanings and constructions of social reality. In a study of pharmacy students' experiences of pharmacy education, the authors[5] described their approach as phenomenological in that the researcher was interested in the meaning a person attributes to his or her reality, his or her world and his or her relationships. Thus the objective of the study was to gain insight into the current education paradigm as experienced by the students.[5]

Social constructionism has also provided a basis for research. In these studies, phenomena are assumed to be a product of social or cultural practices as opposed to external realities. The focus of research is the identification of reality in terms of these social or cultural constructions. Hence, the methodological approaches employed may share features of an interpretative approach. In a study of interpretative repertoires of medication among the oldest-old, the aim was to look for different culturally shared interpretations that could be identified from participants' accounts of their drug use, and of themselves as users of medical drugs. Social constructionism and discourse analysis were incorporated into the analysis of these narrative interviews. Researchers identified three interpretative repertoires. Respondents (all over 90 years of age) presented themselves as responsible users, as accepting the role of patient and as making their own choices in medical care despite the biomedical facts.[6] A social constructionist approach was employed to analyse the accounting practices used in 'making sense of everyday pain'. The analysis was based on ideas of pain sought through discussions with pain researchers and clinicians, focus groups, and a range of texts (popular, academic and professional). The method employed (Q methodology) involved the generation of a large number of culturally derived statements from which different accounts (or interpretations or constructions) can be identified in terms of their commonality and differences.[7]

A phenomenographic approach was described and adopted in a study of reflections on medicines and medication among people on long-term drug regimens. This approach was distinguished from phenomenology in that the former focuses on, and explains, variation between individuals rather than aiming to identify common distinctive features.[8]

Incorporation of specific theories

Sociological and psychological concepts of health and illness in terms of lay and professional models of health and illness and models of health behaviour are summarised by Bowling.[4] Connor and Norman[9] describe some of the most widely applied social cognition models explaining health behaviour, and they review the applications, strengths and weaknesses of each.

The health belief model

The health belief model, in which action taken is believed to be determined by perceptions of threats of illness and evaluation of alternative behaviours to counteract these threats,[9] has provided a theoretical framework for a number of studies of medication use. In studying associations between health beliefs and compliance of black South African outpatients, questions were devised which corresponded to the constructs of the health belief model. These included patient knowledge of medication, health beliefs regarding medication, perceptions of disease, and importance of regular intake of medication.[10] The health belief model also provided a theoretical framework for an investigation of relationships between health and treatment perceptions (as represented in the health belief model), and the use of prescribed medication and home remedies.[11] Cognitions specified by the health belief model have also been combined with the theory of planned action (in a study to identify predictors of adherence to malaria prophylaxis)[12] and health of locus of control (to distinguish users and non-users of self-care protocols).[13]

Health locus of control

Measures of internal and external locus of control were used to compare users and non-users of self-care protocols. These protocols contained algorithms to aid individuals in taking appropriate action in response to common upper respiratory symptoms. Their purpose was to define when users should care for themselves and when they should seek formal medical care, which would thus promote sensible use of medical services.[13] The internal and external locus of control orientations distinguish beliefs that events (in this case health related) are a result of the individual's own actions (over which they have control) from perceptions that events are a consequence of factors beyond their control. In the evaluation of the self-care protocols two subscales of an established health locus of control instrument (measuring internal locus of control and chance locus of control) were included in a questionnaire.[13] A locus of control measure, distinguishing individuals who believed outcomes resulted from their own behaviour from those who tended to attribute outcomes to external forces such as fate or luck, was included in a study of consumers' decision-making related to over-the-counter medicines.[14]

In a study to develop an instrument that would allow the development of effective intervention strategies to improve the quality of pharmaceutical care in long-term care settings, social learning theory was used to examine the structure of caregivers' beliefs and locus of control.[15] Social learning theory is reported by the authors as stating: 'the potential for a behaviour to occur . . . is a function of the expectancy that the behaviour will lead to a particular reinforcement and the value of that reinforcement'. Locus of control is viewed as a construct taken from social learning theory to describe the range of beliefs about control over the outcomes of life's events. The authors argue the importance of locus of control in designing health interventions. They see the role of caregiver as a lay person making decisions about the care of other people as dissimilar from the usual position of testing individuals for locus of control, but sharing features of the study of locus of control in parents of ill children. Caregivers, like parents, are required to make decisions regarding appropriate medicine use by others. Thus, this study adapted the 'Child improvement locus of control scale', which comprised dimensions of locus of control taking into account the role of the caregiver.[15]

A study comparing Thai consumers' and Thai pharmacists' attitudes and beliefs regarding self-care and responsibility for health incorporated both the multidimensional health locus of control and Krantz health opinion survey.[16] The multidimensional health locus of control instrument employed here included the 'powerful others health locus of control' (a subscale measuring the belief that health professionals control one's health) in addition to the subscales relating to internal locus of control and chance locus of control. The Krantz health opinion survey was designed to measure preferences for different treatment approaches. It comprises two subscales that measure preferences for health related information and behavioural involvement: self-care and active participation in medical care. This measure was used in addition to the multidimensional health locus of control to compare the attitudes of pharmacists and consumers in Thailand.[16]

Theory of reasoned action and theory of planned behaviour

The theory of planned behaviour considers how the influences upon individuals determine their decisions to follow particular courses of action. The theory is an extension of the theory of reasoned action.[9] The theory of planned behaviour concerns an individual's intention or motivation to engage in a behaviour and their perceptions regarding their control over, or ability to engage in, that behaviour.[9]

The theory of planned behaviour and the health belief model were used to investigate cognitive predictors of adherence to malaria prophylaxis regimens by tourists returning from malarious regions. Instruments were modified to refer to malaria prophylaxis. Three health belief model measures were included: perceived side-effects, perceived severity, and perceived susceptibility. Measures representing the theory of planned behaviour were used to assess respondents' attitudes to taking their medication after their return home. These comprised views on perceived approval or disapproval of others regarding taking the medication, perceived behavioural control (how easy or difficult it is to take medication as directed), and respondents' intention to take or not take the tablets after their return home, and were expressed on five, seven-point scales (e.g. ranging good–bad, harmful–beneficial). A model based on theory of planned action explained approximately 60% of variance in self-reported adherence to prophylactic use of mefloquine and 40% among users of chloroquine/proguanil. The authors concluded that interventions targeting key cognitions could enhance adherence.[12]

A theoretical model incorporating variables informed by four theories (theory of reasoned action, theory of planned behaviour, theory of trying, and theory of goal-directed behaviour) was used as a basis for an investigation of factors influencing pharmacists' behaviour regarding the implementation of pharmaceutical care. Thus, the survey instrument included measures of attitude, perceived behaviour control, social norm, behavioural intention and past behaviour, which were operationalised according to frameworks and suggestions of previous theorists and researchers. Researchers noted the limited success of previous attempts to influence pharmacists' consultation activities. They devised their model (pharmacists' implementation of pharmaceutical care model) to aid the designing of successful intervention procedures for the implementation of pharmaceutical care.[17]

Theories relating to behavioural change

Models have also been developed to explain the professional behaviours of pharmacists. In an examination of pharmacists' attitudes, social norms and past behaviour regarding their intentions to try to prevent and correct drug therapy problems, researchers developed an instrument based on the theory of trying. The authors selected this model as it relates to goal behaviours where goals are defined as behaviours for which an individual believes that impediments stand in the way of achievement. They acknowledged similarities between the theory of trying and the theories of reasoned action and planned behaviour, which also perceive behaviour as mediated by intention. The authors discuss the development of their survey instrument to meet the study objectives. This included two items to measure pharmacists' behavioural intention to try (the dependent variable) and questionnaire items for each of the independent variables as required by the model (including attitudes, expectation of success and failure, social norm towards trying, and normative beliefs).[18]

Intention to supply injecting equipment to intravenous drug misusers, attitudes towards its supply, subjective norms and perceived demand were incorporated into a study of pharmacists' services to drug misusers.[19]

A survey instrument based on the 'transtheoretical model of change' was devised to measure pharmacists' readiness to adopt a new standard for assessing the appropriateness of clients' requests for non-prescription medicines. The model proposes a sequence of five stages along a continuum of readiness for change: pre-contemplation, contemplation, preparation, action, and maintenance. The survey instrument focused on respondents' impressions of the positive and negative aspects of the new behaviour to determine the stage of change. Following analysis of data the researchers concluded that pharmacists were unready to become more involved in adopting the new standard: over 57% of respondents scored as pre-contemplators and, therefore, by definition had no intention of engaging in the new behaviour in the foreseeable future.[20] The authors subsequently considered the implications of these findings for pharmacy education.[21] In a case study of events that led up to a change in the use of flucloxacillin in Australia, analysis was conducted within the framework of the transtheoretical model of behaviour change, to provide an understanding of the relationship of events that result in changes in medication use.[22] A stage-of-change model was also used as a basis for training pharmacists to assist people in giving up smoking.[23]

A study of the effects of consultation on consumers' decisions regarding over-the-counter medication purchasing examined factors that predict changes in consumer purchasing decisions, by employing a multivariate model. This was based on a behavioural model in which predisposing, enabling and need factors are assumed to affect a patient's decision to use health services.[14] Researchers also used a locus of control measure (to distinguish individuals who believe that their outcomes are a result of their own behaviour from those who tend to attribute their outcomes to external forces such as fate or luck) as well as the Eysenck personality inventory as a measure of extroversion–introversion tendencies.[14]

A cognitive and interactionist psychology model was employed to investigate factors affecting consumers' attitudes to information provision in pharmacies.[24] These researchers described and used a similar model to analyse pharmacists' perceptions of customers.[25] In these studies participants were shown a series of pre-recorded video-vignettes and data were gathered on their responses, perceptions and judgement regarding each of these.

Theory building

Researchers have employed both survey and qualitative methods (see Chapter 4) in the development of theory in pharmacy practice and related research. In many of these studies, survey and qualitative techniques have been combined. This section focuses on the development and validation of explanatory and predictive models using survey methods. The development and validation of these models usually includes the application of multivariate statistical procedures. In particular, regression methods, factor analysis and measures of internal consistency of scales (Cronbach's alpha) have frequently been employed. Researchers have attempted to explain and/or predict aspects of pharmacists' role orientation, job satisfaction, involvement in professional activities and behaviours from other variables. From the perspectives of patients and the public, studies have addressed their perceptions and use of pharmacy services.

Professional orientation and activities

A theoretical causal model of career commitment was developed through extensive review of the literature on professions and organisations. Measures were drawn from the literature to assess components of the model, which included commitment to organisation, career aspirations and job withdrawal intentions.[26] In another study investigating the effect of role stress, age, salary and educational level on organisational commitment, variables were again selected on the basis of those considered important in theoretical frameworks and findings of other researchers. Thus, scales for organisational commitment, turnover intention and role stress were taken, or adapted, from the literature.[27] For both of these studies data were gathered by questionnaire among groups of pharmacists and the models were tested using path analysis.[26,27] In a study of the dimensions of job satisfaction among Australian pharmacists, researchers identified from the literature the need for assessment of the separate components of facet-free satisfaction (i.e. global satisfaction) and facet-specific satisfaction (satisfaction with respect to specified aspects). Factor analysis was employed to determine underlying dimensions of facet-specific job characteristics.[28] In an investigation of pharmacists' role stress and the work/non-work interface, stressors were identified and measured through a series of rating scales. A separate series of items were developed for: role overload, role ambiguity, role conflict, work–home conflict, and job stress.[29]

`Researchers investigating subjective role orientation, conflict and satisfaction among pharmacy students drew attention to debates regarding the dual nature of pharmacists' roles, which claim that the practice of pharmacy embodies the conflicting values and goals of the professional and business worlds.[30] They cite work by earlier researchers who, accepting the general sociological understanding of the concept of role as an institutional set of behavioural expectations and noting the dual role of organisation of retail pharmacy, set out to study the impact of these seemingly divergent role expectations. They claim that the models developed by others, and subsequently adopted more widely, focus on adaptation to role organisation and do not take into account subjective attitudes and preferences; and they also argue that the possibility of disjunction between actor and role or between subjective attitudes and social expectations was not considered. Working among pharmacy students, they developed an alternative model taking these additional dimensions into account and highlighting the complexity of the relationships between subjective role orientations, career satisfaction and role conflict.[30]

Models have been developed to explain or predict aspects of pharmacists' professional activities. Two such studies have focused on pharmacists' behaviour regarding the provision of pharmaceutical care.[17,31] The first deals with theory of reasoned action, theory of planned behaviour, theory of trying and theory of goal directed behaviour, which provided the framework for the selection of explanatory variables (e.g. measures of attitude, perceived behaviour control, social norm, behavioural intention and past behaviour).[17] The second measured pharmacists' assessments of their own efficacy, beliefs, evaluations and behaviour control.[31] In both cases the model was developed from data collected in a two-stage postal survey.

Models have also been developed to explain pharmacists' preferences in recommending non-prescription medicines,[32–35] that is, explanatory models of likelihood of recommending specific products. Qualitative interviews with pharmacists enabled the identification of the considerations of pharmacists in making their recommendations. From this a pilot questionnaire was developed which included a comprehensive list of relevant issues. Researchers developed a survey instrument and employed factor analysis to identify underlying dimensions of the decision-making.

A combination of critical incidents technique, semi-structured interview and a psychometric test were employed to test hypotheses regarding the personal and workplace characteristics that distinguish 'leading edge' practitioners from others.[36] In critical incidents technique, respondents are asked to identify and describe in detail occasions or events from their experience relevant to the topic of study. The data are then analysed to identify quantitative and/or qualitative differences between the groups in terms of the types of events, how they were managed, the contexts in which they arose and/or the outcomes. The findings of one study led to the identification of a range of personal attributes and working styles that were typical of 'leading edge' practitioners.[36] An analysis of critical incidents in interpersonal communication in pharmacy practice enabled the identification of pharmacists' conceptualisations of this aspect of practice.[37]

In a study of barriers and facilitators on the self-reported extent of provision of pharmaceutical care services, potential barriers were based on past research and included lack of reimbursement, lack of time, lack of employer encouragement and physician attitude. Perceived facilitators were pharmacist's attitude, pharmacist's confidence, consumer attitude and lack of legal liability.[38]

A model of shared decision-making which included four characteristics deemed as prerequisites was used to assess the extent to which shared decision-making was apparent in doctor–patient communication about drugs. Researchers looked for evidence in transcripts of consultations of involvement by both the doctor and patient, sharing of information by both parties, steps to reach consensus and agreement on the treatment to be implemented.[39] A postal survey was used to test a model for predicting goal directed behaviours of community pharmacists in addressing prescription-related problems.[40]

Application of established measures in explanatory models

Many researchers have adopted measures from the literature that have been validated in terms of the extent to which they reflect social/cultural constructs (possess construct validity) or include the important dimensions of an attribute, issue or situation (possess content validity) (see Chapter 2). These have been included in studies either to describe characteristics of a population or as independent variables to be included in an explanatory model.

Rest's defining issues test is a psychometric instrument that measures an individual's moral reasoning skills according to cognitive development theories. It consists of six moral dilemmas followed by a series of statements. Respondents are asked to assess the importance of each statement in determining what action they would take. Researchers reported that, after controlling for situational variables, pharmacists' moral reasoning accounted for a significant amount of variance in their self-reported and actual clinical performance.[41] To evaluate pharmacy students' perceptions of the relative status of seven health professional groups, researchers employed a survey instrument based on a measure and theory developed by Furnham. The instrument comprised eight bipolar scales representing pairs of attributes on which respondents rated pharmacists and other health professional groups.[42]

A descriptive analysis of pharmacists' leadership styles employed a commercially produced measure, which contained 12 leadership situations in which respondents select a typical action from four alternatives which represent four styles.[43] A study of job satisfaction among Jordanian pharmacists used the job descriptive index to measure satisfaction.[44] An instrument from the literature was also employed to investigate the extent of pharmacists' business versus professional orientations.[45]

In a survey of stress and the effect it was having on job satisfaction among community pharmacists, measurements were made using the job satisfaction scale from the occupational stress indicator, which measures both mental and physical symptoms of stress.[46] Other researchers have investigated entrepreneurial orientation and its effect on the provision of innovative pharmacy services. A multidimensional measure was employed and factor analysis was used to confirm that a pharmacy's entrepreneurial orientation comprised these dimensions. The researchers reported a positive association with provision of new pharmacy services.[47] A study of personality preferences of lecturers and students at a pharmacy school used the Myers–Briggs type indicator, from which respondents' preferences were categorised according to four characteristics. These preferences were then related to academic performance.[48]

Patients' perspectives regarding pharmacy services

Hedvall and Paltschik,[49] recognising a shift from a business to a service orientation in pharmacy, developed a framework to characterise the type of pharmacy services desired by different groups of clients. From the literature they identified a conceptual model of service quality as well as studies that provided a basis for the development of a survey instrument. Respondents were then asked to rate their opinions of pharmacy services on seven-point semantic differential rating scales. The data were analysed to distinguish different customer groups in terms of the type of pharmacy services they desired.

To investigate factors influencing the quality and commitment of patients to pharmacies or pharmacists, a model was developed using literature sources. Data were obtained by postal survey to 800 individuals in the USA. Seven relationships were investigated in the model, which was composed of five constructs. The model was tested using path analysis. The authors concluded that the perceived expertise of the pharmacist was an important factor influencing the development of a quality relationship, as opposed to the frequency with which the pharmacist interacts with the patient. They also discussed assumptions in the theory (e.g. that patient perceptions of quality are important for commitment in the relationship) and measurement error for the study constructs.[50]

The 'beliefs about medicines' questionnaire was developed to assess commonly held beliefs about medicines. It comprises two sections. The first section includes items that assess representations of medication prescribed for the personal use of the individual. This comprises two factors relating to beliefs about the necessity of prescribed medication and concerns about adverse effects. The second section, relating to beliefs about medicines in general, also comprises two factors, concerning beliefs regarding the harmful effects of medicines and beliefs that medicines are overused by doctors. The two scales were derived from a pool of items representing commonly held beliefs about medicines. Both the development of the questionnaire and its validity among different groups have been described.[51]

In a study of elderly consumers' perceptions of risk of mail order pharmacies, measurement of perceived risk was based on an established model that included several dimensions which might affect a consumer's decision on whether or not to use a mail order pharmacy: financial risk, convenience risk, social risk, psychological risk, and performance risk. The components were measured by responses to series of items on five-point Likert scales, anchored by 'very likely' and 'very unlikely' or 'very important' and 'very unimportant', with a midpoint labelled as 'undecided'.[52]

Patients' preferences regarding therapeutic outcomes were assessed by analysing their responses to hypothetical therapeutic scenarios. The survey instrument consisted of three pairs of scenarios with different types of outcome, from which the authors suggested patients' willingness to accept therapies that carried uncertain outcomes depended on whether these outcomes were favourable or unfavourable.[53]

Analytical procedures in the development of models

Research, either incorporating established theories or described as theory building, has involved a range of methodological approaches and, consequently, analytical procedures. In survey data, the investigation of associations between variables may be a first step in investigating and proposing relationships between them. If there are no observable statistically significant associations between variables in a data set, then it is unlikely that change in one of the variables is dependent on corresponding change in the other. However, if an effect is small, it may not be apparent in a small data set.

Associations between variables in a data set, however, may not indicate causal relationships. Levels of statistical significance, prior planning of statistical analyses to limit the number of tests, procedures that check that relationships between variables of interest are independent of confounding variables, and assurances that relationships are not influenced by either response bias or other features of the research methodology are important considerations when interpreting possible meanings of output from statistical procedures.

The development of explanatory or predictive models depends on the identification of relationships between variables such that a change in the value of one variable (an independent variable) results in a corresponding change in another (the dependent variable).

Bivariate procedures are commonly employed in the initial investigations of relationships between variables. The most appropriate tests (in particular, whether parametric or non-parametric procedures should be employed) will be determined by the structure of variables and/or the distribution of data. Bivariate procedures that are commonly employed include: chi-square tests, t-tests, Mann–Whitney U-test, analysis of variance, Kruskal–Wallis, and parametric (e.g. Pearson's) and non-parametric (e.g. Spearman's) correlations.

Multivariate statistical procedures

In the building of models, multivariate procedures are often employed. For example, CHAID (chi-square automatic interaction detection), was employed in a study to describe the population characteristics of a community pharmacy's clientele. This enabled the identification of subgroups within each variable predictive of use of pharmacy services.[54] Procedures that have most commonly been applied are discussed below.

Multiple regression

Regression analysis has been widely used to study the relationships between variables and in model building in pharmacy studies. The development of explanatory or predictive models depends on the identification of causal relationships between variables in the model. In regression analysis, the researcher aims to build a model in which the value of one variable (the independent variable) is explained or predicted from the values of one (simple regression) or more (multiple regression) dependent variables. In multiple regression an equation is obtained in which the dependent variable is expressed as a function of the dependent variables plus a constant. Details of the statistical techniques involved in multiple regression have been discussed in many texts. In particular, there are many publications which have been designed for use with the statistical software packages (e.g. SPSS: Statistical Package for Social Sciences), which include explanations of the procedures and are commonly used by researchers. In the development of conceptual models or instruments, some researchers have combined multiple regression analysis with data reduction methods such as factor analysis.

It is important to ensure that the assumptions of multiple regression procedures (in terms of the underlying structure of the data set) are met. The relationships between the independent and the dependent variable(s) are assumed to fit a linear model. If the relationships may be better explained by an alternative model, then some transformation of the data may be required prior to the regression analysis. It is also important to ensure normality and equality of variance of the independent variables for any given value of the dependent variable. This is commonly done by analysing the residuals. These relate to that part of the variance that is not explained by the model. If the model provides a better fit (i.e. a good fit is when the values predicted by the model are close to the observed values) for some values of the dependent variable than for others, then this will be apparent on inspection of the distribution of the residuals against the predicted values. For example, in a study to establish determinants of patients' role orientation for pharmacist consultation, the researchers reported that an investigation of the residuals of the regression analysis indicated that the assumptions for regression analysis were not violated, and therefore no transformation of the variables was required.[55] In the study, data were gathered in a population-based survey on a series of experientially based factors (e.g. past experience regarding consultations with pharmacists) and individual traits (selected by the authors: need for cognition, involvement with medications, self-perceived medication knowledge). These data were then included in a multiple regression analysis to identify the effects of these factors on patient role orientation. The results indicated that all the independent variables had a statistically significant influence on patient role orientation.[55]

In an examination of pharmacists' attitudes, social norms and past behaviour regarding their intentions to try to prevent and correct drug therapy problems, researchers developed a model based on the 'theory of trying'. This included measures of pharmacists' behavioural intention to try (the dependent variable), as well as measures to assess attitudes, expectation of success and failure, social norm towards trying and normative beliefs (independent variables). Multiple regression was employed to predict 'intention to try' from the independent variables and led to the development of a causal model.[18] In the development of the components of the model, reliabilities (Cronbach's alpha) were calculated for the constructs with multiple measures, and confirmatory factor analysis was also used to examine the dimensionality of attitudes.

Multiple regression procedures were combined with factor analysis to identify and explain pharmacists' preferences for recommendations of non-prescription products.[32,33] Following identification of the dimensions of pharmacists' preferences, explanatory models of the likelihood of recommending specific products were developed using multiple regression.[32] If cases with missing values are excluded from the data set, this can reduce the statistical power of the procedure. To maximise the number of cases on which a model is based, missing values were replaced with sample means.[32]

The applicability of the model based on the theory of planned behaviour and the health belief model to investigate cognitive predictors of adherence to malaria prophylaxis regimens by tourists returning from malarious regions was assessed using hierarchical multiple regression. Adherence between groups was compared using t-tests.[12]

Logistic regression

Logistic regression is employed when the dependent variable takes on two nominal values. Thus, in a study to identify pharmacist characteristics that were associated with participation in a project to improve care of elderly patients, logistic regression enabled the development of a model of participation versus non-participation as a function of pharmacists' role orientation and other variables.[56] Logistic regression was also employed to identify factors predictive of changes in consumers' purchasing decisions regarding non-prescription medicines. Using this technique researchers identified one 'enabling' variable (availability of generic medicines) and four 'need' factors that were significant predictors of the consumer's decision to purchase a different product from that intended.[14]

In a study to identify factors predictive of antacid use, data were collected on health-related variables (e.g. symptoms and self-perceived health), life style (e.g. smoking and drinking) and socio-demographic characteristics (e.g. education, age, sex). Separate analyses were performed for men and women. This was carried out in three steps: first, with health-related variables, then with life style and socio-economic factors, and finally with both sets of variables in the same regression. Three logistic models were generated based upon the odds ratios for each variable as a predictive factor.[57] Logistic regression has also been used to identify factors associated with non-prescription and alternative medicine use by people with HIV disease.[58]

Discriminant analysis is a statistical procedure that may provide an alternative to logistic regression. In this procedure, independent variables are combined into a new variable, such that the new variable discriminates between individuals in terms of the dependent variable. In this way, a combination of independent variables (the discriminant function) is identified, which distinguishes between sets of cases.[59]

Path analysis

Path analysis is an application of multiple regression that has been used in the development of models in studies among pharmacists and patients. In a study of the effect of role stress, age, salary and educational level on organisational commitment, path analysis was described as 'a graphic representation of one or several sequential multiple regression analysis results'.[27] The steps include the development of a causal model, establishing a pattern of associations between variables in the sequence, and calculating path coefficients for the basic model. Path analysis allows for the assessment of both the direct effect (i.e. not mediated by intervening variables) of a dependent variable on an independent variable, as well as independent effects (i.e. those mediated by other variables in the path). Variables were selected on the basis of those considered important in theoretical frameworks and findings of other researchers. Scales for organisational commitment, turnover intention and role stress were adapted from the literature. A model was constructed which hypothesised positive or negative causal relationships between variables. These were then explored using path analysis, which estimated the magnitudes of the effects of different variables on each other. This was then presented in a diagram of the model, which included the standardised regression (path) coefficients. Each coefficient indicates the extent of effects of an independent variable on a dependent variable. If a dependent variable is affected by more than one independent variable, the standardised coefficients can be used to compare the relative contribution of each of the independent variables. Both the direct and indirect effects were quantified. Three multiple regression analyses were performed in which organisational commitment, future ambiguity (e.g. regarding job security) and salary were the dependent variables respectively.[27]

A theoretical causal model of career commitment, including commitment to organisation, career and job withdrawal intentions, was again developed through a review of the literature on professions and organisations. The authors identified a series of models that had previously been tested using path analysis. They used these in combination with findings of other researchers to develop their own causal model of career commitment and withdrawal intentions. Data were gathered in an eight-page questionnaire sent to a sample of over 2000 pharmacists. Path analysis was employed to test the model. This involved a separate regression analysis for each dependent variable, each variable being regressed on that which preceded it in the model. Again, direct and indirect effects of the components of the model were identified.[26]

Path analysis was also applied to investigate factors influencing the quality and commitment of patients to pharmacies/pharmacists. A model composed of five constructs was developed, taking into account previous studies in the literature, and data were obtained in a postal survey to 800 individuals in the USA. Relationships between variables in the model were investigated, from which the authors concluded that the perceived expertise of the pharmacist was an important influence on the development of a valued relationship.[50]

Factor analysis

Factor analysis has been extensively used in the development of survey instruments and theoretical models.[7,15,17,18,28,30–35,38,46,47,49,51,55,60–66] It is a data reduction technique in that it is used to reduce a large number of variables to a smaller number of underlying dimensions or factors. Many texts have described the analytical processes and alternative procedures that may be employed. Techniques commonly included are:

principal components analysis to identify the underlying variables (or components); varimax rotation to achieve a solution in which there is minimal correlation between factors; and acceptance of factors with eigenvalues of at least 1. The eigenvalues indicate the proportion of variance explained by any factor.

Based on the relationships (correlations) among variables in the data set, the technique derives a smaller number of underlying factors. Correlations of each variable in the data set with each of the factors are represented by a factor loading. If a successful solution is found, each factor reflects a distinct group of variables in the data set. Ideally, each variable will have a high factor loading on one factor, and a low factor loading on the others. The group of variables that have high factor loadings on a given factor are believed to be measuring the same underlying construct or attribute. Thus, the factors together represent the underlying dimensions or components of the full data set. This technique is seen as valuable in distinguishing the components that determine people's attitudes or behavioural patterns. From a comprehensive list of issues important to individuals in their decision-making, attitudes can be reflected by a smaller number of underlying dimensions. Once identified these dimensions may then form the underlying structure of a measurement instrument or conceptual model.

Factor analysis was used to assess the influence of barriers (e.g. lack of reimbursement, lack of time, lack of employer encouragement and physician attitude) and facilitators (e.g. pharmacist's attitude, pharmacist's confidence, consumer attitude and lack of legal liability) on the self-reported extent of provision of pharmaceutical care services.[38] It has also been applied to survey data to identify the underlying dimensions determining pharmacists' attitudes to injecting drug misusers,[62] and to identify the dimensions of entrepreneurial orientation among community pharmacists.[47]

Factor analysis and multiple regression procedures have been employed to identify and explain pharmacists' preferences for recommendations of non-prescription products.[32–35] In a series of qualitative interviews, researchers identified a comprehensive list of factors taken into account by pharmacists in making their product recommendations for coughs and colds. These were incorporated into a pilot questionnaire and factor analysis was employed to reduce these variables to a smaller number of underlying dimensions of pharmacists' preferences.[33] These factors were then entered as independent variables into a multiple regression analysis to develop explanatory models of the likelihood of recommending specific products.[32] Roins *et al.*[34,35] employed a similar approach in a study of pharmacists' recommendations of analgesics for simple, tension and migraine headaches. The results of the factor analysis identified sets of variables (loading onto each factor) relating to distinct dimensions, for example clinical influences, products influences, external influences (self-use and colleagues) and business influences (e.g. on-shelf).[34]

In an exploration of relationships between subjective role orientation, career satisfaction and role conflict among pharmacy students, researchers developed a model using correlation matrices and factor analysis. In a questionnaire, students expressed their preferences regarding daily tasks of pharmacy. Using Pearson correlation coefficients for each pair of tasks, researchers identified distinct groups of tasks preferred by different groups of students. This analysis revealed three distinct orientations of students to their roles: clinical, traditional, and managerial. These findings were confirmed in a factor analysis in which the groups of variables representing each orientation were found to have high factor loadings on three respective factors.[30]

An investigation of factors influencing pharmacists' behaviour regarding the implementation of pharmaceutical care, based on the theory of trying included measures of attitude, perceived behaviour control, social norm, behavioural intention and past behaviour, which were operationalised according to frameworks and suggestions of previous theorists and researchers. The reliability of the measures was checked using Cronbach's alpha; confirmatory factor analysis was used to assess convergent and discriminant validity.[17]

A causal model to predict pharmaceutical care behaviours from pharmacists' self-efficacy, beliefs, evaluations and behaviour control was undertaken by sending an attitude survey to pharmacists, followed by a behavioural survey two weeks later. Descriptive analytical procedures were employed to compare respondents' attitudes with reported behaviour. The analysis also included a principal components analysis which identified three components (behaviours). A causal model was then constructed by ordering the five attitudinal facets to be predictive of behaviours.[31] In a study of community pharmacists' professional role orientation measures included personal agreement with statements (self-perceived norms) and application of statements to the average pharmacist (perceived group norms). Factor analysis was used to derive a meaningful professional orientation scale.[63]

Factor analysis and cluster analysis were combined in an analysis of pharmacy services and clientele. These procedures enabled identification of the styles of pharmacy services that different groups of customers preferred, and how groups of customers (which held these different preferences) may be distinguished. The rationale for conducting a factor analysis (using principal components procedure) was to reduce the variable set to a smaller number of underlying dimensions. This revealed eight principal components reflecting dimensions or characteristics of pharmacy advisory services. Pharmacy customers' scores relating to each of these eight factors were then used as input for the cluster analysis. This analysis distinguished four clusters (or groups) of respondents in terms of their preferences regarding pharmacy services. The groups were described as follows: the contented pharmacist-dependent customer; the independent customer; the information seeker; and the discontented customer.[49] Factor analysis was also used to identify underlying dimensions of consumer satisfaction and loyalty to community pharmacies with different levels of drug information provision.[65]

In a study of everyday pain, employing Q methodology, accounts of pain were identified from a range of sources (e.g. discussions with pain researchers and clinicians, focus groups and various texts). From these accounts a large number of statements reflecting differing perspectives were derived. Statements were sorted to obtain a final Q set (80 statements). In the analysis (which include principal components procedure), eight factors (or patterns of association) were identified, reflecting cultural perceptions of everyday pain.[7]

The underlying factor structure of the beliefs about medicines questionnaire was verified by principal components analysis. Analysis was undertaken to establish whether the factor structure obtained in one illness group was replicated when repeated on data obtained among people from other groups.[51] The first stages in the development of a survey tool to explore patients' perceptions of their prescribed drugs and need for information comprised semi-structured interviews from which the emergent themes formed the basis of a survey tool. Factor analysis was used to identify the underlying dimensions.[66]

Cronbach's alpha

Cronbach's alpha is frequently employed as a measure of reliability or internal consistency.[12,15,17,29,34,35,55,60,67–69] It is used when a series of items in a questionnaire is intended as a measure of a single underlying construct. In such cases the responses to individual items would be expected to correlate. Cronbach's alpha is a measure (between 0 and 1), based on these correlations, which indicates the extent to which the items can be viewed as measuring a single construct. Values above 0.7

or 0.8 are generally considered acceptable. The technique has been used as a check on the construct validity of multi-item measures[12,29] and, in combination with factor analysis, to confirm the internal consistency of variables contributing to each extracted factor.[15,55]

In a study of consumers' perceptions of access to medications and regulatory options, Cronbach's alpha was used to determine the internal consistency of items that formed a scale to measure each of a series of constructs. Initially values of below 0.7 were obtained. To improve the internal consistency of scales, items were removed in turn from each scale and those that contributed to poor reliability were removed. This resulted in a series of scales for which a Cronbach's alpha of at least 0.9 was achieved.[69]

In an investigation of pharmacists' role stress and the work/non-work interface, stressors were identified and measured through a series of rating scales. A separate series of items was developed for: role overload, role ambiguity, role conflict, work–home conflict, and job stress. Each series of items was then tested for internal reliability using Cronbach's alpha.[29] In a study in which the 'Child improvement locus of control scale' was adapted for use in a study of caregivers of adults, construct validity was demonstrated by both factor loadings and Cronbach's alpha.[15]

Generalisability theory

Generalisability theory is an application of analysis of variance, which establishes the reliability of measurements. It enables the identification of sources of error in any assessment procedure. If the sources of error can be identified and quantified then subsequent assessments can be designed to take these into account. Its main application has been in studies in which assessments are made which may be based on an individual's terms of reference (rather than objective criteria). Thus, it has a useful application in the evaluation of health care.

Generalisability theory has been employed to improve the reliability of measures that include a subjective component or value judgement.[70–74] It is an application of analysis of variance in which the sources of variance are quantified. For example, variation in assessments may be a result of factors such as differences of opinion of individual assessors, varying expectations of assessors from different backgrounds (e.g. professional groups), variation due to type of problem, or poor reliability of measurement scales. Generalisability theory comprises two stages. In the first stage (called the G-study), analysis is conducted which identifies and quantifies the sources of variance attributable to each of a range of different factors (main effects in the analysis of variance) and also the interactions between them (e.g. one group of assessors may consistently score a particular type of problem poorly). The second stage (the D-study) is a series of calculations based on the results of stage one. The D-study provides the researcher with revised values for each of the sources of variation for a series of study designs (e.g. for differing numbers of assessors involved in the assessment procedure). Thus, the researcher can then modify the assessment procedure to one in which unwanted sources of variation are taken into account.

In a study of the assessment of student performance in a practice-based clinical pharmacy course, tutors marked (giving scores to) course-work by their own students with whom they were paired, as well as work from other students on the course. The G-study showed that an important source of variance in the scores achieved by students was the interaction between tutors and students. This was apparent from the high value for the component of variance 'student–tutor interaction'. It was found that individual tutors tended to give higher marks to assignments of their own students than to other students. By contrast, overall variation (average marks) assigned by different tutors was small. The components of variance for the main effects and interactions identified in the G-study provided the basis for the D-study. In the D-study, generalisability coefficients for a range of alternative assessment procedures were calculated. From these a more reliable (and therefore fairer) assessment system was identified.[73] Generalisability theory has also been applied to assessment of advice-giving in community pharmacy settings[72] and in scoring the severity of medication errors in hospitals.[74]

Conclusion

Statistical techniques are powerful in evaluating complex mathematical relationships among variables, which is fundamental to the development of explanatory models. However, theory building in research is common to diverse methodologies. It has been a feature of qualitative approaches as well as survey research. Research employing qualitative methods is reviewed in the next chapter.

References

1.   Norgaard L S, Morgall J M, Bissell P. Arguments for theory-based pharmacy practice research. *Int J Pharm Pract* 2000; 8: 77–81.

2. Hassell K. The impact of social change on professions – gender and pharmacy in the UK: an agenda for action. *Int J Pharm Pract* 2000; 8: 1–9.

3. Jones P. *Studying Society: Sociological Theories and Research Practices*. London: Collins Educational, 1993.

4. Bowling A. *Research Methods in Health*. Buckingham: Open University Press, 1997.

5. Rothmann J C, Gerber J J, Lubbe M S, *et al*. Pharmacy students' experiences of the contents of pharmacy education: a phenomenological study. *Int J Pharm Pract* 1998; 6: 30–7.

6. Lumme-Sandt K, Hervonen A, Jylha M. Interpretative repertoires of medication among the oldest-old. *Soc Sci Med* 2000; 50: 1843–50.

7. Aldrich S, Eccleston C. Making sense of everyday pain. *Soc Sci Med* 2000; 50: 1631–41.

8. Fallsberg M. Reflections on medicines and medication: a qualitative analysis among people on long-term drug regimens. [Dissertation.] Linkoping: Linkoping University, 1991.

9. Connor M, Norman P, eds. *Predicting Health Behaviour: Research and Practice with Social Cognition Models*. Buckingham: Open University Press, 1995.

10. Kruger H S, Gerber J J. Health beliefs and compliance of Black South African outpatients with antihypertensive medication. *J Soc Admin Pharm* 1998; 15: 201–9.

11. Brown C M, Segal R. The effects of health and treatment perceptions on the use of prescribed medications and home remedies among African American and White American hypertensives. *Soc Sci Med* 1996; 43: 903–17.

12. Abraham C, Clift S, Grabowski P. Cognitive predictors of adherence to malaria prophylaxis regimens on return from a malarious region: a prospective study. *Soc Sci Med* 1999; 48: 1641–54.

13. Scott D M, Woodward J M B. The influence of locus of control and perceived susceptibility to illness on family managers' self-care chart use. *J Soc Admin Pharm* 1992; 9: 21–8.

14. Nichol M B, McCombs J S, Johnson K A, *et al*. The effects of consultation on over-the-counter medication purchasing decisions. *Med Care* 1992; 30: 989–1003.

15. Hartzema AG, Godbout N, Lee S D, Konrad R. Measuring health locus of control among caregivers in charge of medication administration in long-term care settings. *J Soc Admin Pharm* 1990; 7: 84–92.

16. Charupatanapong N, Chairojkanjana K, Tanapaisalkit A. Comparison of attitudes and beliefs about self-care and personal responsibility for health held by consumers and pharmacists in Thailand. *Int J Pharm Pract* 1996; 4: 103–8.

17. Odedina F T, Segal R, Hepler C D, *et al*. Changing pharmacists' practice pattern. *J Soc Admin Pharm* 1996; 13: 74–88.

18. Farris K B, Kirking D M. Predicting community pharmacists' intention to try to prevent and correct drug therapy problems. *J Soc Admin Pharm* 1995; 12: 64–79.

19. Rees L, Harding G, Taylor K M G. Supplying injecting equipment to drug misusers: a survey of community pharmacists' attitudes, beliefs and practices. *Int J Pharm Pract* 1997; 5: 167–75.

20. Taylor J, Berger B, Anderson-Harper H, Grimley D. Pharmacists' readiness to

assess consumers' over-the-counter product selections. *J Am Pharm Assoc* 2000; 40: 487–94.

21. Taylor J G, Berger B A, Anderson-Harper H M, Pearson R E. Pharmacist readiness for greater involvement in OTC product selection: implications for education. *Am J Pharm Educ* 2000; 64: 133–40.

22. Roughead E E, Gilbert A L, Primrose J G. Improving drug use: a case study of events which led to changes in use of flucloxacillin in Australia. *Soc Sci Med* 1999; 48: 845–53.

23. Sinclair H K, Bond C M, Lennox A S. The long-term learning effect of training in stage of change for smoking cessation: a three year follow-up of community pharmacy staff's knowledge and attitudes. *Int J Pharm Pract* 1999; 7: 1–11.

24. Franzen S, Lilja J, Hamilton D, Larsson S. How do Finnish women evaluate verbal pharmacy over-the-counter information? *J Soc Admin Pharm* 1996; 13: 99–108.

25. Lilja J, Larsson S. 'Mental mirrors' of pharmacists: how do pharmacists perceive their over-the-counter customers? *Int J Pharm Pract* 1993; 2: 136–41.

26. Gaither C A, Mason H L. A model of pharmacists' career commitment, organisational commitment and career and job withdrawal intentions. *J Soc Admin Pharm* 1992; 9: 75–86.

27. Kong S X, Wertheimer A I, McGhan W F. Role stress, organisational commitment and turnover intention among pharmaceutical scientists: a multivariate analysis. *J Soc Admin Pharm* 1992; 9: 159–71.

28. Ortiz M, Walker W L, Thomas R. Job satisfaction dimensions of Australian community pharmacists. *J Soc Admin Pharm* 1992; 9: 149–58.

29. Gaither C A. An investigation of pharmacists' role stress and the work/nonwork interface. *J Soc Admin Pharm* 1998; 15: 92–103.

30. Hornosty R W. Subjective role orientation, conflict and satisfaction among pharmacy students. *J Soc Admin Pharm* 1990; 7: 14–25.

31. Farris K B, Schopflocher D P. Between intention and behaviour: an application of community pharmacists' assessment of pharmaceutical care. *Soc Sci Med* 1999; 49: 55–66.

32. Emmerton L, Benrimoj S. Factors influencing pharmacists' preferences for non-prescription cough suppressants. *J Soc Admin Pharm* 1994; 11: 78–85.

33. Emmerton L, Gow D J, Benrimoj S I. Dimensions of pharmacists' preferences for cough and cold products. *Int J Pharm Pract* 1994; 3: 27–32.

34. Roins S, Benrimoj S I, Carroll P R, Johnson L W. Factors used by pharmacists in the recommendation of active ingredient(s) and brand of non-prescription analgesics for simple, tension and migraine headaches. *Int J Pharm Pract* 1998; 6: 196–206.

35. Roins S, Benrimoj S I, Carroll P R, Johnson L W. Pharmacists' recommendations of the active ingredient(s) of non-prescription analgesics for a simple, tension and migraine headache. *J Soc Admin Pharm* 1998; 15: 262–74.

36. Blenkinsopp A, Allen J, Platts A. Leading edge practitioners in community pharmacy: approaches to innovation. *Int J Pharm Pract* 1996; 4: 235–45.

37. Morrow N C, Hargie O D W. An investigation of critical incidents in interpersonal communication in pharmacy practice. *J Soc Admin Pharm* 1987; 4: 112–18.

38. Venkataraman K, Madhavan S, Bone P. Barriers and facilitators to pharmaceutical care in rural community practice. *J Soc Admin Pharm* 1997; 14: 208–19.

39. Stevenson F A, Barry C A, Britton N, *et al*. Doctor–patient communication about drugs: the evidence for shared decision-making. *Soc Sci Med* 2000; 50: 829–40.

40. Farris K B, Kirking D M. Predicting community pharmacists' choice among means to prevent and correct clinically significant drug therapy problems. *J Soc Admin Pharm* 1998; 15: 69–82.

41. Latif D A, Berger B A, Harris S G, *et al*. The relationship between community pharmacists' moral reasoning and components of clinical performance. *J Soc Admin Pharm* 1998; 15: 210–224.

42. Collins D M, Benson H E A, Occhipinti S, *et al*. The impact of professional socialisation on pharmacy students' role perceptions. *Int J Pharm Pract* 1999; 7: 182–7.

43. Ibrahim M I M, Wertheimer A I. Management leadership styles and effectiveness of community pharmacists: a descriptive analysis. *J Soc Admin Pharm* 1998; 15: 57–62.

44. Sadik F, Reeder C E, Saket M, *et al*. Job satisfaction among Jordanian pharmacists. *J Soc Admin Pharm* 1992; 8: 46–51.

45. Carlson A M, Wertheimer A I. Occupational inheritance and business orientation in pharmacy. *J Soc Admin Pharm* 1992; 9: 42–8.

46. Willett V J, Cooper C L. Stress and job satisfaction in community pharmacy: a pilot study. *Pharm J* 1996; 256: 94–8.

47. Doucette W R, Jambulingam T. Pharmacy entrepreneurial orientation: antecedents and its effect on the provision of innovative pharmacy services. *J Soc Admin Pharm* 1999; 16: 26–37.

48. Rothmann S, Basson W D, Rothmann J C. Personality preferences of lecturers and students at pharmacy school. *Int J Pharm Pract* 2000; 8: 225–33.

49. Hedvall M-B, Paltschik M. Developing pharmacy services: a customer-driven interaction and counselling approach. *Serv Ind J* 1991; 11: 36–46.

50. Worley M M, Schommer J C. Pharmacist–patient relationships: factors influencing quality and commitment. *J Soc Admin Pharm* 1999; 16: 1557–73.

51. Horne R, Weinman J, Hankins M. The beliefs about medicines questionnaire: the development and evaluation of a new method for assessing the cognitive representation of medication. *Psychol Health* 1999; 14: 1–24.

52. Carroll N V, Fincham J E. Elderly consumers' perceptions of the risks of using mail-order pharmacies. *J Soc Admin Pharm* 1993; 10: 123–9.

53. Eraker S A, Sox H C. Assessment of patients' preferences for therapeutic outcomes. *Med Decision Making* 1981; 1: 29–39.

54. Tully M P, Temple B. The demographics of pharmacy's clientele: a descriptive study of the British general public. *Int J Pharm Pract* 1999; 7: 172–81.

55. Schommer J C, Sullivan D L, Haugtvedt C L. Patients' role orientation for pharmacist consultation. *J Soc Admin Pharm* 1995; 12: 33–42.

56. Pendergast J F, Kimberlin C L, Berardo D H, McKenzie L C. Role orientation and community pharmacists' participation in a project to improve patient care. *Soc Sci Med* 1995; 40: 557–65.

57. Furn K, Straume B. Use of antacids in a general population: the impact of

health-related variables, lifestyle and socio-demographic characteristics. *J Clin Epidemiol* 1999; 52: 509–16.

58. Smith S R, Boyd E L, Kirking D M. Non-prescription and alternative medication use by individuals with HIV disease. *Ann Pharmacother* 1999; 33: 294–300.

59. Kinnear P R, Gray C D. *SPSS for Windows Made Simple*. Hove, UK: Psychology Press, 2000.

60. Airaksinen M, Ahonen R, Enlund H. Customer feedback as a tool for improving pharmacy services. *Int J Pharm Pract* 1995; 3: 219–26.

61. Ortiz M, Walker W L, Thomas R. Development of a measure to assess community pharmacists' orientation towards patient counselling. *J Soc Admin Pharm* 1992; 9: 2–10.

62. Harding G, Smith F J, Taylor K M G. Injecting drug misusers: pharmacists' attitudes. *J Soc Admin Pharm* 1992; 9: 35–41.

63. Ortiz M, Walker W-L, Thomas R. Community pharmacists' professional role orientation. *J Soc Admin Pharm* 1992; 9: 97–103.

64. Rupp M T, Segal R. Confirmatory factor analysis of a professionalism scale in pharmacy. *J Soc Admin Pharm* 1989; 6: 31–8.

65. Whitehead P, Atkin P, Krass I, Benrimoj SI. Patient drug information and consumer choice of pharmacy. *Int J Pharm Pract* 1999; 7: 71–9.

66. Duggan C, Bates I. Development and evaluation of a survey tool to explore patients' perceptions of their prescribed drugs and their need for drug information. *Int J Pharm Pract* 2000; 8: 42–52.

67. Gore P, Madhavan S. Credibility of the sources of information for non-prescription medicines. *J Soc Admin Pharm* 1993; 10: 109–22.

68. Krass I. A comparison of clients' experiences of counselling for prescriptions and over-the-counter medications in two types of pharmacy. Validation of a research instrument. *J Soc Admin Pharm* 1996; 13: 206–14.

69. Shefcheck S L, Thomas J. Consumers' perceptions of access to medications and attitudes towards regulatory options. *J Soc Admin Pharm* 1998; 15: 149–63.

70. Cronbach L J, Rajaratnam N, Gleser G C. Theory of generalisability: a liberalisation of reliability theory. *Br J Stat Psychol* 1963; 16: 137–63.

71. Cronbach L J, Gleser G C, Nanda H, Rajaratnam N. *The Dependability of Behavioural Measurements: Theory of Generalisability for Scores and Profiles*. New York: Wiley, 1972.

72. Smith F J, Salkind M R, Jolly B C. Community pharmacy: a method of assessing quality of care. *Soc Sci Med* 1990; 31: 601–7.

73. Smith F J, Jolly B C, Dhillon S. The application of generalisability theory to assessment in a practice-based diploma in clinical pharmacy. *Pharm J* 1995; 254: 198–9.

74. Dean B S, Barber N D. A validated, reliable method of scoring the severity of medication errors. *Am J Health Syst Pharm* 1999; 56: 57–62.

4

Qualitative interviews

Qualitative approaches have gained an increased prominence in health services research in recent years. The superiority of qualitative methods in answering many questions pertinent to the development of effective health services is being conceded. This is apparent from the number of editorials and discussions of qualitative methodology that have appeared in the major health services and pharmacy journals,[1-14] and the increased frequency with which qualitative research studies are published. Although the numbers of qualitative studies are small compared with those using survey methodology, a substantial body of work has been undertaken in pharmacy practice and related settings.

Poor understanding of qualitative methods, resulting in a lack of confidence in their use, may have contributed to the slow acknowledgement of the value of qualitative studies. In this, pharmacy is not alone: in a review of published qualitative research in general practice, a computer database combined with a hand-search of journals identified few relevant papers.[15] Furthermore, the suspicion that doctors and epidemiologists rarely read or cited qualitative medical sociology triggered a systematic review of the literature. This review, which used citation analysis to identify the 'world's top 100 articles', found that citation rates for the qualitative publications were only a fraction of those for high impact biomedical research. The authors also noted that many of the 'qualitative' papers identified were theoretical or historical works, such as Parsons' *The Social System* or Foucault's historical accounts, rather than the result of qualitative field studies.[16]

Despite the comparatively recent recognition of the potential contribution of qualitative work to the knowledge base required to inform health service development, the hand-searches for this review uncovered a substantial body of published work, particularly in the past few years. In the research literature of pharmacy practice, examples of studies indicate that 10–15 years ago a number of enlightened investigators were aware of the strengths of qualitative approaches to address particular problems of pharmacy practice.[17,18] These studies adopted and developed theoretical or conceptual bases to obtain insights into patterns of pharmacists' self-perceptions, and pharmacists' conceptualisations of the interpersonal dimension of practice. The focus of these studies was to investigate self-perception from the pharmacists' perspective rather than to study perceptions from the point of view of the researcher's own beliefs or to attempt to apply models developed by others. Fallsberg[19] undertook an extensive qualitative study into patients' concepts of medicines and their use. This work, involving people taking medication long term, made comprehensive use of conceptual and theoretical frameworks in both designing the study and in the data processing and analysis. These authors were aware that potential readers were likely to be unfamiliar with qualitative approaches and provided good descriptions and discussions of the processes of undertaking qualitative research, including the development of theoretical perspectives. They also displayed an appreciation of the necessary considerations to ensure successful application of qualitative methods.

The most commonly employed qualitative approach in health services and pharmacy practice research is the qualitative interview. Thus, most of the papers reviewed in this chapter involve qualitative, face-to-face interviews with individual respondents, using either an unstructured or semi-structured interview guide. Structured interviews are generally seen as an alternative to the self-completion questionnaire for gathering quantitative data. Research by group interview or focus group, also a qualitative approach, presents its own particular considerations and problems (see Chapter 5).

In undertaking a qualitative study, the principles of the qualitative approach must be considered at all stages, from exploratory or theoretical conception to data collection and analysis. In addition, given the scepticism with which qualitative methods are sometimes viewed by some researchers in other traditions, concerns regarding validity and rigour must be comprehensively addressed at each stage.

This chapter will discuss the study objectives for which a qualitative approach has been selected, sampling procedures that have been employed, methods of data collection, processing and analysis of data, and how the problems of validity, reliability and generalisability have been managed within the qualitative paradigm.

What is qualitative research?

Qualitative studies are considered most appropriate for 'how?' and 'why?' questions, which explore processes and patterns in people's thoughts and behaviour. For example, qualitative researchers may investigate how people see or interpret events or how they make sense of their experiences and the world around them. They may also be a way of identifying meanings that people attach to events and to establish their priorities and concerns. This sharply contrasts with quantitative research, in which the researcher may be testing a hypothesis, investigating frequencies of events and quantifying relationships between clearly defined variables.

Flexibility of approach and receptiveness to respondents' viewpoints is central to qualitative research. Again, this contrasts with quantitative studies in which the direction and content of the questionnaire are predetermined and standardised by the researchers. Thus, once quantitative survey instruments have been developed (a task that requires expertise and careful and time-consuming fieldwork), the data collection, processing and analysis become to some extent administrative tasks. Qualitative researchers, however, must remain sensitive to the respondents' viewpoints and be prepared to consider new issues and ask questions throughout data collection and analysis. To gain insights into the respondents' interpretations and perceptions of events, experiences and surroundings, qualitative researchers must be attentive to the perspectives of the respondents, and endeavour to leave their own preconceptions behind.

To gain understanding of how people view and interpret phenomena, qualitative work is often undertaken in natural settings. The researcher aims to gather data that enables exploration of the viewpoints of individuals in the context of their circumstances or environment. It also allows the researcher to observe and ask questions that may lead to a deeper understanding of phenomena of interest in the context in which they occur.

In the analysis of doctor–patient interactions to investigate the social organisation of chemotherapy treatment consultations, the author describes the cultural and institutional setting of the research prior to descriptions of the sequences of interaction and analysis of the talk.[20] In a study among young people with thalassaemia and their responses to daily chelation therapy in the context of their lives and relationships, researchers investigated how respondents coped with non-compliance and explored the way that responsibility for chelation therapy is negotiated with parents, and young people's views on the value of such therapy.[21] Similarly, a study that explored the management of asthma and medicines aimed to explore this in the context of maintaining 'ordinariness' in the household.[22]

In a study of children's attitudes and beliefs about medicines, researchers recognised the potential implications of social and cultural contexts and variations in determining beliefs about, and use of, medicines. They acknowledge that the views and behaviours of each child will be distinct, but also that they will be evolving in a way that reflects the socialisation process and in accordance with societal and cultural norms.[23] In conducting research among children, different sociological paradigms have been identified that distinguish a focus on the developmental or socialisation processes from approaches that view children as independent social actors with their own perspectives, meanings and contexts.[24]

The investigation of phenomena in their natural contexts is an essential feature of ethnography, which evolved in cultural anthropology with its focus on small scale societies.[25] One researcher described ethnography as 'learning from people' rather than 'studying people'.[26] While qualitative interviews do not constitute ethnography, in terms of aims and objectives they share some important features, and qualitative interviews are frequently a component of ethnographic research.[26,27]

In his paper 'Overcoming ethnocentrism', the anthropologist van der Geest[28] defines culture as a system of shared meanings. He sees social science and medicine as 'two different cultures into which people are encultured and taught to view the world in a particular way', and claims that ethnocentrism not only causes people to judge others by the standards of their own culture, but also prevents them from understanding one another.[28]

In a study of pharmacy students' experiences of the contents of pharmacy education, Rothmann et al.[29] describe their approach as phenomenological, that is, the researcher is interested in the meaning a person attributes to their experiences, environment or relationships. Thus the objective of this research was to analyse the experiences of pharmacy students and to gain insight into the current education paradigm as experienced by them.[29]

Critical incidents technique, in which the data set is participants' descriptions of relevant experiences, has also been viewed as a part of a phenomenological approach in that the process involves descriptions, analysis and interpretation of individuals' understanding of phenomena in their surroundings.[30] This technique was also employed in a study of 'leading edge' practitioners.[31]

In a number of qualitative studies, researchers have applied principles of social constructionism, in which phenomena are assumed to be a product of social or cultural practices as opposed to external realities (see Chapter 3). In a social constructionist analysis to 'make sense of everyday pain', authors gathered their data from discussions with pain researchers, clinicians and relevant texts from which they derived statements representative of the different interpretations.[32] In a study of narratives of people with epilepsy, Faircloth[33] acknowledged that such narratives (story-telling) 'are a means of production and creation of a life and not simply its representation'. The author suggests that 'stories' and narratives have sometimes been employed as simple representation; that is, people's stories are their interpretation of phenomena rather than 'objective' accounts. However, if constructed, such narratives provide insights into individuals' experiences and problems from their perspective. Principles of social constructionism were also employed in the analysis of a data set consisting of life stories of older people.[34]

Qualitative research is frequently exploratory work that aims to examine and explain relationships between variables. It may be described as hypothesis-generating or theory-building, aiming to predict how people may behave in given situations and/or under particular circumstances. Using qualitative methods, many researchers have attempted to develop hypotheses or apply theoretical perspectives to explain phenomena.[17–19,23,26,35–43]

Studying doctor–patient communication about drugs, researchers employed a four-stage model of shared decision-making: both parties are involved, both parties share information, both take steps to build a consensus about preferred treatment, then an agreement is reached on the treatment to implement.[44] In the analysis of interviews with pharmacists on ethical dilemmas and their resolution, researchers applied concepts of autonomy, beneficence, non-maleficence and justice, looking for evidence that these normative principles underpinned professional responsibilities and obligations.[45] In a study of part-time workers in community pharmacy, Symonds[46] referred to previous work which asked whether part-time work was viewed as a 'bridge' or a 'trap'. She then used her data to expand on this issue and thus develop existing theory and contribute to contemporary debates in employment studies on the reconceptualisation of part-time work.[46]

A distinction between problem-oriented and theory-oriented research has been drawn to illustrate how the former would benefit from the introduction of theoretical perspectives in order to develop the knowledge base of health services research.[47] It was argued that theoretical perspectives could be incorporated at an early stage in the project development rather than being applied to, or derived from, the data set during the data processing and analysis. A case for application of theory to health services research in pharmacy has also been argued by Norgaard *et al.*[48]

Research objectives

The studies included in this review address a wide range of research objectives. However, they all share the central features of the qualitative approach in undertaking detailed work to explore issues from the perspective of respondents, or, as one research paper was entitled, to uncover a 'hidden dimension' of a topic of interest.[49] The objectives of many researchers were descriptive in that they wished to explore and describe particular views or experiences. Thus, the qualitative approach has been used to look at different aspects of professional practice from the point of view of groups of practitioners,[18,26,38,50–56] to gain insights into the controversial relationship between dispensing doctors and prescribing pharmacists,[57] to explore the effect of changing prescribing patterns and policy,[58,59] to investigate service development from the perspective of patients,[60–62] and to compare views about, and use of, medicines between two population groups.[63]

Qualitative studies have also been found to be a valuable adjunct in research areas that traditionally relied on a quantitative approach. For example, in contrast to most studies of adverse events in medical care, which depend on patients' medical notes as a source of data, a study which employed ethnographers trained in qualitative methods to gather data uncovered a greater number and range of events.[64] Qualitative research has also successfully provided insights into explaining phenomena uncovered by quantitative research[65] (see Chapter 7).

A large body of qualitative work into aspects of drug use has been conducted outside pharmacy. The pertinence of many of these studies is now recognised by pharmacy practice researchers. Examples include a study by Stimson,[35] which shows how 'non-compliance' can be explained as a rational approach by patients to the use of their medicines rather than defaulting on the doctor's instructions.[35] A paper by Helman[36] published in 1981, examining the dimensions of meaning that psychotropic drugs can have for those that use them, led to the classification of use into three types, 'tonic, fuel and food,' each of which embodied a different perspective on psychotropic drugs, their symbolic meanings and modes of usage. A paper entitled 'The meaning of medicines: another look at compliance,' published in 1985, focused on patients with epilepsy and presented a patient-centred approach of 'self-regulation' to managing medicines as an alternative to the doctor-centred approach to compliance that prevailed at the time.[37] These descriptive studies were followed by a comparative study to investigate the role of cultural factors in determining 'compliance'.[63] Researchers have highlighted the lack of success in improving medication adherence, despite the vast numbers of studies, and have argued for a qualitative approach to investigate the issue from the viewpoints of patients.[66] The importance of patients' views and experiences uncovered in these earlier studies is now recognised, and further exploration of this topic is currently an attractive and thriving area of qualitative research. In terms of the preparedness of the pharmacy and medical professions to value the perspectives of their clients on health care priorities, particularly those revealed in qualitative studies, these papers were possibly before their time.

Patient participation in decision-making regarding their health care has become an important focus for practitioners and researchers. Examples of qualitative research relevant to these issues includes investigation of patients' unvoiced agendas,[67] shared decision-making,[44,68] misunderstandings in prescribing decisions,[68] talk in chemotherapy consultations,[20] compliance in the context of people's everyday lives,[21] and an exploration of 'knowledge based asymmetry' in, and its impact on, pharmacist–client interactions.[69]

There are many examples of qualitative research that have uncovered perspectives relevant to health policy. For example, a study of elderly people's beliefs about influenza vaccination concluded that few people perceived themselves to be at risk from dying of influenza, and that there was a mismatch between elderly people's perspectives and the British government's focus.[70] The study suggested that evidence that vaccination reduces morbidity from influenza and does not cause colds and influenza should be stressed. In another study, limited knowledge of recommendations regarding folic acid supplements was found to be the reason for low use preconceptually and in early pregnancy.[71] A number of researchers have explored views and perspectives regarding the deregulation of emergency hormonal contraception.[72–75]

The British government is encouraging partnership between health authorities, professionals and the public to improve health status. It is also keen that people should have a role in influencing health service development.[76] To achieve these ends, it is important that health policy makers and professionals understand and value the perspectives, views and concerns of the public and patients.

Populations, settings and samples

Procedures for sampling and the criteria for determining the appropriate sample size differ between qualitative and quantitative studies.[77] In quantitative studies, it is important to select probability samples (simple random, systematic, cluster, stratified samples), so that statistical procedures can be applied to provide generalisations to the population from which the sample was drawn. Because of the detailed and intensive work that qualitative studies entail, sample sizes are necessarily small and the application of mathematical rules to calculate sample sizes is generally inappropriate. Even if random sampling procedures are followed, because of the small sampling fraction and resulting possibility of a high sampling error, the application of probability statistics may be inappropriate. The rationale of qualitative researchers for drawing a random sample is to ensure a degree of representativeness. Although the level of representativeness, diversity or homogeneity may be unquantifiable, researchers may wish to describe their sample in terms of their characteristics and their relevance to the wider population.

Small sample sizes are not necessarily limiting to a qualitative study. A small sample enables detailed work to be conducted, taking into account comprehensive contextual and background information. It allows the investigator to explore contexts in which responses are given, and to identify experiences, concerns and rationales that may be predictive of the views expressed. Large samples may not be required and may hinder detailed exploration and analysis that is required for successful realisation of objectives. A survey of pharmaceutical care provision in NHS hospitals in the UK involved respondents from just eight hospitals. Although the sample of hospitals was small, the researcher was able to undertake intensive work at each site, to include a range of professionals and thus to obtain a comprehensive data set. A larger number of hospitals may have resulted in less complete data being obtained from each site.[52] A large sample (226 home interviews), while providing more extensive information in terms of the numbers of respondents, may not provide the opportunity for detailed consideration of the perspectives of each respondent.[78]

Although there are no universal rules for determining sample sizes in qualitative research, authors must always be able to defend the suitability of their sample size for achieving the objectives of the research. The numbers interviewed in qualitative studies will be governed by the aim of the research. The objective of an exploratory study into influences on pharmacists' preferences for cough and cold products was to identify all possible influences, which would later be used as a basis for a quantitative study. Researchers continued with their interviews until no new influences emerged.[79]

Sample sizes in the studies reviewed here were typically between 15 and 50, although there are examples employing smaller and larger numbers. A study of the European Union's systems of drug approval involved 42 interviews with people who were selected to include industrial scientists, regulatory affairs managers and representatives of trade associations in five countries.[80] Thirty-three individuals with different background characteristics were interviewed in a study of home-coping and work-coping among part-time workers.[67] In-depth interviews with 25 young people with thalassaemia enabled identification of important issues regarding compliance, responsibility for therapy and negotiation with parents in the contexts of their daily lives.[21]

Sampling procedures

Sampling strategies often applied by qualitative researchers include purposive, representative, convenience and theoretical samples.

Purposive samples

Purposive sampling is commonly employed in qualitative studies. This method involves the identification and selection of particular individuals who share characteristics relevant to the study, and whom the researcher therefore believes will be most informative in achieving their objectives. Purposive sampling is 'informed' in that the researchers have preconceived ideas regarding the characteristics of the sample. These may be based on established theories regarding relevant explanatory variables or factors identified during preliminary fieldwork. In the study of the European Union's systems of drug approval, sampling procedures targeted individuals in organisations who were knowledgeable about safety evaluation, licensing and regulatory affairs. Thus the data gathered were informed, rather than random, opinions.[80]

A purposive sample of eight hospitals was chosen for a survey of pharmaceutical care provision in NHS hospitals. These were selected on the basis of pilot work in which they displayed a range of features found to affect the provision of clinical pharmacy services.[52] Purposive sampling procedures were also employed to ensure variability among respondents in year of registration, sex and place of work in a study of attitudes and opinions to pharmaceutical care,[81] and in a study of motivations and barriers to provision of community pharmacy services for drug misusers.[82]

Researchers may believe that their research objectives are best served by a diverse, homogeneous or representative group. For example, to maximise variability in the sample of nurses in an investigation of attitudes and beliefs about medication errors, interviewees were selected by ward specialty and grade.[83] In a study of part-time workers in community pharmacy, interviewees were selected on the basis of gender, age, employment status, location and patterns of working.[67] To study elderly people's beliefs about influenza vaccination, interviews were conducted with equal numbers of vaccinated and non-vaccinated people, to allow the researchers to undertake some comparison of their different perspectives.[70]

Representative samples

A representative sampling procedure was adopted by researchers to investigate illicit drug users' views and experiences of pharmacy services. While unable to include a random sample, researchers were keen to involve respondents from different pharmacies and drug agencies. The quota sampling (see Chapter 1) employed ensured inclusion of a minimum number of respondents from all centres, resulting in an attempt to achieve some degree of representativeness.[84] Twenty customers were recruited from two community pharmacies to explore pharmacist–client relationships. This sample, described as purposive and convenient, is similar to a quota sample in that researchers focused on specific client groups who were recruited at different times of day.[85]

In a study of prescribing in two health authorities, the sample was selected from respondents to an earlier study. However, because the sample did not include any practitioners with responsibility for their own budgets (who researchers believed should be included), an additional group was contacted.[53] To achieve a degree of representativeness regarding social background (assumed likely to be an important determinant of patients' views), a sample for a study on self-reported medication adherence was recruited from two medical practices in socially contrasting areas.[86]

Convenience samples

Convenience sampling involves the selection of those individuals most accessible to the researcher or willing to take part. This is often an easy option for the researcher in terms of travel, time and resource implications, as the efforts of contacting and eliciting co-operation of random or purposive samples can be considerable. In some qualitative studies, especially in very early fieldwork when the researcher is in the process of developing an informed approach to the research, convenience sampling may be justified. However, as with quantitative studies, a convenience sample is likely to be unrepresentative of the population of interest, and may introduce a bias of which the researcher is unaware and therefore unable to take into account when evaluating the results. Similar difficulties can arise when the researcher relinquishes the task of sample recruitment to others, for example, pharmacy staff.[87,88] The benefits to the researcher in terms of 'convenience' have to be contrasted with the potential effect of unknown bias and doubt regarding the validity of the study findings. A 'snow-ball' sampling procedure was adopted by researchers keen to identify and recruit a sample of people with epilepsy independently of a medical setting. The 'snow-ball' sampling technique involved placing advertisements in papers, invitation letters and contacts with self-help groups. The objective of the research was to investigate an alternative patient-centred approach to managing medicines rather than the established doctor-centred approach. The researchers believed that independence of any medical setting was of paramount importance to the study and outweighed the potential bias of a non-representative sample.[37] Although, in common with other convenience samples, this method does not allow for claims about the representativeness of the sample and thus generalisability of the findings, it may achieve insights that researchers believe are only possible with a sample totally independent of any medical setting. Similarly, in an investigation of attitudes of drug misusers to pharmacy services, researchers opted to recruit their sample through staff and poster displays at agency needle-exchange schemes and a rehabilitation unit, rather than through pharmacies.[89]

Theoretical samples

Theoretical sampling has been used to describe an iterative process sometimes employed in grounded theory research. The selection of the sample is based on those concepts that have proven theoretical relevance to an evolving theory.[90] Sampling strategies are iterative in that they are redesigned at each stage of the research to enable successively more detailed examination of emerging theory or perspectives.[77] Iterative theoretical sampling procedures were not detailed by pharmacy practice researchers, even in the cases where authors reported that the research process was guided by principles of grounded theory. However, researchers investigating pharmacists' views of patient communication used insights gained from previous interviews to help select individuals for subsequent interviews.[26] The authors referred to the sample as purposive, but there is overlap in the terminology and the procedure described also displayed features of a theoretical sample.

The sampling procedure adopted in any study may display features of more than one of these sampling types. For instance, to explore pharmacists' experiences of violent crime in the course of their work, those reporting serious events in a questionnaire were identified. From this purposely selected group, the final sample was selected using a random procedure.[91] If the researcher believes that a representative sample will be most effective in achieving their research objectives, a representative sample may be, in effect, a purposive sample.[53] When insights gained from previous research are used to inform sample selection for a subsequent piece of work, a purposive sample may be similar to a theoretical sample.[26]

Response rates

Non-response in studies employing random, representative, quota, purposive procedures introduces a non-response bias. Discussion of follow-up of non-responders to establish differences between the views of responders and non-responders, which may be important for the interpretation of the study findings, was rare. However, many researchers did report response rates, which enables the reader to make some assessment of possible bias.[26,42,56,59,62,91–93]

An incentive (prepaid telephone card on successful completion of the interview) was paid to respondents in a study of drug misusers' experiences of community pharmacy.[89] The practices of general medical practitioners who were interviewed regarding appropriateness of long-term prescribing were offered an honorarium of £50 (80 euros).[94]

Development of the interview guide

The data collection instrument was commonly referred to as the interview guide. In the development of the interview guide for qualitative studies, researchers are concerned with the topic headings (or content) and the extent to which it is structured. In these studies, the researcher aims to identify the perspectives of the respondent. Thus, a typical interview guide will comprise a series of open questions or topic headings. Further questions are then based on the responses to these questions. This contrasts with much survey work, in which all questions (and frequently the response options) are determined in advance by the researcher. Thus, qualitative interviews are sometimes described as respondent-led as opposed to researcher-led, as the issues raised by the respondent are an important determinant of the direction of the interview. Additional questions employed in the interview may be neutral requests for further information, clarification of views expressed, exploration of reasoning behind particular viewpoints, etc. The interview guide may also list a range of neutral probing questions to aid the interviewer in a deeper exploration of the respondent's perspectives.

Authors describe their interview schedules as unstructured or semi-structured. While described in this way, interview schedules will fall somewhere on a continuum from unstructured, in which the interview guide lists a few topic headings which are explored according to the issues raised by the respondent, to interview schedules in which comments and views are sought on issues determined by the researcher. Semi-structured interviews possibly represent a half-way house between providing respondents with opportunities to express their views and obtaining information relating to issues of interest to the researcher. The extent of structuring will also be governed by the degree to which the researcher has preformed ideas regarding the topics on which they want the interviewee's views.

Question order is a consideration in qualitative interviews. Generally, researchers will begin with open questions which allow the respondent to raise the issues that are important to them, before the interviewer introduces more specific questions which direct the thoughts of the respondent on to certain topics. This procedure allows the identification of issues relevant to respondents, which may otherwise not be raised. A study to explore dilemmas facing prescribers of benzodiazepines employed critical incidents technique. In the opening question, respondents were asked to recall and describe a relevant experience. Further questions were devised to ensure specific relevant information was provided.[30]

Many of the studies reviewed here were early explorations of issues for which little work had previously been undertaken – at least from the perspectives of the populations of interest. In these cases, the development of a structured interview schedule would require suppositions regarding the relevant questions and the range of responses. For example, researchers studying patients' perspectives of patient-controlled analgesia felt that quantification of patients' experiences by structured questionnaire would be premature, as assumptions would be made as to the important components of patients' experiences. Thus their interview guide began with an opening question 'How did you feel about your pain relief?' in an attempt to allow patients to raise and discuss issues important to themselves. Later in the interview, they were prompted for comments on specific issues including pain, side-effects, emotional state, the equipment from which the analgesia was delivered and nursing care.[92] This resulted in a view of patient-controlled analgesia from the patients' perspective. Researchers investigating users' views and expectations of pharmacy services employed a semi-structured interview guide in which the topics of interest were specified by the researchers (use of chemists, expectations, views on possible extended role, etc.), although open questions were used.[93]

Where previous work had been undertaken, issues identified as important to the topic area could be used to inform the interview guide in subsequent research. In some cases, the researchers' objectives were to conduct a more detailed examination of issues uncovered in previous research.[52,56,91] In these studies, an interview guide in which the topics are determined by the researcher may be appropriate, while comprising predominantly open questions to encourage respondents to express their views. In a study of chain pharmacist turnover, for which job satisfaction was believed to be an important factor, the domains of the job description index were incorporated into the interview guide.[95] In a study of general medical practitioners' views of the role of pharmacists in promoting the appropriate use of benzodiazepines, the interview guide was informed by the views that had been expressed by pharmacists in a previous study.[56]

By contrast, an unstructured approach was used to explore children's attitudes and beliefs about medicines. To do this, children were asked to draw a picture about an episode when they were sick. The interview was then focused around the child's descriptions and explanations of what they had drawn.[23] A similar approach was used in a study among children with asthma to encourage discussion on their terms.[22]

Leading questions may curb the discussion of controversial or socially unacceptable viewpoints. The phrasing of questions is important. In a study among French hospital pharmacists, the interview guide comprised a series of closed and leading questions. The danger of such questions is that they may influence the responses obtained. However, the style of question could have been distorted by the translation process required for publication in an English language journal.[54] In a study of lay beliefs and use of antihypertensive drug therapy, researchers began their questioning by stating that some people often forgot to take their drugs, in order that people would not feel that there was an expected or acceptable answer. They then asked respondents whether they took their tablets every day or just occasionally, and if they had difficulty in remembering to take the tablets and how often they forgot. This was followed by more detailed questions about drug-taking in the previous week.[63] In a study of pharmacy students' experiences of pharmacy education, Rothmann et al.[29] described non-directive interview techniques which included minimal encouragement, attentive listening, clarification, paraphrasing, reflecting and summarising.

Data collection

Interviews are the most common method of data collection in qualitative studies, but alternatives include focus groups (see Chapter 5) and observation (in particular, participant observation, see Chapter 6). Data sets have also included consultation transcripts, narratives (story-telling by respondents), texts and other documents. In some studies, data obtained in different ways have been combined. For example, in a social constructionist analysis of everyday pain, data sources included interviews, group discussions and texts.[32] In a study of the use of medicinal plants by indigenous groups in Mexico, unstructured interviews were combined with participant observation,[96] and in a study on the impact of hospital pharmacy automation, data were collected in semi-structured interviews and by non-participant observation.[97]

The purpose of qualitative interviewing has been described as to 'grasp the perspectives of another person without placing the interviewer's preconceived categories for ordering the world into the individual's mind'.[98] Whether a semi-structured or unstructured interview guide was used, many authors, in their descriptions of the data collection process, showed how the principles of qualitative method were observed. Examples include: 'the subject was given the opportunity to discuss the topic freely drawing from his or her own experience . . . the length of time and amount of information obtained was dependent largely on the relative importance of that issue to the individual respondent'[95]; the interview procedure allowed the respondents to 'express their experiences in their own terms'[92]; interviews were 'open-ended and interactive . . . the researcher attempted to be sensitive to language used by the respondent and the topics raised by them'[93]; 'an interview guide was devised . . . each patient however set his or her own agenda(s) of what was important to them about their condition and of its meaning in their lives'.[66]

In the vast majority of studies, the interviews were audiotaped and transcribed verbatim. Audiotape recording can only be undertaken if the respondent agrees and this was not reported to be a problem. Manual transcription, occasionally employed, during the interview will usually result in some paraphrasing of responses. This in itself is an interpretative process on the part of the researcher which may preclude an objective analysis. If undertaken by the interviewer, it may also compromise the comprehensiveness of the data, as being preoccupied with transcribing they are less able to pick up and develop issues as they are raised by respondents. Accurate verbatim transcriptions are seen as an essential prerequisite for a detailed and valid qualitative data analysis.

Location of interview

In a large number of the studies reviewed, the interviews were conducted in the respondents' own homes.[39,60,61,63,66,86] The importance of an independent interview setting, in conferring validity to findings, was acknowledged by many researchers whose studies were aiming to explore aspects of use of medicines or pharmacy services from the respondents' point of view. Conducting face-to-face interviews in independent settings presents additional administrative, ethical and logistical problems and has resource implications. In some cases this could not be achieved.[59,99]

Privacy will also be important. In a study of use of medicines for asthma in the context of everyday household management, separate interviews were conducted with children and their parents. As part of the study, both parents and children were also asked to complete a 'timeline', which traced events before and after the last asthma attack. As well as obtaining independent perspectives, comparison of data from parents and children may enable some validation regarding associated events and their timing.[22] Separate interviews enable researchers to investigate the extent to which views, concerns and priorities regarding what may be shared activities differ between these individuals. A study of the impact on the families of people with insulin-dependent diabetes involved interviews with both patients and family members. To ensure that respondents felt able to speak freely, the interviews were conducted independently in separate rooms.[100] The realisation of such conditions will often require both tact and a thoughtful explanation of the goals of the project by the researcher. It may not always be achievable.

There are examples in which interviews have been conducted by telephone. Telephone interviews are generally considered as limiting in the extent to which they are suited to in-depth discussion resulting in detailed data. Studies among community pharmacists of motivations and barriers to providing services for drug misusers,[82] and with general medical practitioners to establish their views of deregulation of emergency contraception, were conducted by telephone. In the interviews with the general medical practitioners, the authors claimed that the methodology enabled an exploration of the respondents' reasoning.[74,75]

Researchers should acknowledge that in-depth interviews may be perceived as intrusive by some respondents. Detailed exploration of problematic situations can be upsetting for interviewees (and sometimes interviewers). In the conduct of the interview, researchers should be sensitive in their questioning. This may be particularly important in research among vulnerable groups including children, elderly people and those very sick. It is an ethical requirement that the respondent is fully informed and aware that the interview can be terminated at any point should they not wish to continue. To fulfil the objectives of a study, the researcher, of course, will hope to obtain complete interviews when possible. Potential participants should also be given time between being informed of the study and the time of the interview to consider whether or not they wish to take part.

In many studies, interviews are conducted in respondents' own homes. Concerns of householders regarding granting entry to their home to a researcher who is unknown to them should be addressed in study protocols. Ethical and safety considerations required that the researcher conducting interviews in the private homes of people with a diagnosis of schizophrenia was in some cases accompanied by a community psychiatric nurse.[99]

Data processing and analysis

Prior to any analysis, the data will be transcribed, generally verbatim from the tape-recording. Contextual data, such as field notes, may also be included.[43] Researchers exploring older women's perceptions of health reported that they also noted details such as the tone of voice, which may be important to ensure correct interpretation of data. However, they did not describe how they transcribed and used this information.[101]

Approaches to data analysis

The objectives of researchers ranged from providing detailed descriptions of topics of interest to the development of hypotheses or theories to explain and account for phenomena uncovered. Organisation of the data into themes to provide an accurate reflection of the views raised by respondents may involve minimal interpretation on the part of the researcher. By contrast, the development of theory requires that, following the categorisation of data, conceptual labels are applied and interpretation is placed on the data.[90]

Qualitative analysis requires that data collection be observant of the principles of the qualitative method; that is, the data collected must be an objective and comprehensive reflection of the issues of interest from the perspective of the respondents. Thus, the extent to which the interview guide and conduct of the interview followed the agenda of the researcher, as opposed to that of the interviewees, may be an important consideration regarding the validity of embarking on a theory-building approach. In cases when data are not collected using a qualitative methodology (e.g. open questions as part of a structured instrument), the application of a qualitative analytical procedure may be questionable.

Analytical procedures

Common to virtually all studies in this review was the development of a coding procedure that was then applied to the transcribed data. Whether or not researchers were to embark on a theory-building process, the coding procedure involved the identification of themes, which were compared, discussed and organised into categories.[86,102,103] Analysis of interviews with community pharmacists and general medical practitioners on the deregulation of emergency contraception was conducted in five steps: familiarisation, identifying a thematic framework, indexing (systematic application of codes), charting (rearranging the data according to the thematic content in a way which allows for across case analysis) and mapping and interpretation.[72] In the analysis of data based upon the recollections of prescribers regarding previous dilemmas, responses (stories) were read 'vertically' (each story or case) and 'horizontally' (responses to each open question, across cases).[30]

A number of studies employed grounded theory methodology for data analysis and provided a good explanation of what this entailed.[23,38,49] Grounded theory methodology was developed by Glaser and Strauss.[104–106] It is an approach to inductive theory building in which the theory is discovered, developed and verified through systematic data collection and analysis.[90] The essence of grounded theory techniques has been described as an approach whereby ideas, themes, hypotheses and eventually theory are allowed to emerge from the analysis of data derived from natural settings.[43]

In exploring children's attitudes to, and beliefs about, illness and medicine, an iterative process of constant comparison was employed in the analysis of data. The author[23] describes how items of data were compared by asking the question: 'How is this instance of X similar to or different from previous instances?' and thus how new categories, or subdivisions of existing ones, emerged as the researcher had increased exposure to the data. The end of the process was marked by the emergence of no new categories.[23] A similar process was described in a study of clinical pharmacy. Here the researcher described the process of grouping together quotes in the interviews that discussed similar concepts. Subcategories were then developed and links between categories identified. Segments of data were re-analysed for their relevance to one or more categories and compared with similarly categorised data. Thus, through a systematic sifting of data and the process of repeated comparison between and within categories, the researcher was able to clarify relationships and structures.[49] These examples also demonstrate the central importance of questioning throughout the analytical process.

Researchers investigating patients' perspectives of patient-controlled analgesia developed a taxonomy of patients' experiences based on themes that recurred in their statements. This led the researchers to challenge whether, from the patient's viewpoint, patient-controlled analgesia was genuinely patient-controlled.[92] The analytical procedures of other researchers also led to the development of hypotheses or theories to describe or explain research findings.[17,18,35–37,42,43,45,55,66,71,72]

A number of researchers made use of established theoretical frameworks in the analysis of their data. In a study of professional socialisation, a theoretical framework for the interpretation of the data was sought in the literature relating to emotion management[43]; a qualitative exploration of pharmacists' perceptions of their customers applied a conceptual basis of cognitive psychology.[42] In an analysis of interviews with pharmacists on ethical dilemmas and their resolution, researchers looked for evidence of knowledge of normative principles (autonomy, beneficence, non-maleficence and justice) underpinning professional responsibilities and obligations.[45]

A wide range of approaches to the analysis of qualitative data has been employed and described by pharmacy practice researchers. An early study which paid great attention to ensuring the validity of the research maintained that there were no universal protocols for the analysis of qualitative data.[26] Indeed, while there are principles that need to be observed, one of the texts frequently cited by authors in the papers reviewed describes, by means of case-studies, how qualitative researchers have faced and addressed unique problems in the analysis of their data.[107]

Theoretical sensitivity (an important component of grounded theory procedures) relies on the researcher's awareness of the subtleties of meaning of data, which will itself depend on their knowledge of the subject areas and experience of the research area.[90] While the perspectives of the researcher and the conceptual frameworks employed will be important features of the analytical process, it is important to demonstrate a systematic and rigorous approach to analysis such that research findings cannot be charged with, or challenged as, being an artefact of the research methodology.

Coding procedures of some sort were implemented by virtually all researchers. A comparative research study into definitions of health showed how the reliability of coding procedures can be confounded by cross-national understandings, use of language and translation. This study demonstrated the need for researchers always to be aware that they bring to the analytical process their own preconceptions.[108] In any study, quantitative or qualitative, researchers must be aware of the part that the methods they choose, and their preconceptions, play in generating the study findings.

Computers in data processing and analysis

Comparatively few authors reported using computer software packages for the analysis of data, and there was little discussion by researchers on their experiences of the use of them. However, computer-aided qualitative analysis is well established and software has been developed to facilitate the coding of data, the retrieval of data once coded and, in some cases, to support the theory-building process. Researchers in this review reported using Ethnograph to index data,[93] Winmax[84,109,110] and Hypersoft[38,111]; probably the most well-known software packages are Ethnograph[112] and QSR NUD*IST (Non-numerical Unstructured Data Indexing, Searching and Theory building).[44,46,81,113] Computer software may be particularly useful in the management of large data sets for which it may be a time-consuming process to sift through data by hand to find and extract relevant sections. They may also have a role in validation in that they can identify efficiently all instances in which a particular word, or topic, was raised. This enables the researcher to check their descriptions of views on the topic across all respondents and identify inconsistencies with their emerging hypotheses or theories.

Reporting the results

Unlike quantitative research, in which the usual convention is to present separately the results and the discussion, the majority of papers (in common with qualitative research in other fields) combined the results with interpretation and discussion. This was usually followed by a conclusion to summarise and emphasise what the authors considered to be the important points.

For studies employing semi-structured interview guides and descriptive analytical procedures, the presentation of the results commonly followed the topic headings of the interview guide. It was also usual practice for the results to be illustrated by quotations from the transcripts. This provides the reader with first hand examples of typical, atypical or interesting viewpoints.

In studies employing grounded theory as a basis for the analysis, the results may include the exposition of a theory.[17,18,35–37,92] In a study which aimed to gain a deeper understanding of non-compliance, the authors presented the findings as a model of decision-making and discussed this with reference to other current theories.[39]

The provision of quantitative assessments of the views expressed is not generally the objective of qualitative research. However, some researchers chose to report the numbers or proportion of respondents who expressed similar or opposing viewpoints.[50,56,87–89,91] As well as providing a sense of the range of opinion, this technique has also been suggested as a way of reassuring the reader that attention has been paid to all views expressed on a particular issue.[114]

Content analysis was employed in a phenomenological study of pharmacy students' experiences of their education. The researchers described the steps they took to analyse, quantify and interpret their data. This combined elements of qualitative and quantitative procedures – defining the universe of the content, categorising and interpreting individual themes or units. The number of respondents who mentioned each specific theme was then counted and themes ranked, based on this frequency.[29]

Qualitative and quantitative techniques were combined in the analysis of data on use of medicinal plants by indigenous groups in Mexico. Authors were able to describe differences and similarities in the health practices of different groups. They also conducted an assessment of homogeneity of practices involving medicinal plants using an 'informant consensus' method which compares reports of use of remedies for a certain illness with reports of all remedies used for this ailment.[96]

A similar issue arises as to the rationale for incorporating qualitative illustrations (usually verbatim quotes) in an otherwise quantitative study. Many researchers include or append open questions to survey research instruments, inviting respondents to provide additional information or to raise any other issues of concern. These responses are generally coded and often presented pseudo-qualitatively, often as quotations.[115-120] This may highlight issues important to respondents and provide interesting explanations or illustrations of responses to closed questions. However, care is required in the analysis and interpretation as this data will not have been gathered in accordance with the principles of a qualitative approach and will rarely be comprehensive.

Validity

The validity of the data refers to the extent to which they are an accurate reflection of the phenomena that are the subject of the research. In quantitative studies, the aim of the researcher is to develop and employ questions that are relevant to the study area and that people answer accurately and reliably. In qualitative work, the study objectives are more likely to be exploratory. Questions are thus generally open-ended to allow respondents to raise the issues that they believe are important to the study area, the role of the interviewer (sometimes also the principal researcher) being to explore these in greater detail. The direction and the content of the interview are therefore guided by the responses of the interviewee rather than following the agenda of the researcher. Thus, if principles of qualitative inquiry are successfully followed, the data should be a true reflection of the perspectives of the respondent on the issue of interest. As a result, the data are sometimes seen as possessing an 'inherent' validity. During the interview, the interviewer clarifies ambiguous responses by asking probing questions; greater discussion of interesting and unexpected replies provide insights into respondents' rationale for their responses in the contexts in which the views are held.

Nevertheless, qualitative data are a product of the views, experiences and perceptions of respondents. They represent subjective accounts. Narratives provided by respondents in qualitative interviews have been described as 'a means of production and creation of a life and not simply its representation'.[33]

Pharmacy practice researchers are aware that bias may creep into the data collection process despite the rigorous application of the principles of qualitative methodology. The potential for bias as a result of the preconceptions of the fieldworker has been identified as one possible problem.[49] Researchers have also acknowledged that issues raised may be a reflection of interviewees' pressing concerns at the time of the data collection,[52] rendering the durability of findings questionable. Whether or not the interviewer is known to the respondent may affect the issues they raise[38] and their willingness to share certain views.[26]

Many researchers have gone to considerable lengths to assure respondents of the confidentiality and independence of their research in an attempt to ensure that respondents feel comfortable in discussing their true feelings. Thus, despite added logistical problems and resource implications, in the interests of validity, researchers addressing aspects of pharmacy practice have, as previously discussed, gone outside pharmacy or medical settings to recruit samples and conduct interviews.

In observing principles of qualitative enquiry in interviews (e.g. non-directive questions, audiotaping, verbatim transcriptions) researchers are endeavouring to ensure that they embark on the analysis with data that are a true and comprehensive reflection of the issues and sentiments expressed by the respondents. However, researchers have also acknowledged problems of ensuring validity in the data processing and analysis. Most studies, whether broadly descriptive or theory-building, involved some coding procedure. This identification of themes and patterns and the application of codes requires some interpretation of the meaning of the data. As a validity check on these interpretative processes, in some studies the coding procedures were undertaken independently by two or more researchers.[29,59,102]

The processes of validation of qualitative analysis are sometimes referred to as communicative validation (in which researchers return to the field to collect additional data to verify or further develop their hypotheses or findings), argumentative validation (in which an attempt is made to use the data set to argue a contradictory viewpoint), or cumulative validation (in which researchers may use the literature to demonstrate how their findings are consistent with existing knowledge of the subject). In a study of community pharmacists' views of patient communication, researchers returned to their population of interest to ask for their views and comments on their preliminary findings. This was done in three ways: sharing of the researchers' interpretations of the categories or themes that emerged with informants, a second brief interview with some pharmacists to clarify or verify various issues emerging from the data, and asking informants to read the analysis and share their reactions to the researcher's interpretations.[26] In a study of relationships between pharmacists and customers, themes were identified in the analysis of data. The data were then reviewed for counter-themes.[85]

As qualitative data analysis is necessarily an interpretative process, some researchers advocate presenting some numerical data in the analysis to assure the reader that the findings presented are representative of the full data set, and that attention has been paid to rare events and deviant cases.[114] Computer packages for qualitative analysis may also be a useful tool for this validation, by identifying all data relating to the issue of interest for inspection by the researcher.

Reliability

In contrast to quantitative research, reproducibility of responses is often not a pertinent issue in qualitative work, in which the data are expected to be context specific, although reproducibility of study findings would be expected. When viewing issues from the perspective of respondents, differences between individuals will be explored in the context of their lives and experiences. Should an individual respondent's views differ on a subsequent occasion, this may not present a problem for the researcher provided that he or she has confidence in the validity of the data. The researcher would not be aiming for consistent interpretations or responses, but to understand the underlying contexts and reasons for differences. Thus differences and inconsistencies meriting further exploration may be illuminating in terms of the objectives of the study and may be valuable in informing the analysis and development of hypotheses or theories.

The issue of reliability has been discussed in relation to aspects of conduct of interviews, data processing and analysis. In addressing consistency between interviewers, researchers studying transcripts of interviews undertaken with elderly people commented that they found no systematic difference between the interviewers in terms of the topics, frequency or amount of discussion in the interviews which related to drugs.[34] To ensure consistency in data processing and analysis, coding procedures were undertaken by two or more researchers independently.[29,59,71,102]

Use of open and non-leading questions is important to ensure the success of qualitative interviews. Audiotape recording of interviews enables the practices of interviewers to be reviewed, including the verification of the questions used. In one study, the questions used by the interviewers were included in the presentation of data.[80]

Generalisability

The research objectives served by qualitative methods are generally to explore and explain phenomena rather than to test the extent to which characteristics apply to a large population. Qualitative researchers are generally aware of the limitations regarding the generalisation of their findings. Whilst this is not their intention, the context specificity of data does not necessarily preclude the possibility of providing useful insights leading to the development of hypotheses that may have relevance and applicability beyond the sample involved in the research. In a study of children's attitudes and beliefs about medicines, the authors[23] acknowledge that these attitudes and beliefs will be a product of their social and cultural environment. Although not transferable to other social and cultural groups, the findings may provide insights into the formation of children's perceptions and attitudes in the context of the socialisation process.[23]

The extent to which wider generalisation may be argued will, as in quantitative research, be influenced by the sampling strategy and sample size. As with survey research, low response rates may also introduce important bias, jeopardising the validity of the findings. The intensive procedures of qualitative research necessitate small samples. Even if the researcher employs a random sample, the small sampling fraction, and the possibility of sampling error, will limit the validity of generalisations beyond the sample. While they will be subject to sampling error, a random or otherwise representative sample with good response rates would be expected to provide an opportunity for the exploration of the views and experiences relevant to a wider population group than a self-selecting or convenience sample.

A study of community pharmacists' and general practitioners' views on the deregulation of emergency hormonal contraception reported negative attitudes, which the authors contrasted with the views of the participants' professional bodies.[73] With small numbers and limited information on sample selection, it is difficult for the reader to assess the extent to which the findings would be expected to be generalisable. However, in relation to this topic, similar findings were reported in a study which involved randomly selected general medical practitioners.[74]

Conclusion

Many texts on qualitative research have been published. However, a number of publications were cited by many authors as helpful in guiding the conceptual development, conduct and analysis of their research.[90,104-107,121,122] Much high quality and informative qualitative research into many aspects of pharmacy practice and drug use has been undertaken. This has provided insights into issues that could not have been achieved by the more widely employed quantitative approaches. The importance of understanding the views and experiences of health care from the points of view of different population and user groups and the professionals who work in them cannot be overstated. People are being encouraged to take more responsibility for maintaining their health status, and professionals are expected to be accountable to consumers for the services they offer. In the development and delivery of health care, health professionals need to understand the views and concerns of their clients in the context of their social and cultural circumstances to ensure that provision is relevant and sensitive to their outlooks and needs. Qualitative work (e.g. to identify and explore from pharmacists' perspectives, core situations and difficulties regarding patient counselling[123]) may most successfully highlight potential difficulties, constraints and opportunities from the point of view of pharmacists, pharmacy staff and consumers, to identify feasible and effective service development.

References

1. Launso L. The demands for qualitative research are developing. *J Soc Admin Pharm* 1991; 8: 1–6.
2. Smith F J. The practice researcher's toolbox. *Pharm J* 1992; 248: 179.
3. Strong P. The case for qualitative research. *Int J Pharm Pract* 1992; 1: 185–6.
4. Pope C, Mays N. Opening the black box: an encounter in the corridors of health services research. *BMJ* 1993; 306: 315–18.
5. Black N. Why we need qualitative research. *J Epidemiol Community Health* 1994; 48: 425–6.
6. Fitzpatrick R, Boulton M. Qualitative methods for assessing health care. *Qual Health Care* 1994; 3: 107–13.
7. Pope C, Mays N. Reaching the parts other methods cannot reach: an introduction to qualitative methods in health and health services research *BMJ* 1995; 311: 42–5.
8. Mays N, Pope C. Rigour and qualitative research. *BMJ* 1995; 311: 109–12.
9. Britten N. Qualitative interviews in medical research. *BMJ* 1995; 311: 251–3.
10. Cleary P D. Subjective and objective measures of health: which is better when? *J Health Serv Res Policy* 1997; 2: 3–4.
11. Temple B. A moveable feast: quantitative and qualitative divides. *J Soc Admin Pharm* 1997; 14: 69–75.
12. Verbeek-Heida PM. How patients look at drug therapy: consequences for therapy negotiations in medical consultations. *Fam Pract* 1993; 10: 326–9.

13. Scheff T J, Storrin B. Qualitative methods in the health sciences. *Eur J Public Health* 1997; 7: 355–6.

14. Faltermaier T. Why public health research needs qualitative approaches: subjects and methods in change. *Eur J Public Health* 1997; 7: 357–63.

15. Hoddinott P, Pill R. A review of recently published qualitative research in general practice: more methodological questions than answers. *Fam Pract* 1997; 14: 313–19.

16. Chord J A, Lilford R J, Court B V. Qualitative medical sociology: what are its crowning achievements? *J R Soc Med* 1997; 90: 604–9.

17. Sorensen E W. The pharmacist's professional self-perception. *J Soc Admin Pharm* 1986; 3: 144–56.

18. Morrow N C, Hargie O D. An investigation of critical incidents in interpersonal communication in pharmacy practice. *J Soc Admin Pharm* 1987; 4: 112–18.

19. Fallsberg M. *Reflections on Medicines and Medication: A Qualitative Analysis among People on Long-term Drug Regimens.* Linkoping: Department of Education and Psychology, 1991.

20. Diaz F. The social organisation of chemotherapy treatment consultations. *Sociol Health Illness* 2000; 22: 364–89.

21. Atkin K, Ahmad W I U. Pumping iron: compliance with chelation therapy among young people who have thalassaemia major. *Sociol Health Illness* 2000; 22: 500–24.

22. Prout A, Hayes L, Gelder L. Medicines and the maintenance of ordinariness in the household management of childhood asthma. *Soiol Health Illness* 1999; 21: 137–62.

23. Almarsdottir A B, Hartzema A G, Bush P J, *et al.* Children's attitudes and beliefs about illness and medicines. *J Soc Admin Pharm* 1997; 14: 26–41.

24. Lewis A, Lindsay G, eds. *Researching Children's Perspectives.* Buckingham: Open University Press, 2000.

25. Boyle J S. Styles of ethnography. In: Morse J M, ed. *Critical Issues in Qualitative Research Methods.* London: Sage, 1994.

26. De Young M. An inquiry into community pharmacists' views of patient communication. *J Soc Admin Pharm* 1996; 13: 121–30.

27. Hassell K, Noyce P, Rogers A, *et al.* A pathway to the GP: the pharmaceutical 'consultation' as a first port of call in primary health care. *Fam Pract* 1997; 14: 498–502.

28. Van der Geest S. Overcoming ethnocentrism: how social science and medicine relate and should relate to one another. *Soc Sci Med* 1995; 40: 869–72.

29. Rothmann J C, Gerber J J, Lubbe M S, *et al.* Pharmacy students' experiences of the contents of pharmacy education: a phenomenological study. *Int J Pharm Pract* 1998; 6: 30–7.

30. Bendtsen P, Hensing G, McKenzie L, Stridsman A-K. Prescribing benzodiazepines – a critical incident study of a physician dilemma. *Soc Sci Med* 1999; 49: 459–67.

31. Tann J, Blenkinsopp A, Allen J, Platts A. Leading edge practitioners in community pharmacy: approaches to innovation. *Int J Pharm Pract* 1996; 4: 235–45.

32. Aldrich S, Eccleston C. Making sense of everyday pain. *Soc Sci Med* 2000; 50: 1631–41.

33. Faircloth C A. Revisiting thematisation in the narrative study of epilepsy. *Sociol Health Illness* 1999; 21: 209–27.
34. Lumme-Sandt K, Hervonen A, Jylha M. Interpretative repertoires of medication among the oldest old. *Soc Sci Med* 2000; 50: 1843–50.
35. Stimson G V. Obeying doctor's orders: a view from the other side. *Soc Sci Med* 1972; 8: 97–104.
36. Helman C. 'Tonic', 'fuel' and 'food': social and symbolic aspects of the long-term use of psychotropic drugs. *Soc Sci Med* 1981; 15B: 521–33.
37. Conrad P. The meaning of medicines; another look at compliance. *Soc Sci Med* 1985; 20: 29–37.
38. Anderson C. Health promotion by community pharmacists: perceptions, realities and constraints. *J Soc Admin Pharm* 1998; 15: 10–22.
39. Dowell J, Hudson H. A qualitative study of medication taking behaviour in primary care. *Fam Pract* 1997; 14: 369–75.
40. Donovan J L, Blake D R. Patient non-compliance: deviance or reasoned decision-making. *Soc Sci Med* 1992; 34: 507–13.
41. Cotter S M, McKee M, Barber N D. Clinically oriented education provided by the United Kingdom National Health Service hospital pharmacies for hospital health care staff. *J Soc Admin Pharm* 1997; 14: 133–42.
42. Lilja J, Larsson S. 'Mental mirrors' of pharmacists: how do pharmacists perceive their over-the-counter customers? *Int J Pharm Pract* 1993; 2: 136–41.
43. Sleath B. Emotion management techniques used by pharmacy students during pharmacology laboratory: a qualitative study of professional socialization. *J Soc Admin Pharm* 1994; 11: 97–103.
44. Stevenson F A, Barry C A, Britten N, *et al.* Doctor–patient communication about drugs: the evidence for shared decision-making. *Soc Sci Med* 2000; 50: 829–40.
45. Hibbert D, Rees J, Smith I. Ethical awareness of community pharmacists. *Int J Pharm Pract* 2000; 8: 82–7.
46. Symonds B S. Work-coping and home-coping: achieving a balance in part-time community pharmacy. *Int J Pharm Pract* 2000; 8: 10–19.
47. Harding G, Gantley M. Qualitative methods: beyond the cookbook. *Fam Pract* 1998; 15: 76–9.
48. Norgaard L S, Morgall J M, Bissell P. Arguments for theory-based pharmacy practice research. *Int J Pharm Pract* 2000 8: 77–81.
49. Weiss M C. Clinical pharmacy: uncovering the hidden dimension. *J Soc Admin Pharm* 1994; 11: 67–77.
50. Smith F J. Benzodiazepines: community pharmacists' perceptions of their roles and responsibilities. *J Soc Admin Pharm* 1991; 8: 157–63.
51. Keene J M, Cervetto S. Health promotion in community pharmacy: a qualitative study. *Health Educ J* 1995; 54: 285–93.
52. Cotter S M, McKee M. A survey of pharmaceutical care provision in NHS hospitals. *Pharm J* 1997; 259: 262–8.
53. Weiss M C, Scott D. Whose rationality? A qualitative analysis of general practitioners' prescribing. *Pharm J* 1997; 259: 339–41.
54. Auguste V, Guerin C, Hazebroucq G. Opinions and practices with regard to confidentiality in French hospital pharmacies. *Int J Pharm Pract* 1997; 5: 122–7.

55. Lasselain J. Self-perception of occupational roles by community pharmacists in the French health system. *J Soc Admin Pharm* 1991; 8: 130–5.

56. Smith F J. General medical practitioners and community pharmacists in London: views on the pharmacist's role and responsibilities relating to benzodiazepines. *J Interprofess Care* 1993; 7: 37–45.

57. Gilbert L. Dispensing doctors and prescribing pharmacists: a South African perspective. *Soc Sci Med* 1998; 46: 83–95.

58. Dowell J S, Snadden D, Dunbar J A. Rapid prescribing change, how do patients respond? *Soc Sci Med* 1996; 43: 1543–9.

59. Boath E H, Blenkinsopp A. The rise and rise of proton pump inhibitor drugs: patients' perspectives. *Soc Sci Med* 1997; 45: 1571–9.

60. Williamson V K, Winn S, Livingstone C R, Pugh A L G. Public views on an extended role for community pharmacy. *Int J Pharm Pract* 1992; 1: 223–9.

61. Britten N, Gallagher K, Gallagher H. Patients' views of computerised pharmacy records. *Int J Pharm Pract* 1992; 1: 206–9.

62. Morris C J, Cantrill J A, Weiss M C. 'One simple question should be enough', consumers' perceptions of pharmacy protocols. *Int J Pharm Pract* 1997; 5: 64–71.

63. Morgan M, Watkins C J. Managing hypertension: beliefs and responses to medication among cultural groups. *Sociol Health Illness* 1988; 10: 561–78.

64. Andrews L B, Stocking C, Krizek T, *et al.* An alternative strategy for studying adverse events in medical care. *Lancet* 1997; 349: 309–13.

65. Sparks G, Craven M A, Worth C. Understanding differences between high and low accident rate areas: the importance of qualitative data. *J Public Health Med* 1994; 16: 439–46.

66. Adams S, Pill R, Jones A. Medication, chronic illness and identity: the perspective of people with asthma. *Soc Sci Med* 1997; 45: 189–201.

67. Barry C A, Bradley C P, Britten N, *et al.* Patients' unvoiced agendas in general practice consultations: a qualitative study. *BMJ* 2000; 320: 1246–50.

68. Britten N, Stevenson F A, Barry C A, *et al.* Misunderstandings in prescribing decisions in general practice: a qualitative study. *BMJ* 2000; 320: 484–8.

69. Pilnick A. 'Why didn't you say just that?' Dealing with issues of asymmetry, knowledge and competence in the pharmacist/client encounter. *Sociol Health Illness* 1998; 20: 29–51.

70. Cornford C S, Morgan M. Elderly people's beliefs about influenza vaccination. *Br J Gen Pract* 1999; 49: 281–4.

71. Jessa F, Hampshire A J. Use of folic acid by pregnant British Pakistani women: a qualitative study. *Health Educ J* 1999; 58: 139–45.

72. Harper R, Barrett G. Community pharmacist and general practitioner attitudes to the deregulation of emergency contraception. *J Soc Admin Pharm* 1998; 15: 83–91.

73. Barrett G, Harper R. Health professionals' attitudes to the deregulation of emergency contraception. *Sociol Health Illness* 2000; 22: 197–216.

74. Ziebland S. Emergency contraception: an anomalous position in the family planning repertoire. *Soc Sci Med* 1999; 49: 1409–17.

75. Ziebland S, Graham A, McPherson A. Concerns and cautions about prescribing and deregulating emergency contraception: a qualitative srudy of GPs using telephone interviews. *Fam Pract* 1998; 15: 449–56.

76. Department of Health. Our healthier nation: a contract for health (Cm3862). London: Stationery Office, 1998.

77. Marshall M N. Sampling for qualitative research. *Fam Pract* 1996; 13: 522–5.

78. Jesson J, Pocock R, Jepson M, Kendall H. Consumer readership and views on pharmacy health education literature: a market research study. *J Soc Admin Pharm* 1994; 11: 29–36.

79. Emmerton L, Gow D J, Benrimoj S I. Dimensions of pharmacists preferences for cough and cold products. *Int J Pharm Pract* 1994; 3: 27–32.

80. Abraham J, Lewis G. Harmonising and competing for medicines regulation: how healthy are the European Union's systems of drug approval? *Soc Sci Med* 1999; 48: 1655–7.

81. Bell H M, McElnay, Hughes C M, Woods A. A qualitative investigation of the attitudes and opinions of community pharmacists to pharmaceutical care. *J Soc Admin Pharm* 1998; 15: 284–95.

82. Matheson C, Bond C M. Motivations for and barriers to community pharmacy services for drug misusers. *Int J Pharm Pract* 1999; 7: 256–63.

83. Hand K, Barber N. Nurses' attitudes and beliefs about medication errors in a UK hospital. *Int J Pharm Pract* 2000; 8: 128–34.

84. Matheson C. Privacy and stigma in the pharmacy: illicit drug users' perspectives and implications for pharmacy practice. *Pharm J* 1998; 260: 639–41.

85. Abu-Omar S M, Weiss M C, Hassell K. Pharmacists and their customers: a personal or anonymous service? *Int J Pharm Pract* 2000; 2: 135–43.

86. Britten N. Patients' ideas about medicines: a qualitative study in a general practice population. *Br J Gen Pract* 1994; 44: 465–8.

87. Livingstone C R, Pugh A L G, Winn S, Williamson V K. Developing community pharmacy services wanted by local people: information and advice about prescription medicines. *Int J Pharm Pract* 1996; 4: 94–102.

88. Schafheutle E I, Cantrill J A, Nicolson M, Noyce P. Insights into the choice between self-medication and a doctor's prescription: a study of hayfever sufferers. *Int J Pharm Pract* 1996; 4: 156–61.

89. Sheridan J, Barber N. Drug misusers' experiences and opinions of community pharmacists and community pharmacy services. *Pharm J* 1996; 257: 325–7.

90. Strauss A, Corbin J. *Basics of Qualitative Research: Grounded Theory, Procedures and Techniques.* London: Sage, 1990.

91. Smith F J, Weidner D. Threatening and violent incidents in community pharmacies 2. implications for pharmacists and community pharmacy services. *Int J Pharm Pract* 1996; 4: 145–52.

92. Taylor N, Hall GM, Salmon P. Is patient-controlled analgesia controlled by the patient? *Soc Sci Med* 1996; 43: 1137–43.

93. Vallis J, Wyke S, Cunningham-Burley S. Users' views and expectations of community pharmacists in a Scottish commuter town. *Pharm J* 1997; 258: 457–60.

94. Cantrill J A, Dowell J, Roland M. Qualitative insights into general practitioners' views on the appropriateness of their long-term prescribing. *Int J Pharm Pract* 2000; 8: 20–6.

95. Schulz R M, Baldwin H J. Chain pharmacist turnover. *J Soc Admin Pharm* 1990; 7: 26–33.

96. Heinrich M, Ankli A, Frei B, *et al.* Medicinal plants in Mexico: healers' consensus and cultural importance. *Soc Sci Med* 1998; 47: 1859–71.

97. Novek J. Hospital pharmacy automation: collective mobility or collective control? *Soc Sci Med* 2000; 51: 491–503.

98. Spradley J. *The Ethnographic Interview.* New York: Holt, Rhinehart, Winston, 1979; cited in: De Young M. An inquiry into community pharmacists' views of patient communication. *J Soc Admin Pharm* 1996; 13: 121–130.

99. Francis S-A. Medication and quality of life: a study of people with a diagnosis of schizophrenia. [PhD thesis.] London: University of London, 1998.

100. Rajaram S S. Experience of hypoglycaemia among insulin dependent diabetics and its impact on the family. *Sociol Health Illness* 1997; 19: 281–96.

101. Mitchell G. A qualitative study of older women's perceptions of control, health and ageing. *Health Educ J* 1996; 55: 267–74.

102. Wood K M, Boath E H, Mucklow J C, Blenkinsopp A. Changing medication: general practitioner and patient perspectives. *Int J Pharm Pract* 1997; 5: 176–84.

103. Hunter M S, O'Dea I, Britten N. Decision-making and hormone replacement therapy: a qualitative analysis. *Soc Sci Med* 1997; 45: 1541–8.

104. Glaser B, Strauss A. *The Discovery of Grounded Theory.* Chicago: Aldine, 1967.

105. Glaser B. *Theoretical Sensitivity.* Mill Valley, CA: Sociology Press, 1978.

106. Strauss A. *Qualitative Analysis for Social Scientists.* New York: Cambridge University Press, 1987.

107. Bryman A, Burgess R G, eds. *Analysing Qualitative Data.* London: Routledge, 1994.

108. Hak T. Coding effects in comparative research on definitions of health: a qualitative validation study. *Eur J Public Health* 1997; 7: 364–72.

109. Kuckartz U. *Winmax Pro 96. Software for Qualitative Data Analysis.* Berlin: Freie Universität, 1996; cited in: Matheson C. Privacy and stigma in the pharmacy: illicit drug users' perspectives and implications for pharmacy practice. *Pharm J* 1998; 260: 639–41.

110. Matheson C. Views of illicit drug users on their treatment and behaviour in Scottish community pharmacies: implications for the harm-reduction strategy. *Health Educ J* 1998; 57: 31–41.

111. Dey I. *Hypersoft.* Edinburgh: University of Edinburgh 1992; cited in Anderson C. Health promotion by community pharmacists: perceptions, realities and constraints. *J Soc Admin Pharm* 1998; 15: 10–22.

112. Qualis Research Associates. *The Ethnograph v4.0.* Amherst, MA: Qualis Research Associates, 1995.

113. QSR NUD*IST (*Non-numerical Unstructured Data Indexing, Searching and Theory Building*), version 4. London: Scolari Sage Publications, 1998.

114. Seale C, Silverman D. Ensuring rigour in qualitative research. *Eur J Public Health* 1997; 7: 379–84.

115. Gilbert L. The pharmacist's traditional and new roles – a study of community pharmacists in Johannesburg, South Africa. *J Soc Admin Pharm* 1995; 12: 125–31.

116. Cantrill J, Weiss M C, Kishida M, Nicolson M. Pharmacists' perceptions and

experiences of protocols: a step in the right direction? *Int J Pharm Pract* 1997; 5: 26–32.

117. Winit-Watjana W, Greene R. Perceptions of United Kingdom lecturers about teaching pharmaceutical care. *Int J Pharm Pract* 1997; 5: 133–40.

118. Anderson C, Alexander A. Wiltshire pharmacy health promotion training initiative: a telephone survey. *Int J Pharm Pract* 1997; 5: 185–91.

119. Dixon N H E, Hall J, Hassell K, Moorhouse G E. Domiciliary visiting: a review of compound analgesic use in the community. *J Soc Admin Pharm* 1995; 12: 144–53.

120. Wolfson P M, Paton C. Clozapine audit: what do patients and relatives think? *J Ment Health* 1996; 5: 267–73.

121. Miles M B, Huberman A M. *Qualitative Data Analysis: an Expanded Sourcebook*, 2nd edn. London: Sage, 1994.

122. Silverman D. *Interpreting Qualitative Data: Methods for Analysing Talk, Text and Interaction*. London: Sage, 1993.

123. Morrow N, Hargie O. Patient counselling: an investigation of core situations and difficulties in pharmacy practice. *Int J Pharm Pract* 1992; 1: 202–5.

5

Focus groups

Focus groups are a group interview technique for data collection. They are a well-established marketing research tool.[1] In recent years, their use by political parties and various policy making and research bodies in the UK has received wide publicity. Many senior politicians have been prepared to defend their value as a means of gaining insights into people's thoughts and concerns and used this to inform their campaigning and policy agendas. Within pharmacy, focus groups were employed by the Royal Pharmaceutical Society in the development of the Pharmacy in a New Age initiative to inform the professional strategy for pharmaceutical services into the twenty-first century.[2,3]

In health services research, focus groups are becoming increasingly prominent. A number of health services research and pharmacy practice journals have published papers addressing the processes and application of focus groups.[4–13] They are generally viewed as a qualitative research tool and, just as the value of qualitative research has been more widely acknowledged, there has been increasing interest in the application of focus groups in pharmacy practice and health services research. In common with qualitative studies, focus groups are employed to research topics from the perspective of the group participants, to explore their views and experiences, and identify their concerns and priorities which may explain behaviour patterns. For example, data collected in group interviews with health service users in the Gaza Strip, Palestine revealed a perceived inadequate supply of drugs resulting in the purchasing of drugs in private pharmacies.[14]

Group or individual interviews?

Focus groups provide an alternative means of data collection from individual face-to-face interviews. In the pharmacy practice literature there is a huge body of research in which the data were derived through individual interviews with respondents. Recognition of the advantages of focus groups for particular research problems is apparent from the increasing numbers of research papers in which they are employed.

The important distinguishing feature of focus groups is the inter-action among participants. Interaction can be seen as a normal activity in which people discuss issues and form opinions. Thus, the data collected in focus groups (in terms of issues raised and the views expressed) can be viewed as arising in the context of a natural interactive process. The gathering and interpreting of data in its natural context is an important feature that distinguishes qualitative (in particular ethnographic) research. Focus groups may also be employed for their effectiveness in exploring and identifying relevant questions in a research area. Commonly, focus groups are employed in exploratory studies, in which the interaction between individuals provides a stimulus for the generation and discussion of a wider range of ideas and issues than would arise in individual interviews. A study of consumer expectations of community pharmacy services employed group interviews to identify the possible range of responses to issues of interest.[15]

Although a group discussion may result in the identification of many issues, it may be less conducive to examining the thoughts and reasoning of individuals in detail. In an exploration of older women's perceptions of control, health and ageing, the researchers combined three group interviews with ten individual interviews; they found that more in-depth discussions were achievable in individual interviews than in the groups.[16] Also, in group discussions not all participants will comment on all issues.

Place in the research process

Focus groups have frequently been combined with other research methods and incorporated at different stages within a larger study. Many researchers have used focus groups to inform the developmental stages of a research project.[16-20] Capitalising on the strength of groups regarding the identification of a comprehensive range of issues, focus groups have been used to identify key issues of importance to consumers in relation to consumer readership and pharmacy health promotion literature and from this to formulate a research agenda.[18]

Focus groups have also been used to ensure content validity of structured instruments, that is, that all issues important to the population for which it is intended are included, and not just those apparent to the researchers. In the development of a structured measure of patient satisfaction with out-of-hours health care, focus groups were used to identify issues important to patients.[19] Focus groups have also been used to explore lay people's attitudes to the treatment of depression to clarify potential questions for a larger representative survey.[20]

Focus groups have also been used to obtain more detailed data following questionnaire studies. A focus group of 13 pharmacists was convened to inform and complement findings of a study of advice-giving for asthma.[21] Focus groups were used to gain additional information from Norwegian home-care providers regarding drug-related problems among elderly people living at home.[22,23] Group interviews have also been used as a means of obtaining additional data following a survey for which a low response rate had been achieved.[24] In this study, group interviews were employed to explore additional insights and possibly provide an indication of the extent and nature of non-response bias.

There are also examples in the research literature of pharmacy practice and health services in which focus groups were used as the sole method of data collection.[25–31]

Research objectives and settings

Focus groups have been used to investigate a wide range of research topics and in many different settings. There are examples from developing countries[17,32,33] as well as developed countries; among patient groups,[14,18,19,28,30,31,34,35] the public,[16–18,20,24,25,27,29,32] and professionals.[8,21–23,26,31,36–38] Experiences of virtual focus groups, conducted via the Internet, as a qualitative health services research tool have also been reported.[7]

Many studies have been conducted with a view to informing health or pharmacy policy. A number of researchers have addressed a range of health promotion themes.[16–18,25] It is generally acknowledged that, to be effective, health promotion initiatives must be relevant to people's lives, outlooks and priorities. A qualitative approach to explore people's views and beliefs regarding their health is viewed as important information for policy makers.

Focus groups are generally employed as a research tool for exploratory and descriptive studies; however, there are examples of their application to comparative study designs. For instance, they have been applied to compare the beliefs about diarrhoea of educated and less-educated mothers in a developing country[17] and the health beliefs of people from different social backgrounds in the UK.[16]

Focus groups have also been used to address specific practice problems, such as in a review of prescribing,[39] to ascertain why the recommendations of pharmacists made to general practitioners in a collaborative project were not acted upon. In the assessment of a medication appropriateness index, focus groups with patients provided some insights indicating why their perspectives may differ from those of clinicians.[30] They were also used to study the views of patients and health professionals on self-management plans for people with asthma.[31]

Focus groups have been used in the development of consensus guidelines in health care, for example to develop principles of practice and levels of minimal acceptable care.[36] Expert panels have been convened to judge the importance of discrepancies in prescribed medication following hospital discharge,[40] in the assessment of the quality of advice by community pharmacists[41] and to set standards of prescribing performance.[37]

Consensus methods: nominal group and Delphi techniques

Nominal group technique and Delphi methods are structured group consultation techniques. The application of these techniques to pharmacy practice and health services research has been reviewed.[42–45] The typical stages are outlined below.

Nominal group method is a structured group meeting, the aim of which is to generate a comprehensive list of relevant issues on a given topic and, through structured discussion and ranking, to reach a consensus that reflects the views of the participants. The actual procedures employed vary as researchers adapt the technique to their study needs. However, a nominal group meeting typically begins with each participant independently (in silence) writing their own list of issues that they believe are pertinent to the research question. These thoughts are then contributed one-by-one to form a comprehensive list of the thoughts of all group members. A discussion follows in which items on the list are clarified and restructured, if necessary, care being taken to ensure a comprehensive list is maintained. Participants are then asked individually to rank the issues using a scoring system. The group facilitator then sums the ranks from all group members for each item. These results are then presented to the group for discussion. During this discussion, participants have the opportunity to share their views regarding the appropriate ranking of the different issues and to hear the reasoning of others. Following this, the ranking procedure may be repeated, resulting in a final list of issues (probably revised) reflecting the views of the group as a whole.

Delphi technique similarly aims to achieve a consensus. Consultation with study participants is by questionnaire, rather than face-to-face discussion. Delphi consultation is frequently conducted in two rounds. In the first round, respondents' views on a topic will be gathered using a structured instrument. The responses to this will be analysed and the questionnaire re-circulated. In the second round, participants also receive some feedback on the results of the first round, commonly descriptive data (e.g. mean or median scores) related to the responses of all respondents. Participants are then invited to reconsider their responses in the light of responses from the group as a whole.

These techniques were combined in a study to develop valid and reliable indicators of appropriate long-term prescribing.[38] Nominal group technique was used to identify potential indicators of appropriateness of prescribing, which were then assessed in a two-round Delphi process. The nominal group meeting involved nine 'opinion leaders' and prominent academics, the Delphi process, general practitioners and community pharmacists. In the Delphi process, only respondents to the early rounds will be involved in subsequent rounds, thus attrition of the sample can be an issue. In this study of indicators of long-term prescribing, 85% of general practitioners who agreed to take part completed the first round, and 62% completed both rounds. For community pharmacists, 82% completed round one, and 57% rounds one and two.[38] The Delphi technique was also used to identify commonly used prescribing indicators which possessed both face validity and reliability as indicators of quality and cost.[46]

Selecting groups and sampling procedures

The selection of groups and sampling procedures depend on the objectives of the study. The sampling procedures will have implications for the representativeness of the sample and hence the validity of generalising the findings to a wider population.

As many of the studies were small exploratory studies, with the results being used to inform subsequent research programmes or instruments, it is evident that researchers did not necessarily intend wider generalisation of results. However, to ensure the content validity of a research instrument by preliminary consultation in focus groups, it is important to ensure that groups represent, as fully as possible, the differing perspectives of the population.

Some studies, particularly larger ones, have employed random sampling procedures to recruit study groups or participants. A study investigating community perceptions of primary care services in Guinea conducted focus groups in villages selected at random from lists of administrative districts.[32] For population-based samples, researchers in the UK have used electoral registers, which include all people within an administrative district who have registered to vote in elections, all adults over 18 years being eligible to register,[18] or general medical practice registers, in which the vast majority of the British population in an area will be included.[19]

As with other qualitative methods (see Chapter 4), simple random sampling is not always appropriate, because of the small numbers involved, or practical, for example due to non-availability of a sampling frame or the high costs of convening a randomly selected group. Despite this, many researchers have devised sampling strategies aimed at the inclusion of groups and/or participants that are broadly representative of, or reflective of diversity within, a population. A study of attitudes towards ageing and exercise and implications for health promotion adopted a quota sampling procedure to recruit people in different age bands and socio-economic groups into 15 focus groups.[24]

In a study of lay people's attitudes to treatment of depression, eight groups were convened that were 'balanced for age, sex and social class'.[20] For a study of public perceptions of community pharmacy, participants were selected through five different pharmacies in different demographic locations.[27] Selection through different pharmacies may result in the recruitment of individuals from a range of backgrounds, but will be restricted to members of the public who use pharmacies.

Purposive samples have been employed by some researchers. Studies with a theoretical basis or examining hypotheses require the involvement of participants with particular characteristics. A study of older women's perceptions of control and influences had its basis in the theory of health locus of control, the association of which with social class is well established. A purposive sampling procedure, involving the recruitment of participants via a day-centre in an affluent area and a lunch club in a deprived area of Edinburgh, was adopted.[16] While this would allow an exploration of health locus of control theory and social class, the author points out that the sampling procedure may be biased towards more sociable individuals.

Purposive sampling was employed in a study of diabetes and health beliefs in which individuals with particular experiences or characteristics were selected from medical records.[34] A study of nurses' participation in audit purposively selected nurses responsible for managing and supporting audit at an organisational level in 17 health authorities.[26]

A sample of 'high users' of pharmacy services was identified through pharmacists in the West Midlands (UK); researchers in this study also convened a number of population-based groups drawn from electoral registers covering the same areas.[18]

Diversity in or between groups?

Homogeneous groups are generally viewed as more productive in terms of the participation of all group members and the depth of discussion achieved.[1] Consequently, many researchers attempt to convene groups of people who share background characteristics or common experiences, while attempting to achieve diversity between the groups. Thus, studies have involved separate groups for 'high users' of pharmacy services and the general population,[15] for the affluent and less affluent elderly in Edinburgh,[16] separate groups for elderly people, carers, mothers of young children and employed people to follow-up issues in a survey of the public's views of pharmacists' extended roles,[24] educated and un-educated people in a study of beliefs about diarrhoea,[17] people in differ-ent age bands and socio-economic groups in an exploration of health and ageing.[25]

Participants recruited by 'word of mouth' (e.g. a study to explore lay beliefs about diarrhoea) are likely to result in homogeneous groups.[17] The issues raised and views expressed in groups in which participants are from similar backgrounds would be expected to present limitations in terms of generalisability, but may provide the researcher with an opportunity to gain in-depth insights into the perspectives of a defined group and their concerns.

Established groups or groups convened for the purposes of the study?

Some researchers conducted interviews with pre-existing voluntary com-munity groups.[16,24,28] Members of voluntary groups will have some common interests that bring them together. In everyday life people associate with others with whom they share some characteristics regard-ing their background, experiences and attitudes. (This is, of course, also a feature of many groups that are convened only for the purposes of a study.) In qualitative studies, particularly in ethnographic work, estab-lished groups represent existing social contexts in which thoughts are expressed and discussed, and beliefs and ideas are formed. Some quali-tative researchers have recognised the value of these 'natural clusterings which have their own role and relevance'[6] for the research process. Working with these groups provides an opportunity for the exploration of issues in a natural social context rather than an 'artificial' research environment. Thus research conducted this way is 'ethnographic' in that the data are derived in the context of normal social intercourse.

Practical and logistical issues may also enter into decisions of whether to select pre-existing groups or to set them up for the purposes of the study. Research with established groups has been conducted as part of a regular meeting and/or at their usual venue,[28] which may reduce both administrative burden and costs. It may, of course, also present limitations, regarding the control of the researcher in ensuring that conditions such as the venue and room layout are suitable, and in influencing the selection and number of participants.

In convening groups for the purpose of the study, the researcher can ensure a suitable environment and appropriate participant selection (subject to response rates). Many researchers selected individuals and convened groups for the purposes of their studies.[17–20,25–27,34,37,40] These researchers may prefer to retain control over who participates to ensure that the groups are representative, include people with particular attributes, or individuals not known to each other. Financial incentives were sometimes offered.[27]

The effect of group dynamics on the contributions of individuals to a discussion is often raised. In focus group studies, the interaction between group members is fundamental to the research (data collection and analysis), the method presumably being selected because the researchers believe that this interaction would be the most effective way of achieving their research objectives. Group dynamics will operate, whether or not the group members are known to each other.

How many groups?

The number of groups in the studies in this review ranged from one to 21. When a group was convened to perform the function of an 'expert panel,' a single group was usually formed, with careful consideration paid to the group members. In general, fewer groups were involved when the objective of the study was to explore and identify issues leading to the development of a research agenda or questionnaire.

The number of groups may be determined by a desire to ensure all relevant issues will be identified. Five groups were conducted with elderly people to gather their perspectives regarding a medication appropriateness index. After five sessions the authors reported that no new issues emerged.[39] Once no new issues emerge, researchers may believe that they have achieved a comprehensive set of issues regarding the topic of interest.

The minimum number of groups may be determined by the need to include representatives of different population groups. For example, a comparative study of beliefs about diarrhoea involved one group of educated mothers and one of less-educated mothers.[17] A study to follow-up issues in a questionnaire on pharmacists' extended roles involved at least one group for each of four population groups among whom the original questionnaire had been administered.[24] Five groups, corresponding to clients of five pharmacies in different locations, were conducted to investigate public perceptions of pharmacists.[27] In a study comparing the perspectives of people with arthritis, respiratory disease and mental health problems regarding medication, 12 group interviews were conducted, four with each of these chronic illness groups.[28]

Many studies involved larger numbers of groups. Eight groups were conducted to explore lay people's attitudes to the treatment of depression.[20] A study to investigate the impact of focus group discussion on participants' views of priority setting in health care involved a random sample of 60 patients in 10 groups, each of 5–7 people.[35] Fifteen groups were conducted to explore perceptions of ageing and exercise[25] and 21 (totalling 180 participants) to investigate lay people's views of quality in primary care services.[32]

Group size

The most important criterion regarding the numbers of participants should be the effective functioning of the group. All members should have an opportunity to contribute to the discussion. It may also be frustrating for group members if the size of the group unduly restricts their participation. A large group in which many issues are raised may also obstruct in-depth discussion of important issues. In discussing developments in focus group methodology, Krueger[1] discusses how the group size viewed to be optimal has decreased in number. Smaller groups of 5–7 participants are now often preferred (over previous norms of 10–12), as they provide more opportunity for individuals to talk and are easier to set up. The majority of authors of papers in this review reported group sizes of 6–9 participants, the range being from 1 to 11. However, as with the number of groups involved in a study, information on group sizes was not always provided.

The relationship between group size and participation of individuals in discussion was investigated in a study of views of community groups on deregulation of medicines. The study found that the relative contributions of the most active participants were similar, irrespective of group size. Increasing the number of group members was associated with larger numbers of less-active participants.[29] Researchers convening their own groups may have more control over the group size than researchers conducting group interviews with pre-existing groups for which they may have limited control over the numbers who attend.

Conduct of the groups

As is common in qualitative research, many researchers reported the use of an interview or topic guide, to facilitate or stimulate open discussion on pre-identified themes.[20,24,26,32] In any qualitative study, the issues discussed should be those important to the study participants. Thus, researchers exploring people's understanding of ageing and exercise, and relating this to health promotion, emphasised the flexibility of the discussion sequence.[25] A study into the public's perception of pharmacy was guided by a 'trait approach' in which the discussion addressed each of the six professional criteria which comprise this theory in turn.[27]

The importance of encouraging participation by all group members was also raised. Bale's interaction process analysis was applied to transcripts of groups' discussions on the deregulation of medicines. In this analysis, it was found that over 75% of contributions were classified as 'positive' (e.g. agreement, supportive illustrative comments); questions were common at the start of discussions and contributions classified as negative were few.[29] In an attempt to enable wide and varied participation in a study among voluntary groups of people taking long-term medication, authors reported some questions that they used to gain clarification of issues, obtain explanations, establish the extent to which viewpoints were, or were not, shared by other members of the group, and to encourage participants to raise any related issues that they felt were relevant to the discussion. Researchers reported use of prompts such as:

- Would you say more about . . . ?
- Why do you think . . . ?
- What do you think are the reasons for . . . ?
- Has anyone else had a similar experience . . . ?
- Does anyone have a different view . . . ?
- What other issues are important regarding . . . ?

They also reported the questions used to elicit people's views on their desire to be involved in decision-making regarding their medicines.[28]

The facilitator (or moderator) will steer the discussion according to the interview guide, endeavouring to encourage participation by all group members. In most cases, the authors reported that group discussions were audiotaped. For qualitative data analysis, comprehensive verbatim data is generally seen as a prerequisite. A co-facilitator is usually responsible for ensuring successful recording of data and to attend to any logistical problems. Although data gathered in focus groups (as for data gathered by other methods) is anonymised such that individuals are not identifiable in the results, in the analysis of data researchers need to be able to attribute contributions to individual group members. Only by knowing which statements are made by the same or different individuals can researchers, when analysing the data, take into account the characteristics of group interaction or establish how many participants expressed views on particular issues. Thus, the co-facilitator has an important task of note-taking throughout the meeting. The duration of the discussions, for those that were reported, ranged from 40 minutes to 1¼ hours. A study of public perceptions of pharmacy as a profession also reported that meetings were held at a 'neutral location'.[27]

Data analysis

Analysis of focus group data has the extra complication over individual interviews of the added dimension of interaction between participants. This will influence the direction of the discussion in terms of the issues raised and the contributions of group members.

The importance of explicit consideration of group interaction in the research process has been highlighted by Kitzinger[6] who notes that, in reports of research using focus groups, little attempt is made to concentrate on the conversation among participants. Despite awareness by researchers of group interaction as an important element of the research process, and often the reason for the selection of focus group methodology, it is surprising that it has received so little attention in the analysis of data.

In some studies, researchers combined data from focus groups and individual interviews prior to the analysis,[34] thus precluding any possibility of examining the data sets independently and considering the impact of the group or individual contexts in which the data were derived. Thus, the opportunity to consider the role of group interaction in the formation of ideas is lost.

Group dynamics have been addressed by many researchers in different contexts. In relation to group discussions, researchers have identified the process of group polarisation, which has been defined as a 'group produced enhancement of members' pre-existing tendencies'.[47] For example, a group who tend towards a cautious viewpoint would, following group discussion, be expected to display more cautious opinions; whilst in groups whose members were more inclined to accept risks, this tendency would be expected to be enhanced. Various explanations have been suggested. For example, in a group discussion, the opinions and information shared would be expected to favour the dominant viewpoints and people are most likely to be influenced by the opinions of people with whom they identify.[29,47]

An analysis of discussions of community groups on deregulation of medicines explored how interaction between members of the group may influence the data obtained, arguing that these factors should be borne in mind when analysing data. The researcher illustrated how participants' contributions were made in the context of the group process. In the transcripts, the group norms (majority views) were easy to identify which, it was suggested, could be at the expense of alternative viewpoints.[29]

The effect of discussion and deliberation in a focus group on the public's views of priority setting in health care was investigated in a before-and-after study. A random sample of 60 patients from two urban practices were invited to take part in focus group discussions on two occasions. Participants' views were assessed by questionnaire at the start of the first meeting and at the end of the second. The authors concluded that the views of participants were notably different when they had been given the opportunity to discuss the issues.[35]

Data from the different focus groups may be analysed separately, compared and/or combined into one large data set. Texts of group discussions relating to a study into the public's perception of pharmacy as a profession were analysed by theme comparison, looking for commonalities running through the groups and within each group. Quotes were used to illustrate the results under the six headings suggested by the trait approach.[27] Analysis of data from 12 focus groups (four of which were conducted with each of three illness groups) was conducted in three stages initially at the level of individual groups, then with data from all groups with each condition and, finally, comparison of the findings of the three illness groups.[28]

To identify the contributions of individuals in relation to control, health and ageing, in the analysis researchers indicated against each comment whether they were made by a frail or active person and their age.[16] Researchers investigating perceptions of ageing and exercise reported undertaking a content analysis of the data from the 15 groups, the results then being illustrated with quotations from the transcripts.[25] Data from focus groups were sometimes used to illustrate findings from other parts of a research project rather than being analysed in their own right.[22,23]

There were examples of the use of computer-packages for the analysis of qualitative data. Ethnograph[48] was used to assist in data handling of a study of nurses' participation in audit. A coding frame was developed based on the issues emerging from the data. The analysis involved identifying the differences and similarities in the issues that emerged from each group.[26] The computer software package NUD*IST (Non-numerical Unstructured Data Indexing, Searching and Theory building)[49] was used for the analysis of data relating to people's experiences of diabetes.[34] Prior to analysis, data from focus groups were combined with data from individual interviews to form a single data set to explore health beliefs and diabetes. The data were coded into 11 broad categories. Using the cross-referencing facilities of the software the objective of the analysis was to identify constructs (inferences in the data) and to consider and modify these in the light of all the statements made relevant to each of the constructs. NUD*IST was also used in a study among health service users and providers about pharmacy services.[14]

Validity, reliability and generalisability

The validity of research findings refers to the extent to which they are an accurate representation of the phenomena they purport to represent. As with any qualitative method, researchers should ensure that issues important to the participants are raised, and that participants feel able to express their views and influence the direction of the discussion regarding the topic of research. If this is successfully achieved, the data should be an accurate (i.e. valid) reflection of the perspectives of the group. An assessment of the validity of findings of a study that included the development of theoretical constructs relating culture, health beliefs and diabetes was performed by presenting these findings to a smaller group of respondents. This involved a further focus group in which the findings were discussed and the group's responses recorded.[34]

The reliability of a study refers to the reproducibility of the findings. In qualitative research involving focus groups, the content of the group discussions should reflect the varying experiences and outlook of the groups. The researcher should aim to identify and place in context the differences and similarities between the data generated by each group. Thus, in the data collection, reproducibility is not a pertinent concern. Consistency between raters in evaluating the content of focus group transcripts, however, is an issue that should be addressed. Researchers investigating nurses' participation of audit reported that during the analysis they regularly conferred.[26] Independent coding by two or more researchers may also be undertaken.[28] Inconsistency between raters has been highlighted by researchers who demonstrated a lack of agreement between raters in the interpretation and coding of transcripts in what they had believed to be a controlled and structured framework.[5]

The findings of many studies were not intended to be generalised to a wider population. Many were designed as preliminary explorations to identify important issues, preceding a larger quantitative assessment from which generalisations would be made. Generalisability will be determined by the sampling strategies – both sample size and the extent to which the sample is representative of the population.

Ethical issues

Ethical issues were rarely raised in the published papers. Audiorecording the entire group discussion for later transcription is the usual, and generally regarded as an essential procedure in focus group research. The group facilitator will request permission for this, which is usually granted. Authors, in their papers, did not enter into discussions regarding the requesting of permission. Researchers will require consent from all participants. However, difficulties could arise: a sole objector within a group may feel inhibited from speaking out.

There may also be issues which, within a group context, individuals prefer not to discuss. However, if important and relevant issues are not raised, this will affect the comprehensiveness of the data obtained, which could in turn have an impact on the validity of the findings.

To facilitate maximum freedom of expression, researchers investigating the views on guided self-management plans for people with asthma conducted separate focus group discussions with general practitioners, nurses and patients.[31] Researchers examining medical practitioners' attitudes to social and sexual contact between medical practitioners and their patients employed an anonymised telephone-based focus group methodology. The rationale for this was that the traditional focus group does not allow anonymity of the participants and in some situations or topic areas face-to-face group interviews may not be an acceptable procedure, even though data gained by group interaction may be valuable.[8]

All participants have some thoughts regarding the issues that they are prepared to raise and discuss with the group. In a group discussion (in particular in a group in which the participants are known to each other), the research process could lead to the disclosure of information before the group, which other group members view as confidential. Ethical issues from the perspective of the group participants possibly merit more attention in published research than they generally receive.

References

1. Krueger R A. *Focus Groups: a Practical Guide to Applied Research*. London: Sage Publications, 1994.
2. Royal Pharmaceutical Society of Great Britain. Pharmacy in a New Age: council improves information management strategy for pharmacy. *Pharm J* 1997; 258: 436–43.
3. Royal Pharmaceutical Society of Great Britain. *Pharmacy in a New Age: Building the Future: A Strategy for a 21st Century Pharmaceutical Service*. London: Royal Pharmaceutical Society of Great Britain, 1997.
4. Barbour R S. Using focus groups. *Fam Pract* 1995; 12: 328–34.
5. Weinberger M, Ferguson J A, Westmoreland G, *et al*. Can raters consistently evaluate the content of focus groups? *Soc Sci Med* 1998; 46: 929–33.
6. Kitzinger J. The methodology of focus groups: the importance of interaction between research participants. *Sociol Health Illness* 1994; 16: 103–21.
7. Murray P J. Using virtual focus groups in qualitative research. *Qual Health Res* 1997; 7: 542–9.
8. White G E, Thomson A N. Anonymised focus groups as a research tool for health professionals. *Qual Health Res* 1995; 5: 256–61.
9. Tang K C, Davis A. Critical factors in determination of focus group size. *Fam Pract* 1995; 12: 474–5.
10. Kitzinger J. Introducing focus groups. *BMJ* 1995; 311: 299–302.
11. Hassell K, Hibbert D. The use of focus groups in pharmacy research: processes and practicalities. *J Soc Admin Pharm* 1996; 13: 169–77.
12. Khan M E, Manderson L. Focus groups in tropical disease research. *Health Policy Plann* 1992; 7: 56–66.
13. Smith F J. Collecting data: focus groups. In: Harding G, Taylor K, ed. *Pharmacy Practice*. Amsterdam: Harwood Academic Publishers, 2001: ch 27; 573–83.
14. Beckerleg S, Lewando-Hundt G, Eddama M, *et al*. Purchasing a quickfix from private pharmacies in the Gaza Strip. *Soc Sci Med* 1999; 49: 1489–500.
15. Jepson M, Jesson J, Pocock R, Kendall H. *Consumer Expectations of Community Pharmaceutical Services. A Report for the Department of Health*. Birmingham: Aston University/MEL Research, 1991.

16. Mitchell G. A qualitative study of older women's perceptions of control, health and ageing. *Health Educ J* 1996; 55: 267–74.

17. Pitts M, McMaster J, Hartmann T, Mausehahl D. Lay beliefs about diarrhoeal diseases: their role in health education in a developing country. *Soc Sci Med* 1996; 43: 1223–8.

18. Jesson J, Pocock R, Jepson M, Kendall H. Consumer readership and views on pharmacy health education literature: a market research survey. *J Soc Admin Pharm* 1994; 11: 29–36.

19. McKinley R K, Manku-Scott T, Hastings A M, *et al.* Reliability and validity of a new measure of patient satisfaction with out-of-hours medical care in the UK: development of a patient questionnaire. *BMJ* 1997; 314: 193–8.

20. Priest R G, Vize C, Roberts A, *et al.* Lay people's attitudes to treatment of depression: the results of opinion poll for Defeat Depression Campaign just before its launch. *BMJ* 1996; 313: 858–9.

21. Osman L M, Bond C M, Mackenzie J, Williams S. Asthma advice-giving by community pharmacists. *Int J Pharm Pract* 1999; 7: 12–17.

22. Stromme H K, Botten G. Support and service for the drug treatment of older people living at home: a study of a sample of Norwegian home care providers. *J Soc Admin Pharm* 1993; 10: 130–7.

23. Stromme H K, Botten G. Drug related problems among old people living at home, as perceived by a sample of Norwegian home care providers. *J Soc Admin Pharm* 1993; 10: 63–9.

24. Williamson V K, Winn S, Livingstone C R, Pugh A L G. Public views on an extended role for community pharmacy. *Int J Pharm Pract* 1992; 1: 223–9.

25. Stead M, Wimbush E, Eadie D, Teer P. A qualitative study of older people's perceptions of ageing and exercise: the implications for health promotion. *Health Educ J* 1997; 56: 3–16.

26. Cheater F M, Keane M. Nurses' participation in audit: a regional study. *Qual Health Care* 1998; 7: 27–36.

27. Varnish J. Drug pushers or health care professionals: the public's perception of pharmacy as a profession. *Int J Pharm Pract* 1998; 6: 13–21.

28. Smith F J, Francis S-A, Rowley E. Group interviews with people taking long-term medication: comparing the perspectives of people with arthritis, respiratory disease and mental health problems. *Int J Pharm Pract* 2000; 8: 88–96.

29. Smith F J, Analysis of data from focus groups: group interaction – the added dimension. *Int J Pharm Pract* 1999; 7: 192–6.

30. Volume C I, Burback L M, Farris K B. Reassessing the MAI: elderly people's opinions about medication appropriateness. *Int J Pharm Pract* 1999; 7: 129–37.

31. Jones A, Pill R, Adams S. Qualitative study of views of health professionals and patients on guided self-management plans for asthma. *BMJ* 2000; 321: 1507–10.

32. Haddad S, Fournier P, Machouf N, Yatara F. What does quality mean to lay people? Community perceptions of primary health care services in Guinea. *Soc Sci Med* 1998; 46: 381–94.

33. Konde-lule J K, Musagara M, Musgrave S. Focus group interviews about AIDS in the Rakai district, Uganda. *Soc Sci Med* 1993; 37: 679–84.

34. Greenhalgh T, Helman C, Mu'min Chowdhury A. Health beliefs and folk

models of diabetes in British Bangladeshis: a qualitative study. *BMJ* 1998; 316: 978–83.

35. Dolan P, Cookson R, Ferguson B. Effect of discussion and deliberation on the public's views of priority setting in health care: focus groups study. *BMJ* 1999; 318: 916–19.

36. Fardy H J, Jeffs D. Focus groups: a method for developing consensus guidelines in general practice. *Fam Pract* 1994; 11: 325–9.

37. Bateman D N, Eccles M, Soutter J, *et al.* Setting standards of prescribing performance in primary care: the use of a consensus group of general practitioners and the application of standards to practices in the north of England. *Br J Gen Pract* 1996; 46: 20–5.

38. Cantrill J A, Sibbald B, Buetow S. Indicators of the appropriateness of long-term prescribing in general practice in the United Kingdom: consensus development, face and content validity, feasibility and reliability. *Qual Health Care* 1998; 7: 130–5.

39. Goldstein R, Hulme H, Willits J. Reviewing repeat prescribing: general practitioners and community pharmacists working together. *Int J Pharm Pract* 1998; 6: 60–6.

40. Duggan C, Feldman R, Hough J, Bates I. Reducing adverse prescribing discrepancies following hospital discharge. *Int J Pharm Pract* 1998; 6: 77–82.

41. Smith F J, Salkind M R, Jolly B C. Community pharmacy: a method of assessing quality of care. *Soc Sci Med* 1990; 31: 603–7.

42. Cantrill J A, Sibbald B, Buetow S. The Delphi and nominal group technique in health services research. *Int J Pharm Pract* 1996; 4: 67–74.

43. Gallagher M, Hares T, Spencer J, *et al.* The nominal group technique: a research tool for general practice? *Fam Pract* 1994; 11: 325–9.

44. Van de Ven A, Delbecq A L. The nominal group as a research instrument for exploratory health studies. *Am J Public Health* 1972; 62: 337–42.

45. Hunter D, Jones J. Consensus methods for medical and health services research. *BMJ* 1995; 311: 376–80.

46. Campbell S M, Cantrill J A, Roberts D. Prescribing indicators for UK general practice: Delphi consultation study. *BMJ* 2000; 321: 425–8.

47. Myers D G. *Social Psychology*, 4th edn. London: McGraw-Hill, 1993.

48. Qualis Research Associates. *The Ethnograph v4.0*. Amherst MA: Qualis Research Associates, 1995.

49. QSR NUD*IST (*Non-numerical Unstructured Data Indexing, Searching and Theory Building)*, version 4. London: Scolari Sage Publications, 1998.

6

Non-participant and participant observation

Observation provides researchers with the opportunity to document behaviours, activities and events rather than relying on self-reports by individuals, which may, or may not, be accurate representations of those actions or incidents. Observation has been used both as a sole method for a research study and in combination with other methods. In the pharmacy practice literature there are examples of participant and non-participant observation studies, and both quantitative and qualitative approaches.

The observation studies reviewed here include those in which the researcher is present at the study site and for the duration of a study period observes and records details of specific behaviours, activities and/or events. Confusion can arise between health services and epidemiological research in the use of the term 'observation study'. Epidemiologists (or clinical researchers) may use the term to refer to a cohort study in which people are followed-up over a period of time, their progress being 'observed' or monitored and perhaps compared with a control group.

There are examples of both quantitative and qualitative observation studies in pharmacy settings. In a quantitative observational study, the researcher observes and records activities and/or interactions to provide numeric frequencies of these different activities, often possibly with the intention of investigating relationships between them and/or generalising these findings to a wider population.

The objective of the qualitative observation studies is to provide insights into the behaviours of a group of people against the background of constraints, difficulties or facilitative aspects of their environment. The value of this work is that it should be insightful, providing information that is sufficiently detailed to enable problems to be identified. Even though these studies are commonly small scale, they often have some relevance to other populations and settings that share key characteristics. Their application in health care settings have been addressed by researchers.[1–3]

Participant or non-participant observation

Observation studies can be distinguished as participant or non-participant observation. The majority of observation studies that have been undertaken in pharmacy settings are non-participant observation studies; however, there are examples of each.

Non-participant observation studies are those in which the researcher records activities and behaviours of those under study in the capacity of an outside observer. The majority of these studies are quantitative studies gathering descriptive data. The researcher selects study sites and standardises the data collection to enable some quantitative and generalisable statements to be made regarding the activities being observed. There are also examples of qualitative studies involving data collection by non-participant observation.[4,5] In these cases the data gathered are specific to context or situation.

Participant observation is the principal approach of anthropologists who live and participate as members of the communities that they are researching for the duration of the data collection. Participant observation is generally a qualitative technique in that the observations are made and interpreted in the context of the environments and situations in which they occur. By detailed study of a single community, the researcher endeavours to provide insights into the behaviours, actions and interactions of the people under study. The methodology is not designed to produce findings that are generalisable to a wider population, but to explore and attempt to explain behaviours in the context of the studied people's lives, traditions and situations. However, many of the findings of these studies may be transferable to other communities or populations. As such they may provide useful starting points or hypotheses for researchers in other settings.

Whereas in participant observation studies the researcher acts and interacts as a member of the group under study, the non-participant observer endeavours to be as discreet as possible in order not to influence the behaviours of the people they are observing, and thus bias the study findings.

Non-participant observation

Research objectives and settings

There are many examples of studies in which non-participant observation was combined with other methods of data collection.[4-17] In some cases, this was to provide additional data from a different perspective to serve the same or related objectives. For instance, researchers investigating the views of illicit drug users on their treatment also observed the behaviour of users, pharmacy staff and other clients in the pharmacy, in addition to interviewing users on their perceptions and experiences of services.[13] In a study of health promotion activities of community pharmacies, in addition to semi-structured interviews with pharmacists, observations were made in each pharmacy of the presence of leaflet displays, space available and the size of the premises.[14] Non-participant observation formed just one part of a study of pharmacy in private hospitals in Nigeria.[11] Observation has also been used as the sole method of data collection to serve a set of study objectives.[18–34]

Since non-participant observation enables the researcher to gather information on activities and events as they occur, rather than relying on what is reported to happen in self-completion questionnaires or diaries, observation has been used as a method of validating self-reports by checking the extent to which they are a true reflection of actual events.[35] Covert observation methods (e.g. 'disguised shoppers' in which a researcher poses as a client to gather data on pharmacists' responses in a predetermined scenario) were employed to validate responses in a questionnaire designed to investigate the relationship between pharmacists' moral reasoning and components of clinical performance and in which researchers believed that subjects may have been disposed to provide socially desirable responses.[15]

The vast majority of observation studies are descriptive: identifying, counting and characterising events and activities, and investigating associations between variables. Observation techniques have also been used in experimental or hypothesis testing studies[7,33] to assess aspects of outcomes of pharmacy services[36,37] or to evaluate an intervention.[23,38] In a study to assess the effect of a shop-front pharmacist on non-prescription medicine consultations, an observer collected baseline data on these consultations prior to, and following, the placement of a pharmacist in the front of the shop. The study documented an increased proportion of consultations with non-prescription medicine purchases between the study periods.[23]

A large number of observation studies have focused on the professional activities and behaviours of community pharmacists and their staff. Among these studies there are examples from many different countries, indicating the extent to which these issues are of relevance and concern internationally.[5,9,10,20,24,27,38–41] Non-participant observation studies have also been undertaken to document pharmacy activities and aspects of drug use in hospitals.[4,11,29,32,42]

In a number of studies, data have been collected on audiotape. These studies included quantitative and qualitative research investigating aspects of interaction between pharmacy staff and their clients.[7,21,28,30,36,37] This method enables comprehensive data to be collected regarding oral interaction, which can rarely be achieved by manual note-taking. Obviously, non-verbal background information will not be available for inclusion in the analysis unless separately documented.

Observation studies have included time-and-motion and work sampling techniques.[26,31,43-47] The data obtained by these two approaches have been compared[48] and their application in community pharmacy reviewed.[49] Data on the work activities at an ambulatory care pharmacy were collected by the pharmacy staff themselves who were requested to record their activities at random intervals throughout the day. The methods and issues of validity and reliability of these data reflect those for a self-completion survey, rather than observation by a researcher.[43]

Consultations of medical practitioners have been observed to obtain quantitative data on prescribing patterns[18,39] and to investigate factors that influence prescribing of particular drugs.[7]

Sampling procedures

Observation studies are generally labour-intensive in that they require travel to, and the presence of the observer at, the study sites for the duration of the data collection. Sample size and choice of sites will be an important consideration for populations geographically widespread. The resources available to the study may limit the number of settings in which a study can be undertaken. To gather details on the siting and display of confectionery, a researcher visited 35 pharmacies. These descriptive data enabled an assessment of the extent to which advice of the professional body was followed.[34] Provided pharmacies are easily accessible, data collection for such studies may be completed in a relatively short time. The data may be more reliable and valid than in self-reports. Also, researchers should not experience problems of non-response.

When suitable sampling frames are available, adopting a random sampling procedure enables the researcher to generalise the findings to the population from which the sample was drawn, and provide an indication of the likely accuracy of the estimates when applied more widely. Simple, or stratified, random sampling of pharmacies has been conducted by researchers carrying out descriptive observation studies into aspects of community pharmacy services and medicine supplies in many countries,[9,20,26,35,40,41] indicating the general availability of sampling frames. The sizes of samples for these studies ranged from four to 64. The duration of the observation periods ranged from periods of two hours up to a full day, and in some cases there were multiple visits on up to four occasions.

Random sampling procedures were employed by researchers investigating prescribing patterns of general practitioners and paediatricians in an investigation of their management of children with diarrhoea, although the authors reported difficulty in identifying a suitable sampling frame.[18]

In qualitative work, samples are necessarily small to enable detailed investigation. When the sample size is very small, simple random sampling would not be expected to produce a representative sample. However, by stratifying pharmacies according to particular characteristics, researchers can ensure that the sample reflects diversity among potential respondents with respect to particular features. A study of advice in British pharmacies which involved observation in ten pharmacies, employed a sampling procedure, selecting sites from those who agreed to take part, to include different types of pharmacy.[5] To investigate potential conflicts of demand on pharmacists for prescription and non-prescription advice, pharmacists were asked to select two typical half-days when the pharmacy was usually busy. Thus, the study periods were purposively selected to enable exploration of the issue of interest.

A convenience sample was used to investigate factors influencing prescribing. As the authors point out, this self-selecting sample enabled analysis of relationships between variables, but whether the findings would have wider applicability is unclear.[7] In an observational study to evaluate the impact of an education workshop, a number of volunteer pharmacists were recruited.[38] Although employing a self-selecting sample, the study would provide an indication of the value of the workshop among a group of interested individuals and may provide useful data on which to base further educational initiatives.

Experimental study designs require randomisation of participants to intervention and control groups. In health services research, randomisation is often not practicable owing to logistical or ethical considerations. There were few examples of observation studies in which study sites or individuals being observed were randomised. One example in health services research is a study that compared aspects of the quality of life of people in small nursing homes and geriatric hospital wards.

Eligible persons who agreed to take part in the study were randomly allocated to either setting.[33]

Response rates

Response rates in non-participant observation studies refer to the proportion of the sample who agree to allow a researcher to undertake the observation. An attraction of an observation study (for both the researcher and those being observed) is that once the subjects have agreed the researcher takes responsibility for the data collection. From the point of view of the researcher, they then have control over ensuring the completeness and quality of the data. From the perspective of the subject, only limited involvement is required; and, of course, the validity of the data will be enhanced if the subjects are able to continue operating as though the research were not taking place.

In the observation studies reviewed here, researchers reported no difficulties in recruiting their samples. When responsibility for data collection lies with the researcher and procedures are generally designed to cause minimum interference with normal activities of those being observed, potential participants may be more prepared to take part than if the study were to require their time and commitment. Response rates of over 80% were reported by a number of authors.[9,20,40] In a study in which pharmacists were requested to undertake some self-data collection themselves (in addition to observation by an independent researcher), a lower response rate (39%) was achieved.[50] Response rates reported in non-participant observation studies were often greater than those obtained for self-completion questionnaires among similar populations.

People may be less inclined to participate if a sensitive issue is being investigated or if it is thought that the presence of the observer may be unsettling or disruptive to normal activities. In studies involving audio-taping of consultations, some pharmacists were reported to refuse to participate as they felt that customers' privacy would be compromised.[36] Audiorecoding of consultations raises ethical issues from the perspectives of both pharmacists and their clients (see below).

The information given to potential participants at the recruitment stage may also influence participation rates. Attention should be paid to providing a clear description of procedures and demands of the study, including the level and type of involvement required by pharmacists, pharmacy staff, clients and others who may be affected. In planning the data collection, researchers should also show an awareness of activities and pressures in the pharmacy and the impact the study may have.

Potential respondents may also be concerned about confidentiality of data and they should be assured that no individuals or locations will be identifiable in the findings. If the topic of study is presented as non-threatening, this may also have a positive effect on response rates.

Data collection

The feasibility of data collection, in terms of, first, whether or not the observation procedure provides data of the comprehensiveness and quality to meet the study objectives, and, second, the acceptability of the data collection process for personnel at the study sites, should be established in pilot work. Researchers studying counselling activities reported the pre-testing of structured instruments for data collection in a range of pharmacies and experimenting with the position of the observer.[38]

The observer must be situated where he or she can record all relevant data without appearing intrusive or disrupting the activities under observation. A researcher observing pharmacist–client interaction in medicine sales pretended to price-check products to minimise the appearance of 'watching' the consumer, and moved around to less obtrusive positions, but could still see and record relevant data.[24] Observers also considered their dress; some reported wearing non-uniform clothes,[24] or street clothes and carrying a clip-board.[23] These strategies to remain unobtrusive while collecting comprehensive data require some sensitivity on the part of the observer and adaptability to the conditions in different settings. Observers in these studies emphasised the importance of finding a position from which they could adequately see and hear. To ensure that observers would not face the difficulties of collecting unmanageable amounts of data, a preliminary study of the rate of interaction between pharmacists and consumers had resulted in the restriction of data collection to cough/cold and allergy products.[24]

Many researchers studying oral interactions between pharmacists and clients audiotaped consultations.[7,21,28,30,36,37] Radio-microphone apparatus worn by the pharmacist meant that consultations would be recorded irrespective of where they occurred in the pharmacy, without the intrusiveness of a researcher close-by. A possible disadvantage, depending on the study objectives, would be that the apparatus remained with one individual for the duration of the study period. However, audiotaping has been chosen by many researchers who wished to analyse details of consultations, as it overcomes the inevitable difficulties of securing complete verbatim transcripts by note-taking when consultations are complex or inaudible to the researcher.

Quantitative studies generally involved the collection of structured data on variables determined by the objectives of the study on specially designed pre-coded forms.[7,20,38,41] To ensure that the collection of data would be representative of pharmacy practice as a whole, the timing and duration of the data collection periods were often planned to include different times of day and days of the week,[20,27,40] and, in larger studies for which seasonal variation may be important, times of the year.[35]

Fixed interval work sampling techniques have also been employed to provide systematic observational data on pharmacists' activities.[26,31,44,45] In a study of advice with prescription and non-prescription medicines, the observer made a descriptive record at 1-minute intervals of what the pharmacist was doing, resulting in approximately 9000 observations.[31] For investigation into consultations between general practitioners and paediatricians and children with diarrhoea, a quantitative study in which the findings would be generalisable was planned. Each doctor's practice was observed systematically for a given number of hours on particular days, and data collected on the same set of variables for each consultation.[39]

Qualitative studies require the collection of detailed data on behaviours or interactions as they occur, rather than according to a predetermined agenda. In a study to assess the behaviour and treatment of drug users in pharmacies, a qualitative approach to data collection was employed in which researchers took detailed notes of their observations.[13] Some studies in pharmacies entailed the collection of both quantitative and qualitative data.[4–6,8,9] Non-participant observations in ten community pharmacies were combined with interviews and focus groups to investigate the roles and responsibilities of medicines-counter assistants.[5] A study of the impact of hospital pharmacy automation on professional roles was described as ethnographic, as it employed both direct observation of, and interviews with, pharmacy staff.[4] A study to compare quality of life in two health care settings involved the collection of both quantitative and qualitative data. Structured data were collected by logging activities in 15-minute blocks. Unstructured data included descriptions by the observer of the actions of, and interactions between, staff and clients in the two settings.[33]

Validity

A major difficulty of data collection by observation is that the presence of the researcher, and the knowledge that the study is taking place, may influence the behaviours of the individuals being observed. This is commonly referred to as the Hawthorne effect, following the Hawthorne studies which investigated the relationship between physical working conditions and productivity. In these studies, groups of workers were aware that they were being observed and changed their behaviour to the extent that the effects of changes in the working environment were masked.[51]

Ideally, some attempt to establish the extent to which results are biased by the presence of the researcher and the research process should be undertaken. One observational study in community pharmacies attempted to quantify the effect on pharmacists' behaviour of being observed, by examining the extent to which they habituated to the presence of the observer over a period of two weeks. The hypothesis was that reactivity would decrease as subjects adapted to the presence of the observer. In the four target behaviours that were observed, the pharmacists showed different and individual habituation patterns. In some instances no reactive effect was identified. A number of factors were suggested as to how the results might be explained.[22]

The Hawthorne effect was a consideration for many researchers in deciding the duration and number of observation periods. These considerations led researchers to discard data collected in the first 30 minutes of observation of pharmacists' counselling activities.[41] However, the extent of observer effects and the rate of habituation is unclear and may be expected to vary depending on study objectives, populations and settings as well as with the personalities of the observed and observer. Some researchers have attempted to assess the way in which study findings might have been biased as a result of these effects.

In a study of advice with prescription medicines given to clients, the researcher observed all dispensations and completed a checklist for each prescription, recording whether or not the prescription was handed out by the pharmacist or another member of staff, and any information or advice given or requested. To provide some validation, the researcher devised (and agreed with the pharmacists concerned) a method in which the counter assistants in a number of pharmacies would be trained to conduct observation on a limited number of variables on a single day (which would be unknown to the pharmacist) during the following month. This would not provide comprehensive information on all variables included in the main observation study, but it enabled some assessment of the influence of the observer on key variables.[20]

Many authors have discussed ways in which they attempted to minimise the effects of the research process and their presence on the results of their research. These included spending time with the staff prior to commencement of the data collection so they would feel at ease, emphasising the breadth of the data collection required to minimise the extent to which pharmacists might modify their practice, and providing assurances of confidentiality of results, anonymity of data (when this applied) and the importance of continuing with normal activity.

Observation of administration of medication on hospital wards was undertaken in the UK and USA to investigate the frequency of errors.[32] The authors discuss at length the problems of the effect of the observation process on the data. Because of differences in the medication administration processes in the two countries, the potential for influencing events differs. In the USA, the drugs administered were recorded by the researcher at the time of administration and later compared with the original prescription. In the UK, the prescription is used at the time of administration and thus any error is immediately identified by the researcher, who would then feel compelled to intervene. To reduce the likelihood of changes in behaviour, it was agreed that the data collected would remain confidential to the research team. In any observation study there will be greater potential for bias in some variables than others, and in this investigation of the frequency of errors in administration of medicines, the authors rightly point out that changes in behaviour can only affect those errors which are under the control of the health professional administering the drugs – and so, for example, excluded non-availability or poor transcription.[32] Methods of collecting data on medication administration errors have also been addressed in a study comparing 'no blame' self-reporting of errors by hospital nursing staff with a 'disguised-observer' method.[42]

Self-reports may be subject to bias as a result of individuals knowingly misrepresenting activities or events, or unwittingly as a result of poor memory or misconceptions regarding the actual state of affairs. A number of studies have found that data on the frequencies of pharmacist–client consultations collected by observation generally provide lower estimates than data obtained from self-reporting by pharmacists.[30,50]

In some cases, to minimise possible changes in behaviour, researchers deliberately withheld the true objectives of the study from the subjects of their research.[18,29,39] This may improve the validity of the data, but also has ethical implications (see below). A decision has to be made regarding the information that potential participants need in order to make an informed decision of whether or not to participate, while at the same time limiting the tendency for those being observed to modify their behaviour.

Reliability

In terms of reliability, researchers have addressed both consistency in data collection and in ratings between observers. Studies in different settings may present greater potential for inconsistency in data collection processes. Observers investigating errors in administration of drugs in hospitals in two countries worked together to standardise the method, and each collected data in both countries.[32] Researchers who devolved responsibility to pharmacists for audiotaping consultations in their pharmacies provided written instructions to pharmacists regarding the use of the equipment. All pharmacists were responsible for ten hours of data collection. When the researcher is not present it can be difficult to ensure adherence to the instructions. However, the reliability of data coding between the four raters was assessed.[30] Consistency between coders in the coding of transcripts was assessed in a study of prescribing of psychotropics, the coders being blind to key variables related to the study hypotheses.[7] The consistency of ratings between observers in a study of counselling in pharmacies was assessed using a set of pre-recorded video consultations. Each observer rated these consultations and their levels of agreement were compared by calculating the *Kappa* statistic.[50]

Generalisability

As with any quantitative study, the generalisability of the findings of quantitative observation studies depends on the sampling procedures, sample sizes and response rates (assuming the collection of valid and reliable data). Sampling bias is a potential problem of convenience or self-selecting samples (in which participants are those who are willing or choose to take part). Probability samples in which response rates are low may be subject to response bias. In both cases participants may differ from the wider population in ways that are important to the study. In these cases, careful consideration should be given to the generalisation of results. The investigation and management of non-response and potential bias by pharmacy practice researchers is discussed in Chapter 1.

Data analysis

In the analysis of observation data, certain assumptions may be implicit. These assumptions were listed by researchers investigating the rates of interaction between pharmacists and consumers: that the observer did not alter the behaviour of the consumer or pharmacist; that over the course of the study consumers were observed only once, and that observers coded interactions in a similar fashion.[24]

Analytical procedures have been largely determined by the study objectives, whether quantitative or qualitative, and by whether the data were to be combined with data collected by other methods. The most common procedures employed in the analysis of quantitative studies were the investigation of frequencies and tests for association between variables. More sophisticated procedures were sometimes employed, for example, logistic regression was used to establish factors that influence whether patients or prescribers were the initiators of psychotropic drug therapy.[7]

Qualitative data analysis included the application of the principles of grounded theory[6] in which ideas, themes and hypotheses are derived from the data which are coded accordingly. A qualitative non-participant observation study of long-stay institutions provides an example of the use of a theoretical perspective as a basis for observational data analysis. The data were analysed in relation to total institution and disengagement theory, and showed that a hospital ward setting closely conformed to Goffman's concept of the total institution.[52]

Ethical issues

Co-operation of study participants, and obtaining data that accurately reflect activities and behaviours of individuals under observation, are essential for the success of any study. If the topic of study is perceived as sensitive or the method is intrusive, lower response rates may result. These same issues may lead individuals to modify their behaviour. Poor response rates can seriously jeopardise the generalisability of data; modification of behaviour has a similar effect on the validity.

In a study of consultations between children with diarrhoea and medical practitioners, which investigated the management of symptoms, practitioners were told that the study was designed to collect information about paediatric problems presented to them, but not told about the specific aims of the study. This was done to minimise the expected change in behaviour. However, it raises an ethical issue in that while being accepted (presumably) on trust by the practitioner, the researchers themselves were not being honest about their motives and intentions.[18]

In a similar study of drugs supplied from medical practices and pharmacies in India, the researcher introduced herself as a 'foreign doctor interested in the diseases of the area'. To assure readers of the validity of the findings, she pointed out that none of the doctors whose prescribing habits were being studied was aware of the purpose of the visit. The researcher gained access both to observe consultations and to view patients' notes. There was no discussion reported regarding the information supplied to pharmacists or to patients whose notes were viewed.[39]

Had the researchers in these studies been fully informative about their objectives, they may have jeopardised the co-operation of the practitioners and the chance of obtaining valid data. When researching sensitive topics there is possibly a need to compromise between achieving study objectives and adherence to high ethical standards.

Observational data on supply and availability of drugs, purchases of prescription-only medicines and errors were collected in village pharmacies and health centres. Researchers were investigating activities in village pharmacies and patient compliance following implementation of an essential drugs programme in rural Burkina Faso. In an effort not to influence behaviour, the presence of observers in the pharmacies was explained by the fact that patient compliance was being investigated; nurses and pharmacists were not told that aspects of services and performance of the pharmacy would also be investigated. So as not to compromise patient compliance, the researchers reported that patients were not informed about the study. Names and addresses of patients were recorded by a nurse to prevent the patient suspecting a visit by the research team.[16] Again, this illustrates a trade-off between ethical issues and the need to ensure the validity of data.

In a study of prescribing and administration of intravenous drugs, nurse managers and senior clinicians were aware of the study aims, but staff at ward level were told that a study of prescribing and administration of injections was being carried out to understand constraints that staff worked under and to improve provision of information for their needs. The rationale was that if they were aware that error assessment was the aim of the study, this may have resulted in changes in the behaviour of staff, which could invalidate the findings of the study. All data collected were anonymous. Again, a situation arose in which a judgement had to be made regarding the information supplied to participants while ensuring the validity of the data.[29]

Audiotaping of consultations in pharmacies would necessarily be carried out with the knowledge of the pharmacist (who may well be wearing a microphone). Some researchers reported that clients in the pharmacy were informed of the study by a notice prominently displayed. This may have had some effect on the behaviour of both the pharmacists and the clients, although it would be usual to give assurances of anonymity and confidentiality in the hope of causing minimal changes to normal activity. In one study, the researchers reported that the microphone was placed 'out of sight'.[30] In this study, it is unlikely therefore that the behaviour of clients would have been influenced by the research process. If the data collection was both anonymous and confidential, whether or not the researchers behaved unethically towards these participants becomes debatable. Pharmacists invited to participate in research, recognising their duty to their clients, have expressed concerns regarding maintaining the privacy of their clients.[36]

It can also be argued that conducting research for which the findings are of questionable validity is unethical. Thus, in terms of ethical problems, researchers are faced with a potential conflict between achieving their research objectives (which require data that are known to be both valid and reliable), and respecting the rights of participants to be fully informed.

In reviewing and addressing ethical issues in health services research, three approaches (goal-based, duty-based and rights-based) have been distinguished and presented as a framework.[53] The goal-based approach focuses on the value of the outcomes of the research (for which validity of data is essential), that is the importance of the research and the extent to which the objectives will be achieved. The duty-based approach concerns the extent to which the researcher may be compromising his or her own moral standards in behaviour shown towards study participants. Thus, if the researcher has to be untruthful or contravene his or her own moral standards in order to achieve the study objectives, the research (irrespective of the goals) may be unethical. In a rights-based approach, the researcher considers the extent to which the autonomy of prospective participants is respected, for example, the individual should be able to make an informed choice regarding whether or not to participate in the research.[53]

This framework has been developed for wide application to medical, health services and social research. In relation to observation studies, potential conflicts between goal-, duty- and rights-based morals have been quite explicit. Some researchers may believe that achieving their goals, which treats the safeguarding of valid data as paramount, justifies lack of information provision and/or deceiving participants.

Non-participant observation studies are a popular and valuable method of obtaining data for research on topics of importance to the future of pharmacy, documenting what actually goes on rather than what people report. Many studies present potential or actual conflicts and compromises between safeguarding the rights of study participants to make informed decisions about their involvement, while not jeopardising the validity of research.

Participant observation

Few participant observation studies have been reported in the research literature of pharmacy practice. These studies are generally qualitative, descriptive studies, undertaken in single settings, the objective being to interpret behaviours in the contexts and situations in which they occur.

The objective of one such study was to describe emotion management techniques used by pharmacy students while working with live animals in pharmacology laboratory practical classes. The researcher was a student in the class who observed other students. As is usual for participant observation, data were recorded as fieldnotes. The data collection and analysis were guided by the principles of grounded theory.[8] In a study of the use of medicinal plants in Mexico, quantitative data were supplemented and illustrated by data gathered by participant observation, in particular in relation to healers, healing sessions and self-treatment.[54]

A study of the impact of patient counselling displayed some features of participant observation. The researcher took on the role of a pharmacy consultant in the collection of data. In this role, the researcher documented need for, and uptake of, advice with medicine purchases. In terms of assessing the effects of advice on purchasing behaviour, the researcher acknowledged that this methodology would not produce generalisable results.[25]

A number of covert observation studies into advice from pharmacy staff on minor ailments have been undertaken by both consumer organisations and pharmacy practice researchers.[55–57] These studies share some characteristics of participant observation studies in that the researcher takes on the role of a client. They differ from participant observation studies in the anthropological tradition in that they do not follow the principles of qualitative inquiry. Both the methodological rigour and the ethical issues (these studies were covert) surrounding these studies have been questioned.[58]

The feasibility of participant observation as a pseudo-patient in a hospital in Ghana was investigated by the anthropologist van der Geest and Sarkodie.[59] In discussing the study, they raise practical, methodological and ethical considerations. Although well placed to make insightful observations, the researcher would not share the full experiences of the patients (e.g. concerns of illness and recovery, medication taking).

Van der Geest and Sarkodie also question the ethics of recording details of the activities of individuals, such as visitors to the ward, who were not aware of the researcher's status, objectives and activities.[59]

Conclusion

There are few examples in the pharmacy practice research literature of participant observation studies. Participant observation offers great potential for gaining insights into aspects of health care and the use of medicines in the context of people's situations, environments and everyday lives.

References

1. Helman C. Application of anthropological methods in general practice research. *Fam Pract* 1996; 13: S13–6.
2. Mays N, Pope C. Observational methods in health care settings. *BMJ* 1995; 311: 182–4.
3. Bowling A. *Research Methods in Health*. Buckingham: Open University Press, 1997.
4. Novek J. Hospital pharmacy automation: collective mobility or collective control. *Soc Sci Med* 2000; 51: 491–503.
5. Ward P K, Bissell P, Noyce P R. Medicines counter assistants: roles and responsibilities in the sale of deregulated medicines. *Int J Pharm Pract* 1998; 6: 207–15.
6. Hassell K, Noyce P, Rogers A, *et al*. Advice provided in British community pharmacies: what people want and what they get. *J Health Serv Res Policy* 1998; 3: 219–25.
7. Sleath B, Svarstad B, Roter D. Physician vs. patient initiation of psychotropic prescribing in primary care settings: a content analysis of audiotapes. *Soc Sci Med* 1997; 44: 541–8.
8. Sleath B. Emotion management techniques used by pharmacy students during pharmacology laboratory: a qualitative study of professional socialization. *J Soc Admin Pharm* 1994; 11: 97–103.
9. Gilbert L. The pharmacist's traditional and new roles – a study of community pharmacists in Johannesburg, South Africa. *J Soc Admin Pharm* 1995; 12: 125–31.
10. Calva J, Bojalil R. Antibiotic use in a periurban community in Mexico: a household and drugstore survey. *Soc Sci Med* 1996; 42: 1121–8.
11. Erhun W O, Ademola-Oresanya Y. Pharmacy practice in private clinics in Nigeria. *J Soc Admin Pharm* 1991; 6: 136–40.
12. Brendstrup E, Launso L. Evaluation of a non-drug intervention programme for younger seniors. *J Soc Admin Pharm* 1993; 10: 23–5.
13. Matheson C. Views of illicit drug users on their treatment and behaviour in Scottish community pharmacies: implications for the harm reduction strategy. *Health Educ J* 1998; 57: 31–41.

14. Moore S, Cairns C, Harding G, Croft M. Health promotion in the high street: a study of community pharmacy. *Health Educ J* 1995; 54: 275–84.
15. Latif D A, Burger B A, Harris S G, *et al.* The relationship between community pharmacists' moral reasoning and components of clinical performance. *J Soc Admin Pharm* 1998: 15: 210–24.
16. Krause G, Benzler J, Heinmuller R, *et al.* Performance of village pharmacies and patient compliance after implementation of an essential drugs programme in rural Burkina Faso. *Health Policy Plann* 1998; 13: 159–66.
17. Bekerleg S, Lewando-Hundt G, Eddama M, *et al.* Purchasing a quickfix from private pharmacies in the Gaza Strip. *Soc Sci Med* 1999; 49: 1489–500.
18. Nizami S Q, Khan I A, Bhutta Z A. Drug prescribing practices of general practitioners and paediatricians for childhood diarrhoea in Karachi, Pakistan. *Soc Sci Med* 1996; 42: 1133–40.
19. Benjamin H, Smith F J, Motawi A. Drugs supplied with and without a prescription from a conurbation in Egypt. *East Mediterranean Health J* 1996; 2: 506–14.
20. Aslanpour Z, Smith F J. Oral counselling on dispensed medication: a survey of its extent and associated factors in a random sample of community pharmacies. *Int J Pharm Pract* 1997; 5: 57–63.
21. Smith F J. Community pharmacists and health promotion: a study of consultations between pharmacists and clients. *Health Prom Int* 1992; 7: 249–55.
22. Savage I. Observing pharmacists at work: quantifying the Hawthorne effect. *J Soc Admin Pharm* 1996; 13: 8–19.
23. Stevenson M, Taylor J. The effect of a front-shop pharmacist on non-prescription medicine consultations. *J Soc Admin Pharm* 1995; 12: 154–8.
24. Taylor J, Suveges L. Selection of cough, cold and allergy products: the role of consumer–pharmacist interaction. *J Soc Admin Pharm* 1992; 9: 59–65.
25. Nichol M B, McCombs J S, Boghassian T, Johnson K A. The impact of patient counselling on over-the-counter drug purchasing behaviour. *J Soc Admin Pharm* 1992; 9: 11–20.
26. Fisher C M, Corrigan O I, Henman M C. A study of community pharmacy practice: pharmacists' work patterns. *J Soc Admin Pharm* 1991; 8: 15–24.
27. Fisher C M, Corrigan O I, Henman M C. A study of community pharmacy practice: non-prescribed medicine sales and counselling. *J Soc Admin Pharm* 1991; 8: 69–75.
28. Smith F J. Referral of clients by community pharmacists in primary care consultations. *Int J Pharm Pract* 1993; 2: 86–9.
29. Hartley G M, Dhillon S. An observational study of prescribing and administration of intravenous drugs in a general hospital. *Int J Pharm Pract* 1998; 6: 38–45.
30. Blom L, Jonkers R, Kok G, Bakker A. Patient education in 20 Dutch pharmacies: analysis of audiotaped contacts. *Int J Pharm Pract* 1998; 6: 72–6.
31. Savage I. Time for prescription and over-the-counter advice in independent community practice. *Pharm J* 1997; 258: 873–7.
32. Dean B S, Allan E L, Barber N D, Barker K N. Comparison of medication errors in an American and British hospital. *Am J Health Syst Pharm* 1995; 52: 2543–9.

33. Clark P, Bowling A. Observational study of quality of life in NHS nursing homes and a long-stay ward for the elderly. *Ageing Soc* 1989; 9: 123–48.

34. Dowey J A, Brand V. The display of confectionery in pharmacies: the need for an ethical debate. *Pharm J* 1998; 262: 262–3.

35. Smith F J, Salkind M R. Factors influencing the extent of the pharmacist's advisory role in Greater London. *Pharm J* 1990; 244: R4–7.

36. Wilson M, Robinson E J, Blenkinsopp A, Panton R. Customers' recall of information given in community pharmacies. *Int J Pharm Pract* 1992; 1: 152–9.

37. Evans S W, John D N, Bloor M J, Luscombe D K. Use of non-prescription advice offered to the public by community pharmacists. *Int J Pharm Pract* 1997; 5: 16–25.

38. Berardo D H, Kimberlin C L, Barnett C W. Observational research on patient education activities of community pharmacists. *J Soc Admin Pharm* 1989; 6: 21–9.

39. Greenhalgh T. Drug prescription and self-medication in India. *BMJ* 1987; 25: 307–21.

40. Benjamin H, Smith F J, Motawi A. Community pharmacists and primary health care in Alexandria, Egypt. *J Soc Admin Pharm* 1995; 12: 3–11.

41. Krska J, Kennedy E J, Milne S A, McKessack K J. Frequency of counselling on prescription medicines in community pharmacy. *Int J Pharm Pract* 1995; 3: 178–86.

42. McNally K, Sunderland V B. No-blame medication administration error reporting by nursing staff at a teaching hospital in Australia. *Int J Pharm Pract* 1998; 6: 67–71.

43. Nickman N A, Scheider J K, Knick K A. Work activities at an ambulatory care pharmacy with an integrated model of pharmacy practice. *Am J Health System Pharm* 1996; 53: 397–402.

44. Rutter P M, Hunt A J, Darracott R, Jones I F. A subjective study of how community pharmacists in Great Britain spend their time. *J Soc Admin Pharm* 1998; 15: 252–61.

45. Rutter P M, Hunt A J, Darracott R, Jones I F. Validation of a subjective evaluation study using work sampling. *J Soc Admin Pharm* 1999; 16: 174–85.

46. Savage I. The changing face of pharmacy practice – evidence from 20 years of work sampling studies. *Int J Pharm Pract* 1999; 7: 209–19.

47. Emmerton L, Becket G, Gillbanks L. The application of electronic work sampling technology in New Zealand community pharmacy. *J Soc Admin Pharm* 1998; 15: 191–200.

48. Finkler S A, Knickman J R, Hendrickson G, *et al*. A comparison of work-sampling and time-and-motion techniques for studies in health services research. *Health Serv Res* 1993; 28: 577–97.

49. Emmerton L, Jefferson K. Work sampling observation of community pharmacies: a review. *Int J Pharm Pract* 1996; 4: 75–8.

50. Raisch D W. Patient counselling in community pharmacy and its relationship with prescription payment methods and practice setting. *Ann Pharmacother* 1993; 27: 1173–9.

51. Moser C A, Kalton G. *Survey Methods in Social Investigation*. Aldershot: Gower Publishing Company, 1971.

52.   Clark P, Bowling A. Quality of everyday life in longstay institutions. *Soc Sci Med* 1990; 30: 1201–10.

53.   Botros S. Ethics in medical research: uncovering the conflicting approaches. In: Foster C, ed. *Manual for Research Ethics Committees*. London: Centre for Medical Law and Ethics, King's College London, 1997.

54.   Heinrich M, Ankli A, Frei B, *et al*. Medicinal plants in Mexico: healers' consensus and cultural importance. *Soc Sci Med* 1998; 47: 1859–71.

55.   Consumers' Association. Pharmacists: how reliable are they? *Which? Way to Health* 1991; December: 191–4.

56.   Anderson C W, Alexander A M. Response to dysmenorrhoea: an assessment of knowledge and skills. *Pharm J* 1992; 249: R2.

57.   Ferraz M B, Ronaldo B P, Paiva J G A, *et al*. Availability of over-the-counter drugs for arthritis in Sao Paulo, Brazil. *Soc Sci Med* 1996; 42: 1129–31.

58.   Alexander A. The 'agent provocateur' study as a research tool. *Pharm J* 1991; 247: 154–5.

59.   Van der Geest S, Sarkodie S. The fake patient: a research experiment in a Ghanaian hospital. *Soc Sci Med* 1998; 47: 1373–81.

7

Triangulation

There are many examples of studies where pharmacy practice researchers have combined different types of data, methods and approaches within a single research project. The choice of methods made by health services and pharmacy practice researchers is generally governed by data requirements for fulfilling research objectives and practical considerations in conducting research. This chapter demonstrates how a variety of approaches and methods have been combined for different purposes in a variety of study designs in pharmacy research. Studies include both qualitative and quantitative interviews, questionnaire surveys and interviews, focus groups prior to, or following, a survey, and observation studies combined with a range of other techniques.

Triangulation has been defined as the combining of different types of approach, methods and/or data within the same research study. The term derives from surveying, where different bearings are used to achieve a more reliable estimate of the true position.[1] In health services research, triangulation is employed to provide different perspectives of phenomena, obtain data on a range of issues in relation to a research question, and to assess and demonstrate the validity of research findings.

Triangulation is a common practice in health services, pharmacy practice, social science and, to a lesser extent, clinical research. However, concerns have been expressed over combining methods underpinned by different philosophical assumptions within the conceptual framework of a single study: in particular, qualitative and quantitative approaches, which are characterised by important epistemological and methodological distinctions.

Qualitative research is context-specific in that the researcher aims to collect and interpret data and to describe or explain phenomena in the light of the situations, backgrounds and circumstances in which they occur. No attempt is made to standardise settings to enable comparisons or generalisations; the aim of the research will commonly be to identify differences and attempt to explain them in terms of context-specific factors. In contrast, quantitative research involves the collection of data within a predetermined and standardised framework, devised by (and in accordance with the perspectives of) the researcher. By standardising frameworks and procedures for data collection and analysis, the quantitative researcher would anticipate reproducible findings, generalisable to locations other than those where the study was conducted. However, although reproducible, quantitative methods may lack the flexibility required to provide an accurate reflection of the relevant issues in different settings.

Triangulation is commonly employed in the validation of data, the argument being that using a variety of methods helps overcome the shortcomings of any particular one. Discrepancies uncovered by comparing data collected by different methods may enable the researcher to identify possible biases. However, the extent to which inaccuracies in one method are likely to be complemented by the accuracies of another has been questioned.[2] Furthermore, many social scientists claim that combining approaches or methods ignores the influences of the methodological contexts in which the different data sets are obtained, these contexts being important to the interpretation of the data.

This 'purist' view is not without its critics. Atkinson,[3] in discussing 'some perils of paradigms', challenges the notion of distinguishing qualitative and quantitative methods in the context of distinct research paradigms. He claims that the qualitative paradigm, if it exists, is characterised by a great deal of diversity with no single set of theoretical or methodological presuppositions. He argues that paradigms (although variously defined) cannot be characterised by methods alone, and that qualitative methods in all their diversity, and often in conjunction with quantitative measurement, serve the development of concepts and theories. Moreover, Silverman[2] has argued that presenting frequency data alongside qualitative discussions can aid the interpretation of data.

Temple,[4] acknowledging the differing epistemological positions of, on the one hand, a positivist (scientific) world view concerned with quantification and, on the other, a context-specific social reality in which the qualitative researcher is a part, argues the need for the researcher to be explicit in distinguishing whether it is data, methods or approaches that are being combined.

Health services research and pharmacy practice methods are often distinguished as quantitative or qualitative: for example, survey research is generally a quantitative procedure and participant observation is usually qualitative. Interview techniques may be structured or unstructured, distinctions that are broadly taken to correspond to quantitative and qualitative methodologies, respectively. Pharmacy practice researchers commonly adopt or adapt the methods that best serve their purpose. For example, interviews are most commonly described as 'semi-structured' (i.e. falling somewhere between these two extremes) as this approach is frequently the most appropriate means of fulfilling the research objectives. Qualitative research is often exploratory in its objectives and is sometimes used to generate hypotheses while quantitative studies are designed to test them. Thus, quantitative and qualitative methods, because of their different applications, are frequently viewed as complementary.[5]

Health services and pharmacy practice research is an applied discipline in which authors select and justify their approaches and methods in terms of serving their study objectives. In describing their choice of methodology, they are generally guided by pragmatism rather than the theoretical concerns of mixing methods with differing philosophical assumptions. Nevertheless, the influence of methodological issues in the research process is usually acknowledged.

In reviewing research into consultations between clients and health professionals, many authors have asserted the value of employing different conceptual frameworks for identifying and achieving research objectives. Interactions between professionals and clients are central to health care, and researchers have undertaken large-scale quantitative studies. At the same time, many researchers have pointed out that interactions are complex and context-specific and hence should also be studied by methods that allow for elucidation of the different levels of explanation.[6–8]

Numerous studies have focused on the measurement and/or determinants of compliance or adherence. In many of the 'compliance' studies the patient has been regarded as a passive recipient of instructions, while non-compliance was seen as 'defaulting' from instructions. This view has given way to the concept of adherence, which acknowledges patients' active role in decision-making about their drugs.[9–13] Pill counts, and more recently the development and use of electronic devices that record openings of a container, have been criticised because they do not enable the researcher to address the role of socio-cultural contexts and patients' health beliefs in decision-making about drug use. (They are also of questionable reliability as a measure of drug-taking for compliance studies.) Our changing notions of compliance, adherence or concordance (partnership between health professionals and clients in decisions) result in re-framed objectives that require different methodological approaches. Thus, many researchers examining 'adherence' have employed qualitative methods that enable an examination of the contexts and belief systems which influence drug use from the perspective of respondents. The different methodologies are not necessarily complementary, but they reflect alternative epistemologies, which will have an impact both on the methods selected for a research study and consequently on the study findings.

Comparing methods

Thus, are research findings an artefact of the research process? It cannot be disputed that, at least to some extent, study findings will be determined by the methodology. What researchers find will depend on what they look for, where they look, the information they choose to document and the analytical procedures they select.

Aside from the conceptual frameworks, perspectives and decisions of researchers, all methods present their own logistical and practical strengths and weaknesses which have an impact on the reliability and validity of data (e.g. 'Hawthorne' effects[14] in observation data, memory effects in the collection of retrospective data, missing entries in diaries).

Ortiz et al.[15] compared the data on advice-giving in community pharmacies collected by different methods and found that, in general, self-completion questionnaires overestimated the frequency and duration of episodes, while diaries tended to overestimate the duration but underestimate the frequency; direct observation was believed to have little impact on activities. Other researchers have also found that pharmacists' self-reports tend to provide higher estimates of frequencies of interactions than data obtained by non-participant observation.[16,17]

A study of medication administration errors compared data from 'no blame' self-reports of hospital nursing staff with data gathered by a 'disguised observer'. Researchers concluded that the former system had advantages in terms of costs (being less labour intensive) but that error rates were considerably lower than found by non-participant observation.[18]

A comparison of work-sampling and time-and-motion studies found that the assessments of time spent on the different tasks depended on which method was employed.[19] Thus, the interpretation of the findings of any research should be in the light of the actual methods employed in executing the research, as well as the theoretical perspectives and assumptions (epistemology) of the researcher.

Combining methods for validation

Given the inevitable impact of the methodology on the study findings, some attempts should be made by the researcher to assess the extent to which data are an accurate reflection of the phenomena under study (i.e. to assess their validity). As in navigation, from where the term triangulation derives, comparing the data from different sources is common as a means of confirming the accuracy of research findings.

Researchers investigating the relationship between community pharmacists' moral reasoning and components of clinical performance suspected that respondents might be inclined to provide socially desirable responses in a questionnaire survey. Covert observation was employed to assess whether or not this was the case.[20] In an investigation of pharmacy services in Nigeria, in which data were collected by questionnaires to pharmacists and physicians, observation of some facilities was conducted to provide some validation.[21] Similarly, observation in a small number of sites was undertaken to validate data collected by pharmacists in self-completion questionnaires to study the relationship between prescription payment methods, practice settings and counselling in community pharmacies.[22] To validate data on advice-giving in pharmacies by a non-participant observer, a method of obtaining comparable data by a covert technique was devised. The procedure, agreed with each pharmacist, involved a member of counter staff who was trained to collect limited structured data on advice-giving by the pharmacist in a set period, the actual timing being unknown to the pharmacist.[23] In medical research, general medical practitioners' self-reports in questionnaires have been shown to be inconsistent with data derived from the contents of patients' medical notes. This led researchers to conclude that when gathering data in self-completion questionnaires, the validity of responses to specific questions should be assured prior to their incorporation into a survey instrument.[24] To examine children's attitudes and beliefs about medicines, the results of different methods (drawings by the children who then described and discussed what they had drawn in an open interview, and data from structured interviews) were compared to establish whether or not they supported the same conclusions. When differences were found the researcher theorised about the possible reasons for the differences, which could be either methodological or substantive.[25]

The difficulties of achieving valid estimates of public satisfaction with health services have been extensively discussed in the health services research literature[26,27] (see Chapter 9). Use of different measures has been shown to produce dissimilar results.[28] Researchers have combined various approaches and methods to develop instruments and test their validity. These include comparing questionnaire scores with open-ended questions, relating satisfaction scores with time until the termination of a health insurance contract (assuming that dissatisfied people would terminate sooner), and discriminant validity tests to establish specificity of the instrument for health care (rather than picking-up a person's generalised disposition towards being satisfied or dissatisfied).[29]

Content validity

Content validity refers to the extent to which a study instrument (e.g. questionnaire, interview schedule, proforma for data collection) gathers data on all the relevant issues. Omitting to collect information on events and viewpoints important to the issue under study will result in an incomplete and therefore inaccurate representation of those issues. To ensure the content validity of research instruments, many researchers have conducted preliminary fieldwork to facilitate the identification of all the relevant issues. This commonly involves a smaller exploratory qualitative study prior to the development and application of a structured instrument in a larger sample. A series of qualitative interviews was conducted with a convenience sample of 28 pharmacists to ensure inclusion of all the relevant issues in a survey instrument designed to identify the dimensions of pharmacists' preferences for cough and cold products.[30] Similar procedures were employed to identify factors important to pharmacists when recommending active ingredient(s) and brands of non-prescription analgesics for simple, tension and migraine headaches.[31,32] Researchers employing the health belief model as a theoretical framework to examine the effects of health treatment perceptions on the use of prescribed medicines and home remedies conducted a series of seven in-depth interviews to identify domains for a structured survey instrument.[33] A literature review combined with open-ended interviews with a convenience sample of 24 pharmacists provided the basis for a survey instrument to predict community pharmacists' intentions to try to prevent and correct drug therapy problems.[34] A survey of pharmacists' attitudes, beliefs and practices regarding services to drug misusers involved an initial inductive approach using qualitative methods prior to the design of a postal questionnaire.[35] To assess the motivators and barriers to the implementation of prescription monitoring and review services by community pharmacists, researchers conducted a systematic review of the literature to aid the development of questionnaire statements for a postal Delphi survey.[36]

Focus groups are an effective method for the generation of a wide range of thoughts and ideas in relation to a topic of interest. There are a number of examples of their use by pharmacy practice researchers in the initial exploratory phases of research projects. They were also employed in the preliminary fieldwork of a study of consumers' use and expectations of pharmacy services, to assist in the development of a research agenda and of structured instruments for use in home interviews and as a self-completion survey.[37,38] Eight group discussions were convened to clarify potential questions for a subsequent house-to-house survey of lay people's attitudes to the treatment of depression.[39]

'Experts' have also been used to inform survey instruments. To address seamless care issues (smooth transfer between the hospital and community sectors in the delivery of health care) semi-structured interviews were conducted with ten hospital pharmacists purposively selected as having the greatest knowledge of, and involvement in, pharmaceutical care of patients discharged from hospital. A structured questionnaire was then developed to assess the awareness, and seek the views, of community pharmacists on seamless care issues. The rationale of the researchers was that the prerequisites for smooth transfer between the sectors depend on their initiation by the hospital.[40] Although the questionnaire may effectively cover issues from the perspective of hospital professionals, it will not necessarily include issues of importance to the provision of seamless care from the perspective of community professionals. A panel comprising experts in pharmacy practice, pharmacy education and regulation was convened to identify domains for a survey instrument to examine the opinions of pharmacy regulators at state level on responsibility of pharmacists for pharmaceutical care outcomes.[41]

A postal questionnaire investigating pharmacists' and pre-registration pharmacy graduates' views of proxy consultations (those with a representative of the patient rather than the patient his/herself) was based on data gathered in 12 qualitative interviews with pharmacists. As well as providing insights into the important issues, these interviews influenced sample selection by suggesting that pre-registration graduates would be a relevant group.[42]

Complementarity

Combining data or methods to serve an objective

Many researchers have employed a range of approaches or methods within a single study to provide a more comprehensive or a complete picture of the topic of interest. In some cases, data sets were combined prior to analysis, while in other cases data obtained by different methods were analysed independently and the findings compared.

For example, to examine existing activities of pharmacists and explore their perceptions of their present and future roles from different angles, observation in community pharmacies was combined with structured interviews with pharmacy staff.[43] To examine the role expansion of community pharmacy in South Africa in the context of professional dominance and boundary encroachment, a mixture of qualitative and quantitative methods was used, including interviews with key informers, documentary analysis of public reports and minutes of meetings and questionnaire surveys.[44] A similar triangulated approach was employed to explore professional relationships in the context of dispensing doctors and prescribing pharmacists,[45] and to research the role of training in transforming community pharmacy.[46] To describe the pattern of antibiotic use in a community in Mexico City, interviews were conducted with housewives in 1659 randomly selected households who were asked about the presence of certain symptoms and the use of drugs. An observational study of sales of anti-microbials from pharmacies was also conducted, which included interviews with clients following a purchase.[47] To assess compliance, researchers gathered data from patients' notes on the number of scheduled appointments that were kept and also asked patients in a questionnaire to report the number of days in the previous week they had taken their medication.[48]

Methods or alternative sources of data may also be combined to provide additional contextual data on the population of interest, and/or to compare the characteristics of a sample with a wider population. A qualitative study of the treatment and behaviour of illicit drug users in pharmacies involved semi-structured interviews with users of pharmacy services. Observational data, in the form of field notes, were also collected in pharmacies. In the analysis and presentation of the results these data were used to illustrate the interview findings.[49] In an interview study of health promotion activities in community pharmacies in which pharmacists' perceptions of the barriers and constraints were examined, the interviewers also collected structured observational data, such as the presence of leaflet displays and space available.[50] Group interviews and observation were employed in a study of patterns of health seeking behaviour and use of pharmacies.[51] Interviews, focus groups and observation were combined to study the roles of medicines-counter assistants in the sale of deregulated medicines.[52] Participant observation (especially of healers' healing sessions and self-treatment) provided additional data to illustrate and supplement data from interviews regarding the use of medicinal plants.[53]

Ethnographers aim to gather comprehensive data that enables them to explore issues and phenomena in the natural settings and contexts where they occur. A range of methods was employed to provide an ethnographic description of pharmacies and pharmacy-related behaviour in Bombay. These included semi-structured interviews with pharmacy owners, observation in six pharmacies, drug sales data, exit interviews with 150 customers, and in-depth interviews with medical representatives. The combination of methods enabled a description of activities and pharmacy-related behaviour in relation to aspects of social, cultural and economic contexts. Researchers were also able to compare pharmacy managers' perceptions on issues related to promotion and supply of medicines with observed practices.[54] An ethnographic study in three hospitals was conducted to examine the relationship between new technology and pharmacy's changing role in the division of labour in health care. The study combined direct observation and semi-structured interviews with pharmacy, nursing, administrative staff and trade union officials representing workers. Interviews were designed to provide informants with the opportunity to raise wide-ranging impacts of changes.[55]

The theoretical basis of a study may determine the data and methods required. The theory of reasoned action, which specifies the relationships among beliefs, attitudes, behavioural intentions and behaviour, provided the theoretical basis to explore factors associated with antibiotic prescribing. This theoretical framework requires data on a range of variables obtained from different sources. Thus, face-to-face interviews with a small number of physicians were followed by a mailed questionnaire to collect attitudinal, normative and socio-demographic data, which were combined with antibiotic prescribing data necessary to test the theory.[56]

A study to identify the characteristics of 'leading edge practitioners' combined qualitative and quantitative techniques within a single interview. The critical incident technique was employed at the start of an interview in which respondents were asked to select and relate 'stories' from their experience as a practitioner. This was followed by a structured interview schedule and a psychometric test.[57]

In studies of pharmacists' roles and responsibilities regarding prescribing and use of benzodiazepines, interview schedules were developed to investigate the views of both pharmacists and general medical practitioners. The research instruments also combined open questions, which allowed respondents to express their own views and relate their experiences, with a structured questionnaire to enable summaries and comparisons of the views of professional groups.[58,59]

Combining methodologies to serve related objectives

In some cases, the findings of two studies provide different perspectives on the topic of interest. A second study may be conducted to follow-up issues identified in earlier work, or the two studies may run concurrently.

Questionnaires were used to compare the view expressed in UK guidelines that emergency contraception is reliable and safe, with views of women attending family planning clinics. Semi-structured interviews were also conducted with a population subgroup who were attending for emergency contraception. The two parts of the study covered similar topics, but the interviews enabled a more detailed exploration of issues such as sources and use of information and beliefs about the risks of using emergency contraception.[60]

Research into domiciliary visiting by pharmacists in relation to compound analgesic use comprised two studies to investigate different aspects of the topic of interest. Interviews with patients in their own homes were followed by a postal survey among doctors to elicit their views on domiciliary visiting by pharmacists.[61] Similarly, to investigate the role of pharmacists and general medical practitioners in the management of dermatological conditions, interviews were conducted with people buying skin products in the pharmacy. General medical practitioners were requested to complete daily records of people seen with skin conditions. The information from the two sources can be viewed as complementary in that they provide pictures of different aspects of management of skin conditions in primary care. However, the two surveys related to different population and/or symptom groups and health care contexts, so will not necessarily be comparable.[62]

A survey was undertaken to provide quantitative information regarding the frequency and nature of violent incidents in pharmacies and associated factors.[63] This was followed by an interview study that enabled more detailed descriptions of events, their physical and psychological effects, and their impact on the working lives of pharmacists.[64]

Following the implementation of an essential drugs programme in Burkina Faso, West Africa researchers investigated two different impacts, the performance of village pharmacies and patient compliance with prescribed medicines. To obtain the required information, data were gathered by non-participant observation in the pharmacies for one study objective and for the second objective in home interviews with patients.[65] A pharmaceutical needs assessment in a pharmacy setting was conducted in four stages with different methods at each stage. This involved the application of a range of research methods to aid the development of a pharmaceutical service tailored to local needs. The research began with semi-structured interviews (to identify respondents' unprompted thoughts) with individuals from groups on whom the service would impact. This was followed by a postal survey, which was based on information collected in the interviews, to different groups. Open forum meetings were then held to feedback findings, and in the final stage consensual agreement was reached on an overall priority league table of both professionals' and patients' perceived needs.[66] To obtain comprehensive data, an investigation of hospital pharmacy educational services combined a nation-wide survey with a literature review and interviews with selected staff.[67]

Clinical areas and techniques

Research approaches and methods have also been combined to provide complementary data in clinical studies and investigations of drug use.

Data from three sources were combined to study blood pressure control and self-reported compliance. Community pharmacy records were used to recruit patients to the study, identify the prescriber and obtain medication histories. Medical records were used for data on blood pressure control and prescribed medicines, and questionnaires to patients were used to obtain demographic and personal information related to the study's dependent variables.[68] Morbidity data and drug utilisation data were combined to evaluate trends in drug consumption and assess costs in Bulgaria.[69]

To study antihypertensive drug prescribing habits in the Netherlands, 'paper patients' presented to general medical practitioners revealed differences in drugs used to treat male and female patients, which were then verified from prescription data collected from 80 computerised community pharmacies. The authors discuss the strengths of combining the two methods: 'paper patients' to address issues with respect to specific categories of patient and prescribing data enabling examination of large groups, but not necessarily in relation to particular diagnoses.[70]

In a study to investigate factors that influence whether patients or physicians initiate psychotropic drug therapy, consultations between physicians and patients were audiotaped and participants also asked to complete questionnaires. The combined data set enabled the researchers to relate participants' self-reports or perceptions, 'what they say, they do', with their actual behaviour.[71]

One study of adverse events in medical care employed ethnographers to gather data, in addition to the more traditional method of reviewing patients' notes. Researchers demonstrated how a combination of the two approaches uncovered a greater number and wider range of events.[72] A randomised, controlled trial looking at side-effects of psychiatric treatment also demonstrated the value of concurrent qualitative research. The qualitative data in this study also highlighted some of the difficulties, ethical and practical, of recruiting patients to, and conducting, randomised controlled trials.[73]

Service evaluation

Studies evaluating pharmacy and related health services are reviewed in Chapters 8 and 9. However, in the evaluation of health care interventions or different treatment options, researchers frequently wish to ensure that the impact of the processes and outcomes of care are assessed from different perspectives. Thus, evaluation studies will often require the application of a range of research methods and/or approaches. For example, an evaluation of a non-drug intervention programme for senior citizens combined qualitative and quantitative approaches, which included structured questionnaires, qualitative interviews, and diaries maintained by participants.[74] To assess the value of professional meetings between pharmacists and general medical practitioners to discuss prescribing, a questionnaire survey to participating pharmacists and general medical practitioners was supplemented by a series of semi-structured interviews with a smaller group of pharmacists and general medical practitioners to provide more detailed data.[75] Three studies to assess the outcomes following advice-giving in community pharmacies involved observation (with or without audiotaping) to gather data on the intervention, followed by questionnaires or telephone interviews with clients to investigate subsequent actions and outcomes. These included assessments of the extent to which clients could recall information,[76] the extent to which advice was reported to have been followed,[77] and whether or not advice to see a general practitioner resulted in a consultation.[78]

Logistical considerations

The optimal methods for any study are those that provide the necessary data and are efficient, acceptable and workable for both the researchers and the study participants.

Three different methods were employed to assess the acceptability to patients of specific prescribing changes. Following generic substitution, acceptability was assessed by postal questionnaire, as this would enable a large number of people to whom the change had applied to take part. Face-to-face interviews were conducted with a smaller number of people who had had a therapeutic switch in their medication from cimetidine to ranitidine; this allowed a more detailed examination of patients' feelings than would have been possible in a postal survey. Telephone interviews were conducted with patients or parents/carers who had been switched from a beclometasone diskhaler to a metered-dose inhaler and spacer.[79]

Focus groups have been combined with individual interviews to explore beliefs about influences on health.[80,81] The former were found to be more successful in generating a wide range of responses and ideas, while the latter allowed more detailed exploration of particular issues with individuals.[80] Focus groups have also been used to provide additional data following a questionnaire survey for which a disappointing response rate had been obtained.[82]

To assess the pharmaceutical needs of blind and partially-sighted people, interviews were considered the most appropriate means of data collection. The study also included a postal survey to pharmacists contracted to the local health authority.[83] In a study of patients' perspectives on the use of proton pump inhibitors, in-depth interviews were conducted in patients' own homes, at the workplace, in the surgery or by telephone.[84] Flexibility regarding the setting for the data collection may be an important factor in maximising response rates, which in turn enhances the validity of any study. Researchers, however, must be aware that interview setting could influence the issues raised and discussed by respondents. For example, in a study in which non-responders to a postal questionnaire were interviewed by telephone, the researchers believed that some bias was introduced by the change in method of data collection.[85]

Identification of a population of interest is an essential early stage of any research project. If no sampling frame (list of all members of the population of interest) exists, the selection of a representative (preferably random) sample is difficult. To overcome these problems, some researchers have conducted a screening survey to identify their population prior to the conduct of the main study. A telephone survey was conducted to identify health maintenance organisations that operated drug formularies; this was followed by a mail survey to gather data on the organisations and their use of formularies.[86]

Study design

Morgan[87] discusses the possible designs of studies that involve a combination of methodological approaches. He identifies four basic designs, depending on whether the principal method is quantitative or qualitative, and whether the complementary method occurs as a preliminary or as a follow-up stage to the principal method. In the pharmacy practice literature there are examples of all these designs. In addition, there are also studies in which two approaches were employed concurrently, or in which the different stages may assume similar importance.

A preliminary qualitative stage (e.g. to ensure content validity) prior to a larger quantitative approach is common in health services research. However, there are also examples of studies in which issues identified in a large quantitative study were subsequently explored using a qualitative approach. In a study in which community pharmacists and general medical practitioners completed diaries reporting interprofessional contact, the issues that emerged were followed-up in semi-structured interviews.[88] Group interviews were conducted following a questionnaire study examining the assistance and support with medicines provided to elderly people by home care providers. The groups provided more detailed information regarding some of the issues raised; the data obtained from the groups were used to elaborate on the questionnaire findings.[89,90] The responses to a postal questionnaire on asthma advice-giving by community pharmacists were subsequently discussed in a focus group of 13 pharmacists from a range of settings.[91] Observation of community pharmacists' referral practices when advising on common ailments was followed by the development of an instrument to investigate the views of general medical practitioners on these practices.[92,93]

Data analysis

The differing epistemological positions and resultant methodological approaches of quantitative and qualitative research will determine the appropriate analytical procedures. Data sets obtained by different methods may be combined prior to analysis or analysed independently.

In studies that combined quantitative and qualitative approaches, the analysis of data from each, as expected, was analysed independently. For example, a study examining the attitudes and beliefs of children about medicines involved both structured and qualitative interviews. The findings of each method were analysed and presented separately and then compared. The results of both were presented under headings relating to the research questions. In general, the findings of the two methods concurred; however, differences in coverage would be expected to occur in that in the unstructured interviews issues would only be discussed if the child raised them.[25]

In a study of the characteristics of 'leading-edge practitioners,' qualitative coding procedures were applied in the analysis of 'critical incidents' in which respondents related stories from their experiences while quantitative statistical procedures were employed in the analysis of structured interview data, including the Kirton adaptation innovation inventory.[57] The analysis of an observational study, which involved the collection of both qualitative and quantitative data, included a quantitative comparison of activities and interactions in two different settings,[94] and a qualitative theoretical analysis based on Goffman's institution theories.[95]

In some cases, researchers included open questions in an otherwise structured instrument to ensure respondents had the opportunity to raise issues important to themselves. Open questions may provide some qualitative insights into the perspectives of respondents, or oversights of the researcher. However, the use of open questions in this way does not concur with the principles of qualitative inquiry and qualitative analytical procedures would not generally be employed. Most commonly, responses to open questions have been used just to illustrate or elaborate on the quantitative findings.

In studies where a range of qualitative methods is used, the data sets may be combined prior to analysis. For example, a qualitative study to describe emotion management techniques used by pharmacy students working with live animals in a pharmacology laboratory combined participant observation (data collected as field notes) and interviews. Qualitative analytical procedures were applied to the entire data set.[96]

Within the research and related literature of pharmacy practice there are many examples of studies in which a range of methods and approaches have been combined. A wide variety of combinations of methods and approaches within different study designs have been employed for different purposes. Although concerns are expressed over mixing different approaches within a single research study, in health services and pharmacy practice research the methods selected are usually those that will be most effective, efficient and workable in achieving the study objectives. In their reports, researchers generally justify their choice of methods and discuss the implications of methodological issues in the context of their research.

References

1. Silverman D. *Interpreting Qualitative Data*. London: Sage Publications, 1993.
2. Silverman D. *Qualitative Methodology and Sociology*. Aldershot: Gower Publishing Co., 1985.
3. Atkinson P. Some perils of paradigms. *Qual Health Res* 1995; 5: 117–24.
4. Temple B. A moveable feast: quantitative and qualitative divides. *J Soc Admin Pharm* 1997; 14: 69–75.
5. Smith F J. The practice researcher's toolbox. *Pharm J* 1992; 248: 179.
6. Charon R, Greene M G, Adelman RD. Multidimensional interaction analysis: a collaborative approach to the study of medical discourse. *Soc Sci Med* 1994; 39: 955–65.
7. Hassell K, Noyce P, Rogers A, *et al*. Advice provided in British community pharmacies: what people want and what they get. *J Health Serv Res Policy* 1998; 3: 219–25.
8. Pilnick A. Advice-giving in community pharmacies: a response concerning methods for future research. *J Health Serv Res Policy* 1998; 3: 97–9.
9. Stimson G V. Obeying doctor's orders: a view from the other side. *Soc Sci Med* 1972; 8: 97–104.
10. Conrad P. The meaning of medicines; another look at compliance. *Soc Sci Med* 1985; 20: 29–37.
11. Morgan M, Watkins C J. Managing hypertension: beliefs and responses to medication among cultural groups. *Sociol Health Illness* 1988; 10: 561–78.
12. Donovan J L, Blake D R. Patient non-compliance: deviance or reasoned decision-making. *Soc Sci Med* 1992; 34: 507–13.
13. Royal Pharmaceutical Society of Great Britain. *From Compliance to Concordance*. London: RPSGB, 1997.
14. Moser C A, Kalton G. *Survey Methods in Social Investigation*. Aldershot: Gower Publishing Co., 1971.
15. Ortiz M, Walker W-L, Thomas R. Comparisons between methods of assessing patient counselling in Australian community pharmacies. *J Soc Admin Pharm* 1989; 6: 39–48.
16. Smith F J, Salkind M R. Factors influencing the extent of the pharmacist's advisory role in Greater London. *Pharm J* 1990; 244: R4–7.

17. Fritsch M A, Lamp K C. Low pharmacist counselling rates in the Kansas city, Missouri, metropolitan area. *Ann Pharmacother* 1997; 31: 984–91.

18. McNally K, Sunderland V B. No-blame medication administration error reporting by nursing staff at a teaching hospital in Australia. *Int J Pharm Pract* 1998; 6: 67–71.

19. Finkler S A, Knickman J R, Hendrickson G, *et al.* A comparison of work-sampling and time-and-motion techniques for studies in health services research. *Health Services Res* 1993; 28: 577–97.

20. Latif D A, Berger B A, Harris S G, *et al.* The relationship between community pharmacists' moral reasoning and components of clinical performance. *J Soc Admin Pharm* 1998; 15: 210–24.

21. Erhun W O, Ademola-Oresanya Y. Pharmacy practice in private clinics in Nigeria. *J Soc Admin Pharm* 1991; 6: 136–40.

22. Raisch D W. Patient counselling in community pharmacy and its relationship with prescription payment methods and practice setting. *Ann Pharmacother* 1993; 27: 1173–9.

23. Aslanpour Z, Smith F J. Oral counselling on dispensed medication: a survey of its extent and associated factors in a random sample of community pharmacies. *Int J Pharm Pract* 1997; 5: 57–63.

24. Eccles M, Ford G A, Duggan S, Steen N. Are postal questionnaire surveys of reported activity valid? An exploration using general practitioner management of hypertension in older people. *Br J Gen Pract* 1999; 49: 35–8.

25. Almarsdottir A B, Hartzema A C, Bush P J, *et al.* Children's attitudes and beliefs about illness and medicines: a triangulation of open-ended and semi-structured interviews. *J Soc Admin Pharm* 1997; 14: 26–39.

26. Carr-Hill R A. The measurement of patient satisfaction. *J Public Health Med* 1992; 14: 236–49.

27. Williams B. Patient satisfaction a valid construct? *Soc Sci Med* 1994; 38: 509–16.

28. Cohen G, Forbes J, Garraway M. Can different patient satisfaction survey methods yield consistent results? Comparison of three surveys. *BMJ* 1996; 313: 841–4.

29. Etter J-F, Perneger T V. Validating a satisfaction questionnaire using multiple approaches: a case study. *Soc Sci Med* 1997; 45: 879–85.

30. Emmerton L, Gow D J, Benrimoj S I. Dimensions of pharmacists' preferences for cough and cold products. *Int J Pharm Pract* 1994; 3: 27–32.

31. Roins S, Benrimoj S I, Carroll P R, Johnson L W. Factors used by pharmacists in the recommendation of active ingredient(s) and brand of non-prescription analgesics for simple, tension and migraine headaches. *Int J Pharm Pract* 1998; 6: 196–206.

32. Roins S, Benrimoj S I, Carroll P R, Johnson L W. Pharmacists' recommendations of the active ingredient(s) of non-prescription analgesics for a simple, tension and migraine headache. *J Soc Admin Pharm* 1998; 15: 262–74.

33. Brown C M, Segal R. The effects of health and treatment perceptions on the use of prescribed medication and home remedies among African American and white American hypertensives. *Soc Sci Med* 1996; 43: 903–17.

34. Farris K B, Kirking D M. Predicting community pharmacists intention to try

and prevent and correct drug therapy problems. *J Soc Admin Pharm* 1995; 12: 64–79.

35. Rees L, Harding G, Taylor K. Supplying injecting equipment to drug misusers: a survey of community pharmacists attitudes, beliefs and practices. *Int J Pharm Pract* 1997; 5: 167–75.

36. Tully MP, Seston EM, Cantrill JA. Motivators and barriers to the implementation of pharmacist-run prescription monitoring and review services in two settings. *Int J Pharm Pract* 2000; 8: 188–97.

37. Jepson M, Jesson J, Pocock R, Kendall H. *Consumer Expectations of Community Pharmaceutical Services. A Report for the Department of Health.* Birmingham: Aston University/MEL Research, 1991.

38. Jesson J, Pocock R, Jepson M, Kendall H. Consumer readership and views on pharmacy health education literature: a market research survey. *J Soc Admin Pharm* 1994; 11: 29–36.

39. Priest R G, Vize C, Roberts A, *et al.* Lay people's attitudes to treatment of depression: the results of opinion poll for Defeat Depression Campaign just before its launch. *BMJ* 1996; 313: 858–9.

40. Brown J, Brown D. Pharmaceutical care at the primary–secondary interface in Portsmouth and south-east Hampshire. *Pharm J* 1997; 258: 280–4.

41. Nau D, Brushwood D. State pharmacy regulators' opinions on regulating pharmaceutical care outcomes. *Ann Pharmacother* 1998; 32: 642–7.

42. Weiss M C, Cantrill J A, Nguyen H L. Pharmacists' and pre-registration pharmacy graduates' views of proxy consultations. *Int J Pharm Pract* 1998; 6: 120–6.

43. Gilbert L. The pharmacist's traditional and new roles – a study of community pharmacists in Johannesburg, South Africa. *J Soc Admin Pharm* 1995; 12: 125–31.

44. Gilbert L. Pharmacy's attempts to extend its role: a case study in South Africa. *Soc Sci Med* 1998; 47: 153–64.

45. Gilbert L. Dispensing doctors and prescribing pharmacists: a South African perspective. *Soc Sci Med* 1998; 46: 83–95.

46. Gilbert L. The role of training in transforming community pharmacy: a case study of pharmacists and students in Johannesburg, South Africa. *J Soc Admin Pharm* 1998; 15: 23–32.

47. Calva J. Antibiotic use in a peri-urban community in Mexico: a household and drugstore survey. *Soc Sci Med* 1996; 42 :1121–8.

48. Kruger H S, Gerber J J. Health beliefs and compliance of black South African outpatients with antihypertensive medication. *J Soc Admin Pharm* 1998; 15: 201–9.

49. Matheson C. Views of illicit drug users on their treatment and behaviour in Scottish community pharmacies: implications for the harm reduction strategy. *Health Educ J* 1998; 57: 31–41.

50. Moore S, Cairns C, Harding G, Croft M. Health promotion in the high street: a study of community pharmacy. *Health Educ J* 1995; 54: 275–84.

51. Beckerleg S, Lewando-Hundt G, Eddama M, *et al.* Purchasing a quickfix from private pharmacies in the Gaza Strip. *Soc Sci Med* 1999; 49: 1489–500.

52. Ward P K, Bissell P, Noyce P R. Medicines counter assistants: roles and responsibilities in the sale of deregulated medicines. *Int J Pharm Pract* 1998; 6: 207–15.

53. Heinrich M, Ankli A, Frei B, *et al.* Medicinal plants in Mexico: healers' consensus and cultural importance. *Soc Sci Med* 1998; 47: 1859–71.
54. Kamat V R, Nichter M. Pharmacies, self-medication and pharmaceutical marketing in Bombay, India. *Soc Sci Med* 1998; 47: 779–94.
55. Novek J. Hospital pharmacy automation: collective mobility or collective control? *Soc Sci Med* 2000; 51: 491–503.
56. Lambert B L, Warren Salmon J, Stubbings J, *et al.* Factors associated with antibiotic prescribing in a managed care setting: an exploratory analysis. *Soc Sci Med* 1997; 45: 1767–79.
57. Tann J, Blenkinsopp A, Allen J, Platts A. Leading edge practitioners in community pharmacy: approaches to innovation. *Int J Pharm Pract* 1996; 4: 235–45.
58. Smith F J. Benzodiazepines: community pharmacists' perceptions of their roles and responsibilities. *J Soc Admin Pharm* 1991; 8: 157–63.
59. Smith F J. General medical practitioners and community pharmacists in London: views on the pharmacist's role and responsibilities relating to benzodiazepines. *J Interprofess Care* 1993; 7: 37–45.
60. Ziebland S, Maxwell K. Not a proper solution? The gap between professional guidelines and users' views about the safety of using emergency contraception. *J Health Serv Res Policy* 1998; 3: 12–19.
61. Dixon N H E, Hall J, Hassell K, Moorhouse G E. Domiciliary visiting: a review of compound analgesic use in the community. *J Soc Admin Pharm* 1995; 12: 144–53.
62. Kilkenny M, Yeatman J, Stewart K, Marks R. The role of pharmacies and general practitioners in the management of dermatological conditions. *Int J Pharm Pract* 1997; 5: 11–15.
63. Smith F J, Weidner D. Threatening and violent incidents in community pharmacies: an investigation of the frequency of serious and minor incidents. *Int J Pharm Pract* 1996; 4: 136–44.
64. Smith F J, Weidner D. Threatening and violent incidents in community pharmacies: implications for pharmacists and community pharmacy services. *Int J Pharm Pract* 1996; 4: 145–52.
65. Krause G, Benzler J, Heinmuller R, *et al.* Performance of village pharmacies and patient compliance after implementation of an essential drug programme in rural Burkina Faso. *Health Policy Plann* 1998; 13: 159–66.
66. Williams S E. Bond C M, Menzies C. A pharmaceutical needs assessment in the primary care setting. *Br J Gen Pract* 2000; 50: 95–9.
67. Cotter S M, McKee M, Barber N D. Clinically oriented education provided by United Kingdom National Health Service hospital pharmacies for hospital health care staff. *J Soc Admin Pharm* 1997; 14: 133–42.
68. Gilbert A, Owen N, Samsom L, Innes J M. High levels of medication compliance and blood-pressure control among hypertensive patients attending community pharmacies. *J Soc Admin Pharm* 1990; 7: 78–83.
69. Dimitrova Z D, Getov N, Ivanova A D, Petrova G I. Trends in antidiabetic drugs consumption in Bulgaria. *J Soc Admin Pharm* 1997; 14: 52–6.
70. Paes A H P, Bakker A. Antihypertensives drug prescribing in the Netherlands. *J Soc Admin Pharm* 1993; 10: 171–9.
71. Sleath B, Svarstad B, Roter D. Physician vs. patient initiation of psychotropic

prescribing in primary care settings: a content analysis of audiotapes. *Soc Sci Med* 1997; 44: 541–8.

72. Andrews L B, Stocking C, Krizek T, *et al.* An alternative strategy for studying adverse events in medical care. *Lancet* 1997; 349: 309–13.

73. Anthony P, Lancashire S, Creed F. Side effects of psychiatric treatment: a qualitative study of issues associated with a random allocation research study. *Sociol Health Illness* 1991; 13: 530–44.

74. Brendstrup E, Launso L. Evaluation of a non-drug intervention programme for younger seniors. *J Soc Admin Pharm* 1993; 10: 23–5.

75. Pilling M, Geoghegan M, Wolfson D J, Holden J D. The St. Helen's and Knowsley prescribing initiative: a model for pharmacist led meetings with GPs. *Pharm J* 1998; 260: 100–2.

76. Wilson M, Robinson E J, Blenkinsopp A, Panton R. Customers' recall of information given in community pharmacies. *Int J Pharm Pract* 1992; 1: 152–9.

77. Evans S W, John D N, Bloor M J, Luscombe D K. Use of non-prescription advice offered to the public by community pharmacists. *Int J Pharm Pract* 1997; 5: 16–25.

78. Blenkinsopp A, Jepson M H, Drury M. Using a notification card to improve communication between community pharmacists and general medical practitioners. *Br J Gen Pract* 1991; 41: 116–18.

79. Wood K M, Boath E H, Mucklow J C, Blenkinsopp A. Changing medication: general practitioner and patient perspectives. *Int J Pharm Pract* 1997; 5: 176–84.

80. Mitchell G, A qualitative study of older women's perceptions of control, health and ageing. *Health Educ J* 1996; 55: 267–74.

81. Greenhalgh T, Helman C, Mu'min Chowdhury A. Health beliefs and folk models of diabetes in British Bangladeshis: a qualitative study. *BMJ* 1998; 316: 978–83.

82. Williamson V K, Winn S, Livingstone C R, Pugh A L G. Public views on an extended role for community pharmacy. *Int J Pharm Pract* 1992; 1: 223–9.

83. Grills A, MacDonald A. An assessment of the pharmaceutical needs of the blind and partially sighted in Dumfries and Galloway. *Pharm J* 1997; 259: 381–4.

84. Boath E H, Blenkinsopp A. The rise and rise of proton pump inhibitor drugs: patients' perspectives. *Soc Sci Med* 1997; 45: 1571–9.

85. Sibbald B, Addington-Hall J, Brenneman D, Freeling P. Telephone versus postal surveys of general practitioners: methodological considerations. *Br J Gen Pract* 1994; 44: 297–300.

86. Hanson E C, Shepherd M. Formulary restrictions in health maintenance organisations. *J Soc Admin Pharm* 1994; 11: 54–6.

87. Morgan D L. Practical strategies for combining qualitative and quantitative methods: applications to health research. *Qual Health Res* 1998; 8: 362–76.

88. Kennedy E, Blenkinsopp A, Purvis J. A diary record study of the nature, purpose and extent of communication between community pharmacists and general medical practitioners. *J Soc Admin Pharm* 1997; 14: 143–51.

89. Stromme H K, Botten G. Support and service for the drug treatment of older people living at home: a study of a sample of Norwegian home care providers. *J Soc Admin Pharm* 1993; 10: 130–7.

90. Stromme H K, Botten G. Drug related problems among old people living at home, as perceived by a sample of Norwegian home care providers. *J Soc Admin Pharm* 1993; 10: 63–9.

91. Osman L M, Bond C M, MacKenzie J, Williams S. Asthma advice-giving by community pharmacists. *Int J Pharm Pract* 1999; 7: 12–17.

92. Smith F J. Referral of clients by community pharmacists in primary care consultations. *Int J Pharm Pract* 1993; 2: 86–9.

93. Smith F J. Referral of clients by community pharmacists: views of general medical practitioners. *Int J Pharm Pract* 1996; 4: 30–5.

94. Clark P, Bowling A. Observational study of quality of life in NHS nursing homes and a long-stay ward for the elderly. *Ageing Soc* 1989; 9: 123–48.

95. Clark P, Bowling A. Quality of everyday life in longstay institutions. *Soc Sci Med* 1990; 30: 1201–10.

96. Sleath B. Emotion management techniques used by pharmacy students during pharmacology laboratory. *J Soc Admin Pharm* 1994; 11: 97–103.

8

Evaluation of pharmaceutical services: objectives, designs and frameworks

Chapters 8 and 9 review approaches and methods employed by health services and pharmacy practice researchers in the evaluation of pharmacy services. Chapter 8 discusses the application of different study designs and frameworks to the evaluation of existing and innovative services and interventions; Chapter 9 addresses the methods and measures employed in the evaluation process. Although many of the issues regarding study design and evaluation frameworks may be relevant to clinical trials comparing the efficacy of alternative drug therapies, the focus of this chapter is on pharmacy services. Audit is also excluded, being a cyclical process, consisting of reviewing and monitoring current practice and evaluation (comparison of performance) against agreed predefined standards.[1] Most researchers would distinguish between evaluation and audit, although the latter includes evaluative procedures. However, audit procedures have sometimes been incorporated into service evaluation; for example, an audit tool was used to evaluate prescribing before and after the appointment of a pharmacist in a general medical practice.[2]

Evaluation has been defined as the use of scientific method, and the rigorous and systematic collection of research data, to assess the effectiveness of organisations, services and programmes (e.g. health service interventions) in achieving predefined objectives.[3] This requires the use of an appropriate study design to enable an evaluation independent of confounding factors, the identification and employment of measures pertinent to the objectives of the intervention, and the collection of data that are comprehensive, reliable and valid.

The definition of evaluation of St Leger et al.[4] includes 'the critical assessment on as objective basis as possible, of the degree to which entire services or their component parts fulfil stated goals'. In their definition, the authors draw attention to the need for objectivity, that is, that findings should be, and be seen to be, independent of the judgements and prejudices of the evaluators or interested parties. Many studies evaluating pharmacy services are undertaken and/or commissioned by pharmacists or professional bodies who may have a vested interest in demonstrating particular outcomes. Similarly, individual practitioners identifying needs and developing services to address them will be keen to demonstrate that these initiatives fulfil their objectives. In the published literature, the objectivity of some studies may appear questionable because of an unbalanced statement of the aims of the study. It is not unusual for objectives to be expressed in terms of demonstrating that objectives are met rather than assessing the extent to which they are, or are not, fulfilled. For example, a study that aims to demonstrate that pharmacists can work with general medical practitioners[5] may convey to a reader that the researcher is not as active in seeking data that demonstrates that they cannot. What is important is that researchers are seen to be balanced in their approach to research and that they are receptive regarding negative aspects in any evaluation.

Further bias may arise from the fact that researchers are more likely to submit positive findings for publication than findings that are inconclusive or present an unwelcome message. Publications and conferences to promote professional interests may also be more inclined to include research that presents favourable results. The majority of published papers report results of studies in which pharmacists were found to be effective in achieving their objectives. These positive findings may, of course, be a reflection of the wide-ranging potential value of pharmacy services to health care provision.

Research objectives

In the pharmacy practice research literature there are a large number of studies which evaluate aspects of pharmacy services. These include many assessments of existing services as well as those evaluating innovations in professional practice.

This huge body of literature evaluating established and new services in hospitals and the community covers a wide range of study objectives. In the evaluation of existing services, studies include assessments of pharmacists' involvement in drug therapy decisions and clinical roles[6-9] and aspects of advice-giving.[10-12] A number of researchers have monitored practice following the introduction of new guidelines or recommendations for practice.[13-17] Among service innovations, studies have addressed methods of supply of drugs to hospital wards,[18,19] clinical service developments,[20-26] discharge services and primary/secondary care interface initiatives,[27-34] methods of provision of advice on prescribing,[35-38] collaboration between health professionals,[5,37,39-41] health promotion activities[2,42–47] and repeat dispensing by community pharmacists.[48] Numerous studies have considered direct costs and/or financial implications of service development.[49–65] In particular, cost containment is an important objective of many interventions to influence prescribing.[5,49,55,56,66,67] Many researchers have evaluated training initiatives,[35,68–81] including continuing education by teleconference.[82] Consumer satisfaction is viewed as an important indication of the success of health care programmes. Consequently consumers' perspectives of services are frequently incorporated into service evaluation[26,61,83–93]; in some cases being a principal outcome measure.

Some studies focusing on service innovation are described as feasibility studies, that is, the assessment of aspects of the practicalities of offering a new service or the achievement of specific goals, prior to recommendations for more extensive service provision. Feasibility studies have assessed the practicalities or effectiveness of service provision,[24,94–99] the accuracy of clinical measures[23,94,95] or acceptability of procedures to pharmacy staff, clients or other practitioners.[25,31,94,96]

Study design

An appropriate study design is fundamental for ensuring the objectivity of the evaluation process and the validity of its outcomes. The study designs that have been used in the evaluation of pharmacy services include randomised controlled trials, quasi-experimental designs, before-and-after studies, cohort studies (with or without a control group) and descriptive studies.

The objectives of evaluation studies are sometimes expressed as hypotheses. Although hypothesis testing requires an experimental design, this has been undertaken by randomised controlled trials, quasi-experimental designs and within descriptive studies. In other studies, the evaluation may be based on documentation of the processes of service delivery, and experiences of participants in a programme.

Randomised controlled trials (RCTs)

In the evaluation of health care, RCTs are viewed as a 'gold standard'. This is an experimental design that includes randomisation, whereby each participant has an equal chance of allocation to either an alternative treatment or control group. Randomisation provides a safeguard against the introduction of bias as a result of non-equivalence between groups. The inclusion of a control group enables the researcher to attribute differences in outcomes between the groups to the antecedent intervention. To avoid observer bias, participants and, preferably, professionals will be blind regarding allocation to either intervention or control groups.

However, although considered a 'gold standard', the application of RCTs to the evaluation of health services presents a number of difficulties, and their suitability for this purpose has been questioned.

Holme Hansen and Launso[100] have challenged the appropriateness of RCTs in the assessment of drug technology. In their argument, they cite a definition of technology as 'more than machines or instruments; it is also the knowledge or skills that are necessary for using the apparatus and it is the organisation that ensures the apparatus works'.[101] They discuss how RCTs do not take into account these broader issues in that they use short periods of data collection, specific patient groups and controlled settings that do not reflect the everyday lives of users. They question the generalisability of findings derived from samples drawn from specific patient populations, environments and conditions. Glasgow *et al.*[102] have discussed practicalities and difficulties of conducting RCTs in different settings, enabling demographic patterns, cultural factors and established health professional–patient relationships to be taken into account.

Britton *et al.*[103] acknowledge that, in planning and conducting RCTs, potential subjects will be excluded by design, and centres by practitioners choosing not to participate. The generalisability of findings may be jeopardised by this selective participation in the research and exclusions from it. Following a review of RCTs, Britton *et al.*[103] concluded that most evaluative studies fail to document adequately the characteristics of those who, while eligible, do not take part. Difficulties arise in that both the eligible and participating may differ in important ways from the wider population to whom the results may be assumed to be applicable. However, narrow inclusion criteria may enable improved precision in the results and willing participants may be more co-operative in adhering to protocols, thus providing more complete and reliable data. Thus, there may be a trade-off between the generalisability and accuracy (or internal validity) of results.

The problem of generalisability of the findings was addressed in an evaluation of a health promotion training programme. All pharmacists within one geographical area were invited to participate in this study, and those who accepted were allocated to either the test or the control group. The test group participated in a three-day training programme, and all pharmacists maintained logbooks. All participants in the study were self-selecting, although they were randomised to intervention and control groups. However, to obtain data representative of all pharmacists in the study area and thus improve the generalisability of the findings, the researchers recruited a second control group of non-volunteers.[104–106]

Comparison of outcomes between alternative treatment groups is confined to outcome variables that can be quantified. In many clinical studies, endpoints may be both limited in their number and restricted to those that are quantifiable (e.g. physiological measures). However, in the evaluation of health service programmes, the anticipated outcomes and impacts may be many, and different techniques will be required for their identification and measurement.

In a review of the methodological literature regarding the advantages and disadvantages of RCTs over non-randomised studies, the benefits and shortcomings have been discussed on theoretical, ethical and practical grounds.[107,108] Regarding RCTs in primary care settings, the advantages of a greater representativeness of the patients in the community have been emphasised.[108]

Patient preferences have also been identified as having a potential impact on the outcomes of randomised controlled trials.[109] One study demonstrated that patients randomised to their preferred treatment had improved outcomes when compared with patients randomised to the same group, but who expressed no preference.[110] The role of psychology in influencing the effectiveness of therapy (cf. the placebo effect) has been raised as a potential confounder, particularly in unblinded studies, which may result in RCTs wrongly attributing effects to a treatment option.[109] Researchers have discussed ways of designing trials to enable the effects of patients' preferences to be identified so they can be taken into account in the analysis.[109,110] Patient preferences may present ethical problems in the design of studies that could conflict with the scientific requirements of the research.

The scientific rationale for conducting an RCT is that health care professionals are genuinely unclear regarding the optimal treatment options (i.e. a situation of collective equipoise exists). Under such circumstances, future patients are believed to benefit at no cost to the participants, provided the participants are in personal equipoise and give informed consent on this basis.[111] In the case of the majority of the studies reviewed here, the interventions being evaluated were additional to those that are normally offered as part of health or pharmacy services.

Blinding of participants and researchers regarding their allocation to either the intervention or control group can be one of the most difficult features of RCTs for health services and pharmacy practice researchers to achieve. It may not be possible to shield clients from the knowledge that they are receiving specialist advice. Pharmacists will, inevitably, be aware of their participation in training initiatives. To evaluate the impact of the pharmacy extension programme (PEP) on clients' experiences of medication counselling, an RCT was constructed to test two hypotheses: first, that there is no difference between median frequency of counselling between clients collecting prescriptions at PEP and non-PEP pharmacies, and, second, that there is no difference between the two in the proportion of clients who receive counselling. The experimental and comparison groups were randomly selected and equivalence between them evaluated by comparing, for example, the average number of staff on duty and monthly prescription volume.[84] However, such a study could not be blind. Similarly, to study the impact of counselling areas, the intervention group included pharmacists who took up an offer of a counselling area; the participants may be both self-selecting and mindful of which group they are in.[112]

The difficulties of attributing outcomes to an antecedent intervention was raised in relation to a study evaluating the effects of community pharmacists on general practitioners' prescribing. The objective of the study was to identify changes in prescribing patterns which may have occurred as a result of meetings between individual community pharmacists and general medical practitioners. Even though the study design included a control group, the researchers acknowledge that medical practitioners who meet with pharmacists may also be more responsive to other encouragements to modify their prescribing habits.[66]

In their review of the placebo effect and its hypothetical relationship to adherence and improved patient outcomes, Tucker and Wertheimer[113] point out that all interventions have placebo effects. A randomised placebo-controlled trial design was employed to test the hypothesis that pharmacists can play a role in aiding disease prevention by improving vaccine acceptance rates. Participants were randomly assigned to receive either a letter advising of risks of influenza infection and availability of vaccine, or (the control group) a letter advising recipients to 'poison-proof' their home by returning unwanted medicines. The objective of the letter to the control group was to establish a comparable level of perceived concern by the subject's pharmacist.[114] In an RCT conducted to measure the impact of domiciliary pharmacy visits on medication management in an elderly population, patients were randomly allocated to one of three groups: (a) home visits with counselling, (b) home visits without counselling and (c) traditional pharmacy services, that is, no visits except at the beginning and end of the study. Group (b) was included to determine whether or not the interest of the investigator would result in the control group of patients altering their behaviour.[115] Thus, in both these cases, the investigators were designing their studies to account for the placebo effect.

Despite the difficulties and concerns regarding the application of RCTs in health services research, in addition to the studies mentioned above, RCTs have been combined with a range of methodologies. To compare the effectiveness of small group versus small formal seminar for improving appropriateness of prescribing for children under five with acute diarrhoea, a study was conducted in which six districts were randomly assigned to either one of these groups or the control. The results were monitored by comparing the prescribing patterns.[79] In a study to evaluate two different methods of providing practice-based, antibiotic prescribing feedback, 66 general medical practices were randomised to take part in face-to-face discussions with an advisor or to receive a prescribing analysis workbook. The results were also compared with 23 practices that did not wish to participate.[38] An RCT was conducted to compare verbal and computer counselling on inhaler technique.[116] Patients in one pharmacy were asked to demonstrate their inhaler technique (which was rated using a checklist) and then sequentially allocated to one of the two groups. Following counselling, patients' technique was retested. To assess patient outcomes following counselling, pharmacy clients designated 'intending to buy' were randomly assigned to study or control groups, which determined whether or not they received counselling. All clients were subsequently followed-up with a telephone call.[117]

RCTs have been conducted to compare pain control in patients who did, or did not, receive counselling on patient-controlled analgesia,[118] to assess the effectiveness of a pharmaceutical care model on the management of non-insulin-dependent diabetes[119] and to establish the cost-effectiveness of pharmaceutical intervention to assist people in giving up smoking.[62]

An RCT was conducted to measure the effect of a letter given to hospital patients prior to discharge for them to take to their community pharmacist. The rates of unintentional discrepancies in prescribed medication in the control and intervention groups were then compared in home interviews.[33] A similar study assessed the influence of an individualised information letter to each elderly patient discharged from hospital and also to members of the primary health care team regarding the patient's medication. Again, patients were allocated to test and control groups. Following discharge, patients and health personnel were followed up to establish the value of the letters in influencing the frequency of drug-related problems.[120] In a randomised controlled trial to evaluate the effects of pharmacy discharge planning on medication problems, patients from three wards were randomly allocated to intervention or control groups. Domiciliary visits were conducted at 1, 4 and 12 weeks to assess the impact at different times (including duration of any differences between groups).[34] To evaluate a community pharmacist's interventions regarding drug-related problems resulting from repeat prescriptions, the latter were assigned to a trial (pharmacist intervened) or control (no intervention) group. The resolution of drug-related problems between the two groups was compared.[121]

Quasi-experimental studies

To overcome some of the difficulties presented by RCTs, quasi-experimental designs have sometimes been employed. These studies are adopted when random allocation to alternative intervention or control groups is not possible. Non-random allocation presents the potential problem that the study groups may not be equivalent. Thus, quasi-experimental design is seen as weaker than an RCT, as differences in study outcomes between the groups may be attributable to features other than the intervention under evaluation, that is, as a result of a confounding factor. This is a problem particularly in the evaluation of interventions for which participants are self-selecting, for example, pharmacists who opt for training programmes or medical practitioners who choose to collaborate with pharmacists.

In quasi-experimental designs, random allocation is replaced by 'matching' in an attempt to achieve equivalence of the groups. The most important factors on which to ensure that groups are equivalent are those which are known, or believed, to be associated with the variable under study. Thus, in a trial to evaluate the effect of a pharmacist intervention on prescribing costs in general medical practice, the intervention and control sites were matched on the basis of several characteristics that might be expected to have an influence on changes in prescribing costs (e.g. if they held their own budgets, if they undertook their own dispensing, their list size). In this study, the researchers acknowledged that the findings would not necessarily be replicated in general medical practices that did not want help from practice-based pharmacists.[67] In a study in the Netherlands, assessing the effect on prescribing of co-operation between pharmacists and general medical practitioners, the groups were matched on factors known to influence prescribing.[40] To determine the potential benefits of a clinical pharmacy service to people in residential care, 160 residents in nine residential homes were divided into two groups, matched for age, sex, number of prescription drugs and general categories of drug therapy.[41]

Some of these studies can be described as 'before and after studies with a control group'. For example, a 'smile for sugar-free medicines' campaign was conducted in two health authorities. In the evaluation, two further health authorities were selected as controls, matched for socio-demographic characteristics. The campaign was evaluated by comparing the number of sales and prescriptions for commonly used sugar-free paediatric medicines prior to and following the campaign.[122] To evaluate a vacation training programme, students were divided into two cohorts (training and control) matched in terms of age and gender. The knowledge and skills of all students were assessed and compared before and after the programme.[74]

Before-and-after studies

Before-and-after studies have been used in the evaluation of a number of service initiatives. They involve the collection of structured baseline data, prior to an intervention, for variables on which the intervention is expected to impact, followed by the gathering of further data sets on one or more occasions after the intervention. The before-and-after data sets are then compared.

Before-and-after studies have also been employed in the investigation of the impact of a pharmacist-initiated drug regimen review process on the incidence of drug-related problems in an elderly population[123]; to compare prescribing patterns and costs before and after the introduction of multidisciplinary medication review on a long stay ward[56]; to compare the costs of laxatives prescribed prior to, and following, the introduction of a prescribing policy[55]; and to assess the effect of government recommendations on methadone prescribing.[17] Before-and-after studies have also been used in the evaluation of training initiatives.[68–71,73,75,124]

A potential problem of before-and-after studies that do not include a control group is attributing changes to the intervention, rather than any other circumstances or events. In a study examining whether the introduction of decentralised pharmaceutical care had any effects on the processes of discharge, the authors acknowledged that, in the absence of controls, other unrelated changes might have occurred which could confound the results. They attempted to minimise this by using the same wards, consultant teams, time of year and observer.[27] In another study, prescribing data on four classes of drug were examined before and after presentations to general medical practitioners. Again, although some changes in prescribing were found, the authors pointed out that these might not necessarily have been solely attributable to the project.[125]

Some researchers have designed the data collection to provide evidence to address concerns that changes are attributable to factors other than the intervention. A before-and-after assessment of pharmacists' knowledge formed part of the evaluation of clinical guidelines to ensure appropriate over-the-counter advice in community pharmacies. The evaluation was controlled by the inclusion of questions about symptom management that were not included in the guidelines.[126] The data collection for a study assessing the effect of a shop-front pharmacist on advice on non-prescription medicines was designed with an additional period of 'baseline' observation. The study involved two interventions separated by a rest period. Comparison (control) data were collected (as is conventional) prior to the commencement of the study, and again following the first, but prior to the second, intervention.[127] Were other factors responsible for changes observed, this should have been reflected in the 'control' data.

To consider the extent to which change was sustained following the introduction of new guidelines on antibiotic therapy, data were collected immediately after they were introduced and 10 months later.[128]

In a study of a new health centre pharmacy, researchers planned to conduct an evaluation prior to its establishment and 12 months later. In this case study, the early stages of the evaluation confirmed opportunities for the introduction of new pharmaceutical services, but also identified that there was no strategy for change and that this would be unlikely to happen by chance. The authors commented that in a traditional experiment, researchers would just return 12 months later to document changes and events. However, they adopted an alternative evaluation methodology that included an active decision to intervene. They demonstrated how this alternative evaluation methodology can help provide insights into ways of ensuring more positive outcomes.[129] A case study approach employed in the analysis of events (within the framework of the trans-theoretical model of behavioural change) that led up to changes in use of a drug in Australia was used to provide insights into the impact of these events.[130]

Cohort studies

In cohort studies, participants in a programme are followed-up over a period of time. Thus, in two separate studies, participants in two community pharmacy-based smoking cessation programmes were followed-up.[42,47] In a programme offered by the National Corporation of Swedish Pharmacies, individuals who had participated in 20 groups were subsequently sent a questionnaire to establish smoking status. The descriptive data obtained enabled researchers to explore and identify factors associated with cessation.[47] Clients recruited to a community pharmacy-based smoking cessation scheme in the UK were also followed-up after the end of the scheme to establish change in smoking status.[42] What is difficult to establish in these studies is the extent to which changes were directly attributable to the programme rather than other variables, especially given that participants may have been self-selecting, and results would not be comparable with those of a similar group who did not participate in the programme. Patients who had received advice from a drug information service were followed-up by telephone to gather data on subsequent outcomes. However, the extent to which any actions or outcomes may be attributable to antecedent advice would be difficult to determine.[131] In a study suggesting a favourable impact on the quality of patient care of a clinical pharmacy intervention in a psychiatric hospital, the authors acknowledged the need for a further study with a control group, if the results were to be confirmed.[21] Hospital discharge procedures and shared care initiatives on aspects of drug use and knowledge have also been assessed by subsequent follow-up of patients.[32,132]

Descriptive studies

There are many examples of the application of descriptive studies to the evaluation of service developments in both community and hospital settings.

The majority of studies to evaluate advice-giving in pharmacies are descriptive. A range of methods has been used to gather data on activities (observation, audiotape, researchers posing as clients, self-reports or diaries maintained by pharmacy staff), from which authors have described the advice-giving activities of pharmacists. Many researchers have also attempted to evaluate advice-giving in terms of its quality by, for example, comparing it with predetermined standards or the views of an 'expert panel', or by following-up clients to assess some aspects of the outcomes after advice-giving.[9–11,117,133–135]

A survey of activities of hospital pharmacists in adverse drug reaction monitoring in UK hospitals was conducted prior to the extension of the Committee on Safety of Medicines 'yellow card' scheme to hospital pharmacists. These descriptive data could provide a baseline (cf. a 'before' study).[15] To evaluate the adverse drug reaction reports by hospital pharmacists in the first year of the extension of the 'yellow card' scheme, descriptive data on the number and nature of reports were collected. Researchers also compared the reports from pharmacists with those from doctors,[136] and with subsequent surveys of adverse drug reaction reported by hospital pharmacists.[137] Descriptive data on indicators of availability and quality of key drugs (e.g. if in stock and storage facilities) provided baseline data on pharmaceutical services at primary care clinics.[138]

Evaluation of new initiatives from the perspectives of service users is seen as increasingly important. Many researchers evaluating service innovations gather descriptive data prospectively or retrospectively on the views and/or experiences relating to service users' participation in the programme and/or the outcomes. A study to evaluate a community pharmacy-based interactive patient education programme, which enabled pharmacists to give clients a personalised information letter according to their needs, was evaluated by collecting usage statistics and by surveying opinions of pharmacists and clients.[44–46] In an investigation of the potential role for pharmacists working with general medical practitioners, meetings and interventions with the practice staff and the general medical practitioners were documented.[37] Descriptive data were gathered to assess the value of offering pharmaceutical advice to elderly patients in their own homes on multiple medication, in a collaborative initiative between their pharmacist and general practitioner.[139] The evaluation of a pharmacist's participation as a member of a hospital-based community mental health team included descriptive data that encompassed documentation of all interventions, and noted if these were acted upon.[140] Descriptive data on queries and advice were collected to assess the impact of a drug information service; for each interaction, an assessment was made regarding whether possible drug misadventure had been avoided and, if so, the potential cost savings.[141]

Hypothesis-testing has been built into some descriptive studies. In assessing customers' recall of information after advice in a community pharmacy, researchers examined the hypothesis that customers who took a more active part in discussion, understood and remembered more than those who were more passive. The researchers investigated the association between these variables and also between recall of information given in busy or quiet areas of the pharmacy.[133] Descriptive data were also used to test the hypothesis that standards of prescribing in primary care could be improved by a therapeutics advisory service provided by a consultant clinical pharmacologist and a clinical pharmacist.[142]

In descriptive studies, hypothesis testing involves applying statistical procedures for association among variables in the data set. Some caution must be exercised in that, in most descriptive studies, data are collected on a large number of variables. By setting a conventional 5% level of statistical significance, many statistically significant associations will appear within a data set. These associations may just appear by chance, or may reflect some underlying trends in the data. It is important that hypotheses are stated in advance of any wider exploration of the data. Although descriptive studies can be used to identify associations among variables, caution is required before claiming that these may be causal. Exploratory analysis of descriptive data is sometimes viewed as hypothesis-generating rather than hypothesis-testing.

Frameworks

Study design and frameworks for evaluation (i.e. what is to be evaluated) are both determined largely by the study objectives. However, decisions have to be made by the researcher regarding the aspects of a programme that should be assessed as part of the evaluation and from whose perspective it should be undertaken. The evaluation may focus on a single endpoint (e.g. the evaluation of a therapeutic drug monitoring service in community pharmacy by assessing the proportion of patients with serum concentrations within a given range[23]) or include a wide range of issues (e.g. a study to evaluate a non-drug intervention programme for 'younger seniors' combined clinical measures, psychological tests and participants' views[143]). It may include variables important to policy makers (e.g. costs), health professionals (time, resources), clients (satisfaction, response to their priorities), and also indirect effects on other professionals or informal carers.

Structure–process–outcome

A framework for the assessment of health care interventions has been presented by Donabedian[144] based on the separate consideration of the structures of services, processes in their delivery and the outcomes of care. The difficulties of measuring outcomes has frequently led researchers to evaluate services in terms of the structure and the process components, a relationship between these components and outcomes being assumed.

Structure

Donabedian[144] argues that structural features (appropriate resources and system design), although not a measure of quality of care in themselves, provide the context in which care is delivered and as such may be an important influence on the process of care and hence its quality. Donabedian also views appropriate structures as the most important means of protecting and promoting good quality care. Thus, without appropriate structures and processes based on the best available evidence, optimal outcomes (attributable to the intervention) would be unlikely to result.

Structural characteristics have been part of the evaluation of both hospital[19,145] and community-based[112,146–148] pharmacy services. For the evaluation of the impact of structural factors (e.g. features of buildings, environment, organisation and staff), many of which are fixed, RCTs are generally not appropriate. Bowling[2] suggests that the most suitable approach is a descriptive survey in which data are collected within an experimental design to compare these factors in relation to outcome.

This approach was used to identify whether the management of medicines was improved by registration of a home with a community pharmacy. The study compared practices in 42 registered and 40 non-registered homes. Given that randomisation for the purposes of the study would not be possible, the higher standards of medicines management found in homes registered could be due to greater awareness of the staff and not a result of the pharmacy service. In this study, data were collected in interviews, which would provide an opportunity for researchers to explore the extent to which findings may have been attributable to the pharmacist's role.[146] In a study to examine the relationships between practice setting and community pharmacists' interactions with prescribers, researchers compared chain and independent pharmacies. Again, this study design enabled an investigation of associations among variables and the generation of hypotheses regarding causal relationships by controlling or matching for other variables.[147]

Process

Improving processes of care may be seen as an essential prerequisite for optimal outcomes, justifying the assessment of processes independently of outcomes. Moreover, the purpose of some interventions is to improve aspects of processes of delivery of health care. The objective of the implementation of a new patient-oriented pharmacy service was, among other things, to improve service delivery. Thus, the appropriate outcome measures would be expected to relate to processes of care.[26]

Many evaluation studies in the pharmacy literature focus on the processes of care. Measures to evaluate pharmacists' involvement in drug therapy decisions in a UK hospital related to the types of intervention and levels of involvement.[6] Data on the activities of nurses and pharmacy technicians were collected to assess a ward-based pharmacy technician service.[149] In research into prescription interventions in community pharmacies in New Zealand, descriptive information was gathered on the action taken by pharmacists (rather than outcomes of these actions).[8] In the evaluation of a model of collaboration between pharmacists and general medical practitioners, researchers documented inter-professional meetings and activities following the implementation of the model.[150] Many educational initiatives among pharmacy personnel have been evaluated in terms of their effect on the knowledge and skills base of the staff concerned rather than a measure of their consequences for clients.

Studies evaluating aspects of community pharmacy advisory services frequently focus on aspects of the processes of advice-giving.[10,11,134] Analysis is based on descriptive data regarding aspects of the content of advice and features of the communication. Just as suitable structural features may be important prerequisites for a satisfactory delivery of health care, the processes of advice-giving (style and conduct of the interaction) may be seen as important requirements for the achievement of desirable outcomes. Many researchers have compared processes of advice-giving with what would be considered good practice (i.e. likely to lead to desirable outcomes). Thus, in assessing advice-giving, the processes have been assessed as a proxy for outcomes. This involves explicit or implicit assumptions regarding the relationship between the processes (e.g. quality of advice) and expected health outcomes. However, from the perspective of clients, the structure (e.g. privacy) or processes of care (e.g. appropriate questions) may themselves be important aspects (and from their perspectives, outcomes) of care. In a review of research into patients' participation in decision-making regarding their therapy, the authors concluded that benefits of participation (in terms of treatment outcomes) had not been demonstrated. However, they did find that patients wanted to be informed and more involved when different treatment options were available. They argued that patient participation (as a process) in consultations was justified on the grounds of patients' wishes and self-determination.[151] Thus, in terms of the preferences and/or goals of patients, participation in decision-making was a desired outcome.

Researchers examining the relationship between appropriateness of prescribing for elderly people and health outcomes identified inappropriate prescribing as a process measure directly related to adverse health outcomes. However, they claimed that existing evidence of the relationship between inappropriate prescribing and health outcomes was sparse, although they cited some examples of studies that have attributed hospital admissions and re-admissions to inappropriate prescribing.[152]

Two descriptive studies of patient medication record systems focused on structural and process features, respectively. The first compared systems held in community pharmacies with contractual requirements,[148] while the second examined and described clinical interventions using patient medication records.[153] To determine the impact of installing consultation areas (a structural feature), researchers documented changes in the processes of advice-giving, including response times and types of question.[112] Structural and process features were also brought together in a study in which researchers hypothesised that hospital pharmacies under the pressure of managed care (working within a particular structure) would be more likely to adopt process innovations to assure more cost-effective service provision.[63] A qualitative study of illicit drug users' views of good and bad pharmacy services identified three broad categories of response: structural factors (e.g. privacy in the pharmacy), process factors (e.g. waiting times), and people factors (e.g. attitudes of staff).[93]

Outcome

The goal of many evaluation studies is to demonstrate whether or not there is any effect on patients' outcomes. The anticipated outcomes will depend on the nature and objectives of the intervention. These may be clinical measures, patterns of adherence, frequency of drug-related problems, which may result in what are sometimes regarded as true outcome measures: changes in health status, quality of life or client satisfaction. Outcomes assessed from the perspective of health professionals have included changes in inter-professional communication, prescribing patterns, job satisfaction, professional satisfaction with services and costs.

In the evaluation of health services it is common for process and outcome measures to be combined. Two studies evaluating initiatives to rationalise prescribing included the measurement of both processes and outcomes. Changes in prescribing on a long-stay hospital ward were assessed in terms of processes (the reduction in the range of drugs used) and outcomes (an improvement or no deterioration in patients' mental health state).[56] Similarly, the evaluation of a pharmaceutical advisory service in a private nursing home included measures of the proportion of medicines administered in accordance with prescribers' wishes (process) and the number of patients free of drug-induced problems (outcome).[154] A comparison of out-of-hours care provided by patients' own general practitioners and commercial deputising services focused separately on the processes of care (including response to call, time to visit, prescribing and hospital admissions)[155] and the outcomes (including health status, patient satisfaction and subsequent health service use).[156]

A number of researchers have investigated outcomes following advice-giving in pharmacies. These have included an assessment of the extent to which clients can recall information or whether their subsequent actions were in accordance with advice given.[117,133,135] In the assessment of outcomes of a programme, the evaluation is often confined to those components that are measurable. While these may be important, they may not take into account wider aspects of the context in which the services are provided. The importance of assessing the outcomes of care in the context of the wide-ranging goals and expectations of clients, health professionals and other stakeholders, many of which may be difficult to quantify, has been explored in the context of the evaluation of pharmacy services.[157]

Attention to the components of structure, process and outcome provides a useful framework for the evaluation of health services. This framework in its totality has also been used to consider the contribution of pharmacists to rational drug use.[158]

Efficacy, effectiveness and efficiency

In the early stages of service development a new initiative will often be provided (and evaluated) in a single setting, involving one or a small number of self-selecting pharmacists. In some respects, the conditions of such an initiative may be ideal in that the practitioners will be enthusiastic and/or selected on the basis of a suitable environment for the provision of a particular service. Study findings that demonstrate that under these circumstances a new intervention meets its objectives cannot necessarily be taken as evidence that in a wider range of settings the results will be reproducible. Studies conducted in one or a few sites and/or involving a few frequently self-selecting personnel may be viewed as evaluating the efficacy of the initiative, that is, under particular circumstances 'can this work?' Once the efficacy of an intervention is established, researchers may then turn their attention to evaluating the effectiveness, that is 'does it work?' when extended to a normal range of practice and working environments.

Efficacy

For any new service, it is sensible and normal practice to perform some evaluation in a limited range of settings. Reflecting this, there are many pilot and small-scale studies in the health services research and pharmacy practice literature. If problems arise in what may be favourable circumstances, then it would be unlikely that an initiative would be effective when implemented more extensively.

Examples include the evaluation of a drug information service provided free to users from a single community pharmacy,[159] a multidisciplinary programme to rationalise prescribing on a long-stay ward,[56] a study to test the hypothesis that standards of prescribing in primary care could be improved by a therapeutic advisory service provided by a consultant clinical pharmacologist and a clinical pharmacist,[142] and the development and assessment of a system of pharmaceutical care to medical progressive care patients in a single facility.[22]

These studies may be described as feasibility studies. They focus on the assessment of specific features or objectives that would be deemed essential for success. For example, prior to sending discharge information to community pharmacists, researchers established the extent to which patients reported using the same pharmacy regularly, and whether community pharmacists were in favour of the development of the scheme.[31] In a study of the use of over-the-counter ibuprofen, researchers commented on the feasibility of pharmacovigilance studies of non-prescription medicines.[160]

Thirty pharmacies were involved in a study to assess the feasibility of blood glucose measurement in community pharmacy. Feasibility was assessed on the basis of the accuracy of measurements made (by comparing measurements of samples by the participating pharmacists and a hospital ward) and by acceptability to the pharmacists.[94] These were seen as essential prerequisites for an effective service. To determine whether it was possible to detect potential problems with medication among asthma patients during routine pharmacy visits, a study was conducted in one pharmacy (with two pharmacists) in a rural town in Finland.[161]

A pilot study in a general medical practice assessed the feasibility of pharmacist involvement in opportunistic biochemical and haematological screening as an early indicator of iatrogenic disease. Although in a single setting, the study concluded that the programme was useful in assessing appropriate use of medication and alerting to potential adverse drug reactions.[95]

In a study to assess the feasibility of community pharmacy provision of a therapeutic drug monitoring service, patients taking theophylline were identified from patient medication records held by the pharmacy and offered the service. An improvement in the proportion of patients with therapeutic serum concentrations over the time period of the study demonstrated that the scheme was feasible.[23] To obtain information on outcomes following advice in the pharmacy, researchers have also investigated the feasibility of requesting pharmacy clients to maintain diaries. Both the acceptability to clients and pharmacists' reasons for non-issue of diaries were investigated.[96]

Effectiveness

In the evaluation of pharmacy services, many researchers have attempted to assess the effectiveness of new programmes in a representative range of practice settings. An evaluation of a community pharmacy-based therapeutic drug monitoring service found no statistically significant differences in the accuracy of measurements in the community pharmacy compared with those carried out by a hospital biochemistry department.[24] Researchers therefore extended the study to patients attending a community pharmacy to address issues of the service provision in a practice setting.[25] Thus, part one of the study demonstrated that an essential element of the service provision could be carried out satisfactorily (efficaciously), while part two extended this to an assessment of the effectiveness in a 'real-life' situation.

To assess whether the provision of training on asthma management can improve the knowledge base of community pharmacists, course participants were asked to demonstrate the use of various inhaler devices on arrival for the course and 3–6 months later in the pharmacy. Conducting the subsequent assessment in the practice setting may assist the researchers in gaining some insight into whether improvements demonstrated in a training environment are transferable to the practice setting.[68] Many education or training initiatives demonstrate an effect on pharmacists' knowledge and/or skills. Less clear is whether or not training affects what happens in practice. To address this problem, researchers evaluating a health promotion training programme compared practices in pharmacies in which the pharmacist had undergone the training with those in a neighbouring area.[162]

Larger studies that include a range of environments and practice settings provide information generalisable beyond the study sites. A study to assess the effectiveness of issuing a letter at discharge for patients to take to their community pharmacist involved over 500 patients distributed between control and intervention groups. Thus, the total sample will have included many and diverse community pharmacies representative of those in the area of the study.[33]

Efficiency

Demonstrating that a particular intervention is effective in meeting its objectives is often insufficient. The prominence of costs in health policy decisions necessitates a consideration of the costs and resource implications of any potential development. Not surprisingly, many evaluation studies in pharmacy include an assessment of costs and/or resource implications of service developments.[49–67]

A range of approaches to comparing the costs of different programmes have been developed by health economists, including cost-minimisation analysis, cost-effectiveness analysis, cost–benefit analysis and cost–utility analysis (see Chapter 9). There are many texts discussing these methodologies and their application in health care settings.[163]

Studies that include an assessment of costs have been conducted in both community and hospital settings. Many relate to costs (or cost savings) associated with drug usage and prescribing initiatives. For some initiatives (e.g. the introduction of prescribing formularies, use of patients' own drugs in hospital), potential financial savings are deemed an important objective. In other studies, costs may be just one of a number of considerations (e.g. the researchers evaluating a repeat prescribing review programme acknowledged that the programme would be expensive in terms of both pharmacists' and medical practitioners' time).[164]

A number of researchers have assessed the costs or cost savings associated with formulary development.[5,55,57,165] Changes in prescribing costs which may have resulted from meetings between general medical practitioners and pharmacists have also been assessed.[66] An investigation of financial savings achieved by changing dosage forms and regimens investigated the efficiency in terms of staff time and material costs.[58] The cost implications of new drug policies and changes in epidemiology of tuberculosis and HIV in Zimbabwe were assessed by comparing the costs of treatments according to the old and new regimens.[60] The cost implications of re-use of patients' own drugs have been assessed by a number of researchers, although the findings have not always been consistent.[51-53]

Appropriateness

An assessment of appropriateness is a common component in the evaluation of health care (including pharmacy) interventions. However, in the context of health care, appropriateness has been variously defined[2] and an interesting debate surrounds its operationalisation in health services research. The potential subjectivity regarding what constitutes an 'appropriate' service is addressed by Buetow et al.[166] who point out that appropriateness lacks a precise conceptual meaning that is uniformly stated and understood. They endeavour to contribute to an understanding and refinement of the construct of appropriateness by discussing how it has been defined and applied in studies of health care in general and prescribing in particular. Liberati,[167] in discussing the measurement of appropriateness of medical procedures, characterises appropriateness as 'a function of its method of construction and when and where it was defined'. He asserts that no research is interpretation-free, observing that the assessment of appropriateness may combine evidence from literature reviews and the opinions of experts. Recognising the difficulties in defining appropriateness, consensus methods (nominal group technique and Delphi method) have been employed to derive and validate indicators of the appropriateness of long-term prescribing.[168] Nominal group technique has also been used to develop a set of criteria for the assessment of appropriateness of advice-giving in community pharmacy.[169]

In discussing the development of a measure of prescribing appropriateness, Fitzgerald et al.[170] distinguish between explicit review methods, that is, standardised guidelines requiring little or no clinical judgement to apply, and implicit methods which focus on the appropriateness of the patient's entire regimen (rather than a single drug or class) and combine the patient's medical history and clinician's judgement and knowledge. In a study of drug prescribing habits related to characteristics of medical practices, researchers identified features of inappropriate prescribing.[171]

To assess the appropriateness of extemporaneous prescribing, prescriptions for extemporaneous preparations were surveyed for therapeutic appropriateness, that is, whether they conformed to recommended treatment for the diagnosis in question according to the medical literature. To assess pharmaceutical appropriateness, researchers used their own criterion of whether or not the product could have been replaced by a commercial alternative.[172] To assess inappropriate prescribing in an elderly population, researchers adopted a subset of criteria from the literature that had been developed by a panel of 'experts' in geriatric medicine and pharmacology.[173] In a study of appropriateness of prescribing in nursing homes, a local expert panel was convened to propose criteria for inappropriate prescribing. The agreed criteria were then applied to residents' drug profiles.[174] Panels of experts have also been involved in assessing the appropriateness of advice given by a drug information service.[131]

Current guidelines were used to assess the appropriateness of the management of oral health problems in community pharmacies.[10] In another study, the referral practices of community pharmacists regarding clients presenting with common ailments (established as part of an observational study[175]) were compared with the views (subsequently surveyed) of general medical practitioners regarding appropriate referral practices.[176] The outcome of a medication review process was investigated regarding the extent to which recommendations met the approval of prescribers.[123]

Acceptability

The acceptability of services (to both providers and consumers) is viewed as an important component of service evaluation. The British Government is keen to ensure that services are responsive to the priorities and needs of patients. An annual survey of users' experiences of the National Health Service forms part of the British Government's strategy of quality assurance in health services.[177]

Client satisfaction, the measurement of which presents many methodological problems, is increasingly used as an indicator of quality in health services. Many researchers in the evaluation of pharmacy interventions or services have solicited the views of participants: professionals and/or clients.[7,74, 85–87, 135, 178–180]

Low response or high attrition rates in a study may be an indication of the questionable acceptability or feasibility of a new service.[5,40,104,106,152] Researchers evaluating pharmacists' roles in formulary development noted that the recruitment of general practitioners and pharmacists to the study was easier than their retention.[5] In a study to evaluate the effectiveness of community pharmacists in supplying advice on smoking cessation, 89% of the clients recruited were from just three of the ten pharmacies originally included.[42] These results may suggest that aspects of the schemes may be insufficiently acceptable to the practitioners and/or their clients, and that to be more effective, programmes require some further refinement.

In a study of clinical pharmacy services in residential homes, experienced medical practitioners rated suggestions made by pharmacists as beneficial and sometimes potentially life-saving, thus meeting clinical objectives. However, the extent to which these same practitioners acted upon the advice did not reflect this apparent positive acceptance. The authors suggested that some questions regarding the acceptability remained unanswered.[41] This study possibly demonstrates the importance of assessing a range of objectives and outcomes when evaluating service development.

Accessibility of the pharmacist to the public is commonly voiced as a strength of pharmacy services that is valued by clients. In a review of non-prescription medicine consultations, Taylor and Greer[181] focus on availability, accessibility and approachability as the important issues and propose operational definitions for each.

Conclusion

The designs and frameworks that have been employed by researchers in the evaluation of existing and innovative pharmacy services are many and varied. The choice of design will depend on the study objectives and what is workable in a practice setting; however, it will also determine the extent to which outcomes can be confidently attributed to the programme under evaluation. Frameworks, such as Donabedian's 'structure, process, outcome', can provide researchers with a useful aid in planning their evaluation and ensuring that all the important features are included in the assessment. Researchers are then in a position to decide the most appropriate methods for gathering data and the selection of measures, which must be relevant and sensitive to the anticipated outcomes.

References

1. Bowling A. *Research Methods in Health: Investigating Health Services and Health*. Buckingham: Open University Press, 1997.
2. Hughes C M, Turner K, Fitzpatrick C, *et al*. The use of a prescribing audit tool to assess the impact of a practice pharmacist in general practice. *Pharm J* 1999; 262: 27–30.
3. Shaw C. Aspects of audit 1: The background. *BMJ* 1980; 280: 1256–8. [As cited in Reference 1.]
4. St Leger A S, Schneiden H, Walsworth-Bell J P. *Evaluating Health Services' Effectiveness*. Buckingham: Open University Press, 1992.
5. Tordoff J M, Wright D. Analysis of the impact of community pharmacists providing formulary development advice to GPs. *Pharm J* 1999; 262: 166–8.
6. Wood J, Bell D. Evaluating pharmacists' involvement in drug therapy decisions. *Pharm J* 1997; 259: 342–5.
7. Baigent B. Evaluation of clinical pharmacy in a mental health unit. *Pharm J* 1993; 250: 150–3.
8. Hulls V, Emmerton L. Prescription interventions in New Zealand community pharmacy. *J Soc Admin Pharm* 1996; 13: 198–205.
9. Caleo S, Benrimoj S, Collins D, *et al*. Clinical evaluation of community pharmacists' interventions. *Int J Pharm Pract* 1996; 4: 221–7.
10. Sowter J R, Raynor D K. The management of oral health problems in community pharmacies. *Pharm J* 1997; 259: 308–10.
11. Ferraz M B, Pereira R B, Paiva J G A, *et al*. Availability of over-the-counter drugs for arthritis in Sao Paulo, Brazil. *Soc Sci Med* 1996; 42: 1129–31.
12. Nichol M B, McCombs J S, Boghossian T, Johnson K A. The impact of patient counselling on over-the-counter drug purchasing behaviour. *J Soc Admin Pharm* 1992; 9: 11–20.
13. Steward M, Gibson S. Evaluation of the Farillon vaccine delivery service to GP practices. *Pharm J* 1994; 253: 650–1.
14. Bangen M, Grave K. Introduction of a standard prescription form for drug prescribing to farmed fish in Norway. *J Soc Admin Pharm* 1995; 3: 159–62.
15. Green C F, Mottram D R, Rowe P, Brown A M. An investigation into adverse drug reaction monitoring by UK hospital pharmacy departments. *Int J Pharm Pract* 1997; 5: 202–8.
16. Lee A, Bateman D N, Edwards C, *et al*. Reporting of adverse drug reactions by hospital pharmacists: pilot scheme. *BMJ* 1997; 315: 519.
17. Strang J, Sheridan J. Effect of Government recommendations on methadone prescribing in south-east England: a comparison of 1995 and 1997 surveys. *BMJ* 1998; 317: 1489–90.
18. Deshmukh A A, Eggleton A G, Monteath A J. Evaluation of ward pharmacy activity and effects of a change in non-stock ward supply. *Int J Pharm Pract* 1995; 3: 236–40.
19. Guerrero R M, Nickman N A, Jorgenson J A. Work activities before and after implementation of an automated dispensing system. *Am J Health Syst Pharm* 1996; 53: 548–54.
20. Radley A S, Hall J. The establishment and evaluation of a pharmacist-developed anticoagulant clinic. *Pharm J* 1994; 252: 91–2.

21. Dorevitch A, Perl E. The impact of clinical pharmacy intervention in a psychiatric hospital. *J Clin Pharm Ther* 1996; 21: 45–8.

22. Smythe M A, Shah P P, Spiteri T L, *et al*. Pharmaceutical care in medical progressive care patients. *Ann Pharmacother* 1998; 32: 294–9.

23. Maguire T A, McElnay J C. Therapeutic drug monitoring in community pharmacy – a feasibility study. *Int J Pharm Pract* 1993; 2: 168–71.

24. Hawksworth G M, Chrystyn H. Therapeutic drug and biochemical monitoring in a community pharmacy: Part 1. *Int J Pharm Pract* 1995; 3: 133–8.

25. Hawksworth G M, Chrystyn H. Therapeutic drug and biochemical monitoring in a community pharmacy: Part 2. *Int J Pharm Pract* 1995; 3: 139–44.

26. Eadon H J, Batty R, Beech E F. Implementation of a patient-orientated pharmacy service. *Int J Pharm Pract* 1996; 4: 214–20.

27. Taheney K, Tyrrell A, Cairns C, Bunn R. Influence of patient focussed care on managing medicines for discharge. *Pharm J* 1999; 262: 368–71.

28. Choo G C C, Cook H. A community and hospital pharmacy discharge liaison service by fax. *Pharm J* 1997; 259: 659–61.

29. Elfellah M S, Jappy B M. Outcomes following discharge prescription monitoring by the ward pharmacist. *Pharm J* 1996; 257: 156–7.

30. Eadon H. Use of pharmacy discharge information for transplant patients. *Pharm J* 1994; 253: 314–16.

31. Cook H. Transfer of information between hospital and community pharmacy – a feasibility study. *Pharm J* 1995; 254: 736–7.

32. Binyon D. Pharmaceutical care: its impact on patient care and the hospital-community interface. *Pharm J* 1994; 253: 344–9.

33. Duggan C, Feldman R, Hough J, Bates I. Reducing adverse prescribing discrepancies following hospital discharge. *Int J Pharm Pract* 1998; 6: 77–82.

34. Shaw H, Mackie C A, Sharki I. Evaluation of effect of pharmacy discharge planning on medication problems experienced by discharged acute admission mental health patients. *Int J Pharm Pract* 2000; 8: 144–53.

35. Sykes D, Westwood P. Training community pharmacists to advise GPs on prescribing. *Pharm J* 1997; 258: 417–19.

36. Corbett J M. The provision of prescribing advice by community pharmacists. *Pharm J* 1995; 255: 555–7.

37. Goldstein R, Hulme H, Willits J. Reviewing repeat prescribing – general practitioners and community pharmacists working together. *Int J Pharm Pract* 1998; 6: 60–6.

38. Braybrook S, Walker R. Influencing prescribing in primary care: a comparison of two different prescribing feedback methods. *J Clin Pharm Ther* 1996; 21: 247–54.

39. Pilling M, Geoghegan M, Wolfson D J, Holden J D. The St Helens and Knowsley prescribing initiative: a model for pharmacist-led meetings with GPs. *Pharm J* 1998; 260: 100–2.

40. Th van de Poel G, Bruijnzeels M A, van der Does E, Lubsen J. A way of achieving more rational drug prescribing? *Int J Pharm Pract* 1991; 1: 45–8.

41. Rees J K, Livingstone D J, Livingstone C R, Clarke C D. A community clinical pharmacy service for elderly people in residential homes. *Pharm J* 1995; 255: 54–6.

42. Bower A, Eaton K. Evaluation of the effectiveness of a community pharmacy based smoking cessation programme. *Pharm J* 1999; 262: 514–5.

43. Morrison A, Elliott L, Cowan L, *et al.* The Glasgow pharmacy summer protection campaign. *Pharm J* 1997; 258: 641–2.

44. Lindsay G H, Hesketh E A, Harden R M. Community pharmacy-based interactive patient education: 1. implementation, 2. pharmacist opinion. *Pharm J* 1994; 252: 541–4.

45. Lindsay G H, Hesketh E A, Harden R M. Community pharmacy-based interactive patient education: 3. Patient acceptability. *Pharm J* 1994; 252: 578–9.

46. Hesketh A, Lindsay G, Harden R. Interactive health promotion in the community pharmacy. *Health Educ J* 1995; 54: 294–303.

47. Isacson D, Bingefors C, Ribohn M. Quit smoking in the pharmacy – an evaluation of a smoking cessation scheme in Sweden. *J Soc Admin Pharm* 1998; 15: 164–73.

48. Dowell J, Cruikshank J, Bain J, Staines H. Repeat dispensing by community pharmacists: advantages for patients and practitioners. *Br J Gen Pract* 1998; 48: 1858–9.

49. Smyth E T M, Barr J G, Hogg G M. Potential savings achieved through sequential, intravenous to non-parenteral, antimicrobial therapy. *Pharm J* 1998; 261: 170–2.

50. Malek M. Glyceryl trinitrate sprays in the treatment of angina: a cost minimization study. *Pharm J* 1996; 257: 690–1.

51. Semple J S, Morgan J E, Garner S T, *et al.* The effect of self-administration and reuse of patients' own drugs on a hospital pharmacy. *Pharm J* 1995; 255: 124–6.

52. Miles S A, Bourns I M. Resource implications of using patients' own drugs at discharge from hospital. *Pharm J* 1995; 254: 405–7.

53. Bowden J E. Reissuing patients' medicines – a step to seamless care. *Pharm J* 1993; 251: 356–7.

54. Hopkinson P, Hutton J. Cost analysis of patient-controlled analgesia. *Pharm J* 1998; 260: 244–6.

55. Patel K. A policy for rationalising laxatives use and expenditure. *Pharm J* 1993; 250: 185–6.

56. Cloete B G, Gomez C, Lyon R, Male B M. Costs and benefits of multidisciplinary mediation review in a long-stay psychiatric ward. *Pharm J* 1992; 249: 102–3.

57. Ferguson B, Luker K, Smith K, *et al.* Preliminary findings from an economic analysis of nurse prescribing. *Int J Pharm Pract* 1998; 6: 127–32.

58. Wallenius K, Tuovinen K, Naaranlahti T, Enlund H. Savings at ward level through simplification of dose schedules. *Int J Pharm Pract* 1996; 4: 55–8.

59. Ryan M, Bond C. Using the Economic Theory of Consumer Surplus to estimate the benefits of dispensing doctors and prescribing pharmacists. *J Soc Admin Pharm* 1996; 13: 178–87.

60. Maponga C C, Nazerali H, Mungwindiri C, Wingwiri M. Cost implications of the tuberculosis/HIV co-epidemic and drug treatment of tuberculosis in Zimbabwe. *J Soc Admin Pharm* 1996; 13: 20–9.

61. March G, Gilbert A, Roughead E, Quintrell N. Developing and evaluating a model for pharmaceutical care in Australian community pharmacies. *Int J Pharm Pract* 1999; 7: 220–9.

62. Sinclair H, Silcock J, Bond CM, *et al*. The cost-effectiveness of intense pharmaceutical intervention in assisting people to stop smoking. *Int J Pharm Pract* 1999; 7: 107–12.

63. Sloan F A, Whetten-Goldstein K, Wilson A. Hospital pharmacy decisions, cost containment, and the use of cost-effectiveness analysis. *Soc Sci Med* 1997; 45: 523–33.

64. Krass I, Smith C. Impact of medication regimen reviews performed by community pharmacists for ambulatory patients through liaison with general medical practitioners. *Int J Pharm Pract* 2000; 8: 111–20.

65. French M T, McGeary K A, Chitwood D D, McCoy C B. Chronic illicit drug use, health service utilisation and the cost of medical care. *Soc Sci Med* 2000; 50: 1703–13.

66. Geoghegan M, Pilling M, Holden J, Wolfson D. A controlled evaluation of the effect of community pharmacists on general practitioner prescribing. *Pharm J* 1998; 261: 864–6.

67. Rodgers S, Avery AJ, Meecham D, *et al*. Controlled trial of pharmacist intervention in general practice: the effect on prescribing costs. *Br J Gen Pract* 1999; 49: 717–20.

68. Wilcock M, White M. Asthma training and the community pharmacist. *Pharm J* 1998; 260: 315–17.

69. Collett J H, Rees J A, Crowther I, Mylrea S. A model for the development of work-based learning and its assessment. *Pharm J* 1995; 254: 556–8.

70. Morrow N C, Benson M A. A self-instructional management course for pre-registration trainees. *Pharm J* 1993; 251: 288–90.

71. Batty R, Barber N, Moclair A, Shackle D. Assertion skills for clinical pharmacists. *Pharm J* 1993; 251: 353–5.

72. Bond C M, Williams A, Taylor RJ, *et al*. An introduction to audit in Grampian: a basic course for pharmacists. *Pharm J* 1993; 250: 645–7.

73. Mottram D R, Rowe P H. Evaluation of the impact of recent changes in postgraduate continuing education for pharmacists in England. *Int J Pharm Pract* 1996; 4: 123–8.

74. Rees J A, Collett J H, Mylrea S, Crowther I. Subject-centred learning outcomes of structured work-based learning in a community pharmacy training programme. *Int J Pharm Pract* 1996; 4: 171–4.

75. Savela E, Hannula A M. Different forms of in-company training and their suitability for pharmacies. *J Soc Admin Pharm* 1991; 8: 76–80.

76. Damsgaard J J, Folke P E, Launso L, Schaefer K. Effects of local interventions towards prescribing of psychotropic drugs. *J Soc Admin Pharm* 1992; 9: 179–84.

77. Totten C, Morrow N. Developing a training programme for pharmacists in coronary heart disease prevention. *Health Educ J* 1990; 49: 117–20.

78. Sinclair H, Bond C, Lennox AS, *et al*. An evaluation of a training workshop for pharmacists based on the Stages of Change model of smoking cessation. *Health Educ J* 1997; 56: 296–312.

79. Santoso B. Small group intervention vs. formal seminar for improving appropriate drug use. *Soc Sci Med* 1996; 42: 1163–8.

80. Sinclair H K, Bond C M, Lennox A S. The long-term learning effect of training in stage of change for smoking cessation: a three year follow-up of

community pharmacy staff's knowledge and attitudes. *Int J Pharm Pract* 1999; 7: 1–11.

81. McPherson G, Davies G, McRobbie D. Pre-registration trainee clinical competence: a baseline assessment. *Pharm J* 1999; 263: 168–72.

82. Savela E, Lilja J, Enlund H. Continuing education by teleconference to remote areas. *J Soc Admin Pharm* 1996; 13: 159–66.

83. Livingstone C R, Pugh A L G, Winn S, Williamson V K. Developing community pharmacy services wanted by local people: information and advice about prescription medicines. *Int J Pharm Pract* 1996; 4: 92–102.

84. Krass I. A comparison of clients' experiences of counselling for prescriptions and over-the-counter medications in two types of pharmacies: validation of a research instrument. *J Soc Admin Pharm* 1996; 13: 206–14.

85. Franzen S, Lilja J, Hamilton D, Larsson S. How do Finnish women evaluate verbal pharmacy over-the-counter information? *J Soc Admin Pharm* 1996; 3: 99–108.

86. Hoog S. Positive and negative incidents perceived by self-care pharmacy customers. *J Soc Admin Pharm* 1994; 11: 86–96.

87. Dowell J S, Snadden D, Dunbar J A. Rapid prescribing change: how do patients respond? *Soc Sci Med* 1996; 43: 1543–9.

88. Rickles N M, Wertheimer A I, McGhan W F. The selective attention model for patient evaluation of pharmaceutical services (SAMPEPS). *J Soc Admin Pharm* 1998; 15: 174–89.

89. Whitehead P, Atkin P, Krass I, Benrimoj S I. Patient drug information and consumer choice of pharmacy. *Int J Pharm Pract* 199; 7: 71–9.

90. Read R W, Krska J. Targeted medication review: patients in the community with chronic pain. *Int J Pharm Pract* 1998; 6: 216–22.

91. Clarke K, Sheridan J, Williamson S, Griffiths P. Consumer preferences among pharmacy needle exchange attendees. *Pharm J* 1998; 261: 64–6.

92. Anderson C. Health promotion by community pharmacists: consumers' views. *Int J Pharm Pract* 1998; 6: 2–12.

93. Matheson C. Illicit drug users' views of a good and bad pharmacy service. *J Soc Admin Pharm* 1998; 15: 104–16.

94. King M J, Halloran S P, Kwong P Y P. Blood glucose measurement in the community pharmacy. *Pharm J* 1993; 250: 808–10.

95. Broderick W M, Purves I N, Edwards C. The use of biochemical screening in general practice – a role for pharmacists. *Pharm J* 1992; 249: 618–20.

96. Cantrill J A, Vaezi L, Nicolson M, Noyce P R. A study to explore the feasibility of using a health diary to monitor therapeutic outcomes from over-the-counter medicines. *J Soc Admin Pharm* 1995; 12: 190–8.

97. Matheson C I, Smith B H, Flett G, *et al.* Over-the-counter emergency contraception: a feasible option. *Fam Pract* 1998; 15: 38–43.

98. Boorman S, Cairns C. Another way forward for pharmaceutical care: a team-based clinical pharmacy service. *Pharm J* 2000; 264: 343–6.

99. Coast-Senior E A, Kronor B A, Kelley C L. Management of patients with type 2 diabetes by pharmacists in primary care clinics. *Ann Pharmacother* 1998; 32: 636–41.

100. Holme Hansen E, Launso L. Is the controlled clinical trial sufficient as a drug technology assessment? *J Soc Admin Pharm* 1989; 3: 117–26.

101. Bemaerkinger til Forslag om lov om et teknologinaevn, lovforslag nr. L 167 (Remarks to Bill to Danish Parliament on a Technology Board, Bill No. L167. Sheet No. 928.)

102. Glasgow N J, Murdoch J C, Baynouna L, *et al*. Doing randomised controlled trials in a developing country: some practical realities. *Fam Pract* 1996; 13: 98–103.

103. Britton A, McKee M, Black N, *et al*. Threats to applicability of randomised trials: exclusions and selective participating. *J Health Serv Res Policy* 1999; 4: 112–21.

104. Ghalamkari H H, Rees J E, Saltrese-Taylor A, Ramsden M. Evaluation of a pilot health promotion project in pharmacies: 1. Quantifying the pharmacist's health promotion role. *Pharm J* 1997; 258: 138–43.

105. Ghalamkari H H, Rees J E, Saltrese-Taylor A. Evaluation of a pilot health promotion project in pharmacies: 2. Clients' initial views on pharmacists' advice. *Pharm J* 1997; 258: 314–17.

106. Ghalamkari H H, Rees J E, Saltrese-Taylor A. Evaluation of a pilot health promotion project in pharmacies: 3. Clients' further opinions and actions taken after receiving health promotion advice. *Pharm J* 1997; 258: 909–13.

107. Abel U, Koch A. The role of randomisation in clinical studies: myths and beliefs. *J Clin Epidemiol* 1999; 52: 487–97.

108. Wilson S, Delaney B C, Roalfe A, *et al*. Randomised controlled trials in primary care: a case study. *BMJ* 2000; 321: 24–7.

109. McPherson K, Britton A R, Wennberg J E. Are randomised controlled trials controlled? Patient preferences and unblind trials. *J R Soc Med* 1997; 90: 552–6.

110. Torgerson DJ, Klaber-Moffett J, Russell I T. Patient preferences in randomised trials: threat or opportunity? *J Health Serv Res Policy* 1996; 1: 194–7.

111. Edwards S J L, Lilford R J, Hewison J. The ethics of randomised controlled trials from the perspective of the patient, the public and health care professionals. *BMJ* 1998; 3: 1209–12.

112. Harper R, Harding G, Savage I, *et al*. Consultation areas in community pharmacies: an evaluation. *Pharm J* 1998; 261: 947–50.

113. Tucker P P, Wertheimer A I. Placebo effect: its role in adherence, treatment effectiveness and patient outcomes. *Int J Pharm Pract* 1995; 3: 68–73.

114. Grabenstein J D, Hartzema A G, Guess H A, Johnston W P. Community pharmacists as immunisation advocates: a pharmacoepidemiological experiment. *Int J Pharm Pract* 1993; 2: 5–10.

115. Begley S, Livingstone C, Hodges N, Williamson V. Impact of domiciliary pharmacy visits on medication management in an elderly population. *Int J Pharm Pract* 1997; 5: 111–21.

116. Stapleton L J, Liddell H, Daly M J. Inhaler technique – a pilot study comparing verbal and computer counselling. *Pharm J* 1996; 256: 866–8.

117. Rantucci M J, Segal H J. Over-the-counter medication: outcome and effectiveness of patient counselling. *J Soc Admin Pharm* 1986; 3: 81–91.

118. Berwick S J, Lanningan N A, Ratcliff A. Effect of patient education in postoperative patients using patient-controlled analgesia. *Int J Pharm Pract* 1994; 3: 53–5.

119. Jaber LA, Halapy H, Fernet M, *et al*. Evaluation of a pharmaceutical care model on diabetes management. *Ann Pharmacother* 1996; 30: 238–43.

120. Cromarty E, Downie G, Wilkinson S, Cromarty J A. Communication regarding the discharge medicines of elderly patients: a controlled trial. *Pharm J* 1998; 260: 62–4.

121. Granas A, Bates I. The effect of pharmaceutical review of repeat prescriptions in general practice. *Int J Pharm Pract* 1999; 7: 264–75.

122. Bentley E M, Mackie I C, Fuller S. Pharmacists and the 'smile for sugar-free medicines' campaign. *Pharm J* 1993; 251: 606–7.

123. Bellingham M, Wiseman I C. Pharmacist intervention in an elderly care facility. *Int J Pharm Pract* 1996; 4: 25–9.

124. Anderson C, Alexander A. Wiltshire pharmacy health promotion training initiative: a telephone survey. *Int J Pharm Pract* 1997; 5: 185–91.

125. Roddick E, Maclean R, McKean C, *et al.* Communication with general practitioners. *Pharm J* 1993; 251: 816–19.

126. Bond C M, Grimshaw J, Taylor R, Winfield A J. The evaluation of clinical guidelines to ensure appropriate 'over-the-counter' advice in community pharmacies: a preliminary study. *J Soc Admin Pharm* 1998; 15: 33–9.

127. Stevenson M, Taylor J. The effect of a front-shop pharmacist on non-prescription medication consultations. *J Soc Admin Pharm* 1995; 12: 154–8.

128. McCaig D J, Hind C A, Downie G, Wilkinson S. Antibiotic use in elderly hospital inpatients before and after the introduction of treatment guidelines. *Int J Pharm Pract* 1999; 7: 18–28.

129. Wilson K A, Jesson J, Staunton N. Evaluation of a new health centre pharmacy: a case study. *Int J Pharm Pract* 2000; 8: 97–102.

130. Roughead E E, Gilbert A L, Primrose J G. Improving drug use: a case study of events which led to changes in use of flucloxacillin in Australia. *Soc Sci Med* 1999; 48: 845–53.

131. Melnyk P S, Shevchuk Y M, Remillard A J. Impact of the dial access drug information service on patient outcome. *Ann Pharmacother* 2000; 34: 585–92.

132. Ashcroft D M, Clark C M, Gorman S P. Shared care: a study of patients' experiences with erythropoietin. *Int J Pharm Pract* 1998; 6: 145–9.

133. Wilson M, Robinson E J, Blenkinsopp A, Panton R. Customers' recall of information given in community pharmacies. *Int J Pharm Pract* 1992; 1: 152–9.

134. Morrow N, Hargie O, Donnelly H, Woodman C. 'Why do you ask?' A study of questioning behaviour in community pharmacist–client consultations. *Int J Pharm Pract* 1993; 2: 90–4.

135. Evans S W, John D N, Bloor M J, Luscombe D K. Use of non-prescription advice offered to the public by pharmacists. *Int J Pharm Pract* 1997; 5: 16–25.

136. Davis S, Coulson R A, Wood S M. Adverse reaction reporting by hospital pharmacists: the first year. *Pharm J* 1999; 262: 366–7.

137. Green C F, Mottram D R, Rowe P H, Brown A M. Adverse drug reaction monitoring by United Kingdom hospital pharmacy departments: impact of the introduction of 'yellow card' reporting for pharmacists. *Int J Pharm Pract* 1999; 7: 238–46.

138. Kishuna A, Smit J. Assessing pharmaceutical services at primary care clinics in Kwa Zulu-Natal: an indicator based approach. *Int J Pharm Pract* 1999; 7: 143–8.

139. Fairbrother J, Mottram D R, Williamson P M. The doctor–pharmacist interface: a preliminary evaluation of domiciliary visits by a community pharmacist. *J Soc Admin Pharm* 1993; 10: 85–91.

140. Kettle J, Downie G, Palin A, Chesson R. Pharmaceutical care activities within a mental health team. *Pharm J* 1996; 257: 814–16.

141. Kinky D E, Erush S C, Laskin M S, Gibson G A. Economic impact of a drug information service. *Ann Pharmacother* 1999; 33:11–16.

142. Wood K M, Mucklow J C, Boath E M. Influencing prescribing in primary care: a collaboration between clinical pharmacology and clinical pharmacy. *Int J Pharm Pract* 1997; 5: 1–5.

143. Brendstrup E, Launso L. Evaluation of a non-drug intervention programme for younger seniors. *J Soc Admin Pharm* 1993; 10: 23–35.

144. Donabedian A. *Explorations in Quality Assessment and Monitoring*, vol 1. *The Definition of Quality and Approaches to its Assessment*. Michigan: Health Administration Press, 1980.

145. Cavell G F, Hughes D K. Does computerised prescribing improve the accuracy of drug administration? *Pharm J* 1997; 259: 782–4.

146. Norman F, Scrimshaw A. Do residential homes benefit from registration with a community pharmacy? *Pharm J* 1994; 252: 97–9.

147. Raisch D W. Interactions between community pharmacists and prescribers: differences between practice settings. *J Soc Admin Pharm* 1993; 10: 42–51.

148. Noble S C, MacDonald A. Monitoring of patient medication records in two Scottish health board areas. *Pharm J* 1992; 249: 406–8.

149. Langham J M, Boggs K S. The effect of a ward-based pharmacy technician service. *Pharm J* 2000; 264: 961–3.

150. Chen T F, Crampton M, Krass I, Benrimoj S I. Collaboration between community pharmacists and GPs: the medication review process. *J Soc Admin Pharm* 1999; 16: 145–56.

151. Guadagnoli E, Ward P. Patient participation in decision-making. *Soc Sci Med* 1998; 47: 329–39.

152. Schmader K E, Hanlon J T, Landsman P B. Inappropriate prescribing and health outcomes in elderly veteran outpatients. *Ann Pharmacother* 1997; 31: 529–33.

153. Rogers PJ, Fletcher G, Rees JE. Clinical interventions by community pharmacists using patient medication records. *Int J Pharm Pract* 1994; 3: 6–13.

154. Deshmukh A A, Sommerville H. A pharmaceutical advisory service in a private nursing home: provision and outcome. *Int J Pharm Pract* 1996; 4: 88–93.

155. Cragg D K, McKinley R K, Roland M O, *et al*. Comparison of out of hours care provided by patients' own general practitioners and commercial deputising services: a randomised controlled trial 1: the process of care. *BMJ* 1997; 314: 187–9.

156. McKinley R K, Cragg D K, Hastings A M, *et al*. Comparison of out of hours care provided by patients' own general practitioners and commercial deputising services: a randomised controlled trial 2: the outcome of care. *BMJ* 1997; 314: 190–3.

157. Watson P. Community pharmacists and mental health: an evaluation of two pharmaceutical care programmes. *Pharm J* 1997; 258: 419–22.

158. Han B-H, Sorofman B A. Toward a theory of pharmacists' contribution to rational drug use. *J Soc Admin Pharm* 1996; 13: 109–20.
159. Muhammed T, Ghalamkari H, Millar G, Hirst J. A community drug information service. *Pharm J* 1998; 260: 278–80.
160. Sinclair H K, Bond C M, Hannaford P C. Over-the-counter ibuprofen: how and why is it used? *Int J Pharm Pract* 2000; 8: 121–7.
161. Narhi U, Vainio K, Ahonen R, *et al.* Detecting problems of patients with asthma in a community pharmacy: a pilot study. *J Soc Admin Pharm* 1999; 16: 127–33.
162. Anderson C. A controlled study of the effect of a health promotion training scheme on pharmacists' advice about smoking cessation. *J Soc Admin Pharm* 1995; 12: 115–24.
163. Drummond M F, Stoddart G L, Torrance G W. *Methods for the Economic Evaluation of Health Care Programmes.* Oxford: Oxford University Press, 1997.
164. Sykes D, Westwood P, Gilleghan J. Development of a review programme for repeat prescription medicines. *Pharm J* 1996; 256: 458–60.
165. Ekedahl A, Petersson B-A, Eklund P, *et al.* Prescribing patterns and drug costs: effects of formulary recommendations and community pharmacists' information campaigns. *Int J Pharm Pract* 1994; 2: 194–8.
166. Buetow S A, Sibbald S, Cantrill J A, Halliwell S. Appropriateness in health care: application to prescribing. *Soc Sci Med* 1997; 45: 261–71.
167. Liberati A. Assessing the appropriateness of care. *J Health Serv Res Policy* 1996; 1: 53–4.
168. Cantrill J A, Sibbald B, Buetow S. Indicators of the appropriateness of long term prescribing in general practice in the United Kingdom: consensus development, face and content validity, feasibility and reliability. *Qual Health Care* 1998; 7: 130–5.
169. Bissell P, Ward P, Noyce P R. Appropriateness measurement: application to advice-giving in community pharmacies. *Soc Sci Med* 2000; 51: 343–59.
170. Fitzgerald L S, Hanlon J T, Shelton P S, *et al.* Reliability of a modified medication appropriateness index in ambulatory older persons. *Ann Pharmacother* 1997; 31: 543–8.
171. Ferguson J A. Drug prescribing habits related to characteristics of medical practice. *J Soc Admin Pharm* 1990; 7: 34–47.
172. Kettis-Lindblad A, Isacson D, Eriksson C. Assessment of appropriateness of extemporaneous preparations prescribed in Swedish primary care. *Int J Pharm Pract* 1996; 4: 117–22.
173. Aparasu R R, Fliginger S E. Inappropriate medication prescribing for the elderly by office-based physicians. *Ann Pharmacother* 1997; 31: 823–9.
174. Lunn J, Chan K, Donoghue J, *et al.* A study of the appropriateness of prescribing in nursing homes. *Int J Pharm Pract* 1997; 5: 6–10.
175. Smith F J. Referral of clients by community pharmacists in primary care consultations. *Int J Pharm Pract* 1993; 2: 86–9.
176. Smith F J. Referral of clients by community pharmacists: views of general medical practitioners. *Int J Pharm Pract* 1996; 4: 30–5.
177. Government White Paper. A first class service: quality in the new NHS 13175. London: Stationery Office, 1998.

178. Burtonwood A M, Hinchliffe A L, Tinkler G G. A prescription for quality: a role for the clinical pharmacist in general practice. *Pharm J* 1998; 261: 678–80.
179. Anderson C. Health promotion by community pharmacists: consumers' views. *Int J Pharm Pract* 1998; 6: 1–12.
180. Whittlesea C M C, Walker R. An adverse drug reaction reporting scheme for community pharmacists. *Int J Pharm Pract* 1996; 4: 228–34.
181. Taylor J, Greer M. NPM consultations: an analysis of pharmacist availability, accessibility and approachability. *J Soc Admin Pharm* 1993; 10: 101–8.

9

Evaluation of pharmaceutical services: methods and measures

A full range of health services research methods has been employed in the evaluation of services. Aspects of the application of the principal methods to the evaluation of existing and innovative pharmacy services are considered here. The evaluation of any service requires measures that are relevant to its objectives and sensitive to the anticipated outcomes. The identification of suitable, valid and reliable measures is both challenging to researchers and essential for the fair and successful evaluation of any programme. This chapter discusses the development and selection of measures which have been employed in the evaluation of pharmacy services.

Methods

Both quantitative and qualitative methods have been applied in the evaluation of pharmaceutical services. Quantitative procedures enable the evaluation of a programme in terms of measurable (quantifiable) variables, such as drug costs, prescribing patterns, numbers of requests for advice and rates of compliance or adherence. Quantitative data are also required for descriptive and comparative statistical procedures, the comparison of outcomes of different programmes and investigations of associations between variables. In these studies, the data are collected within a predetermined, standardised framework devised by the researcher according to specific anticipated outcomes of a programme.

Qualitative approaches, which are often exploratory in nature, have been used to identify and assess the outcomes of programmes from different perspectives, including unforeseen problems and benefits. The application and rationale for the employment of qualitative approaches was described by Watson[1] who evaluated two pharmaceutical care programmes in mental health from the perspective of the individuals involved, both professionals and consumers. Through qualitative methods the researcher established what these stakeholders wanted the programmes to achieve and the criteria they would use to judge success. She pointed out that using this approach a wide range of anticipated and actual outcomes would be identified, and that the findings would be expected to uncover both positive and negative aspects. This contrasts with quantitative approaches in which decisions are taken in advance regarding the relevant outcome(s) and appropriate measures.

Surveys

In terms of evaluation of services, surveys can be an efficient method of gathering data and have been used among pharmacists and their staff,[2–10] as well as other professional groups, in particular medical practitioners[2,4,11–15] and nurses,[14,16,17] but also clients.[3,17–30]

These studies generally focus on opinions and experiences of services from the perspectives of the population surveyed. Data on perceived or actual outcomes of interventions, for example, improved patient knowledge[31] or recall of information following counselling,[26,27,31] and smoking cessation following a health promotion programme,[29] have also been obtained using survey methods among programme participants. An assessment of the contribution of intensive care pharmacists in the UK was based on data gathered in a postal questionnaire regarding the common roles of pharmacists.[32] Structured questionnaires were also used to assess the acceptability and understandability of drug information leaflets.[33]

Interviews

Structured, semi-structured and in-depth interviews have been used in the evaluation of pharmacy services. The advantage of collecting data by structured interview, rather than self-completion questionnaire, is that it provides the researcher with the opportunity to ensure that comprehensive data are gathered and to clarify any ambiguous responses. For example, data on the management of medicines in residential homes were collected in interviews with a senior member of staff. This enabled the researchers to ensure they obtained the comprehensive information required to assess whether or not procedures and activities of medicines management complied with Royal Pharmaceutical Society of Great Britain and local authority guidelines.[34] In general, interview methods are not feasible if the researcher wishes to gain views from a large or widely dispersed sample. However, in the evaluation of some initiatives, structured follow-up interviews have been conducted by telephone.[10,26,35,36]

In semi-structured or unstructured (in-depth, qualitative) interviews, the researcher aims to gather information from the perspective of the respondents, giving them the opportunity to raise issues important to themselves, some of which may not have been apparent to the service providers or the research team. Thus, these interviews may uncover aspects that could otherwise have been missed. Qualitative interview methods have been employed to explore the perspectives of different stakeholders regarding two mental health pharmaceutical care programmes.[1] They were also used to obtain patients' views regarding changes to their prescribed medication.[37] Focus groups have been employed in the evaluation of collaboration between pharmacists and medical practitioners.[38,39]

There are examples of the application of other techniques to evaluate services from the perspective of service users. For example, a cognitive interactional psychology model was applied to analyse how Finnish women assessed the value of information provided by pharmacists. For each of five pre-recorded video-vignettes, women completed a questionnaire assessing the vignette on a number of cognitive scales. The data were used to explore conscious and unconscious cognitive processes employed in assessing the consultations.[40] The application of the 'selective attention model for patient evaluation of pharmaceutical services' has been discussed regarding the evaluation of aspects of community pharmacy services. This framework is based on cognitive psychology research concerning how humans subconsciously process and selectively attend to certain information.[41] Critical incidents technique is also a process intended to identify issues of relevance from the perspective of research subjects. It has been used to identify positive and negative incidents in service provision as perceived by pharmacy customers.[42] A literature evaluation was undertaken to establish how pharmacy services are valued, that is, how the benefits of pharmacy services are perceived and who are the beneficiaries.[43]

Observation

Observation has been employed in the evaluation of services, both as the sole method of data collection and in combination with others. Data from direct observation of the drug administration process in hospitals were used to compare the accuracy of administration using hand-written and computer-generated charts.[44] In a community pharmacy setting, data were collected by observation to evaluate the effects of the location of the pharmacist within the pharmacy on giving advice about non-prescription medicines.[45]

Covert observation, in which the subjects are unaware that they are being observed, and overt observation methods have been used to provide descriptive data for the assessment of quality of advice-giving in community pharmacies,[46–54] and to evaluate training programmes.[55] Observation has been used in combination with other methods to provide a more comprehensive data set on different aspects of a pro-gramme,[1,56] as well as to validate data collected by other methods.[56,57] Descriptive data were maintained on the establishment and operation of a village level treatment facility in Sri Lanka over an 18-month study period, during which a researcher visited to observe the operation and to discuss it with staff and clients.[58]

Analysis of routinely collected data

In the evaluation of many initiatives, researchers have been able to draw on existing data sets (e.g. routinely collected prescription data, reports to official bodies of adverse drug reactions), rather than gathering their own data.[5,12,57,59–70] If a suitable data set can be identified, it may provide a convenient and inexpensive data source. However, because the data have been collected for a different purpose, they often present limitations when used to evaluate specific outcomes of health care pro-grammes. As the researchers do not generally have responsibility for the maintenance of the database, they have to satisfy themselves regarding the completeness and reliability of the information. Researchers also have no control over the variables in the data set; variables that are important indicators of successful outcomes or, more commonly, con-founding variables might not be included. Thus, researchers may be unable to comment on certain outcomes or, because of a lack of relevant contextual information, be unable to draw conclusions regarding the extent to which outcomes are attributable to the intervention. For inter-ventions assessed by comparing before-and-after data, researchers must be satisfied that the data are sufficiently sensitive to pick up changes, especially if they are expected to be small. Prior to any evaluation, careful consideration has to be given to whether or not an existing data set provides the necessary variables, and is sufficiently sensitive and complete.

A study was undertaken to assess the validity and reliability of an electronic, population-based prescription database of dispensed prescriptions.[71] The accuracy was assessed by comparing details from original prescriptions with information on the database. The validity of the information was questioned in that comparison of database records with prescriptions submitted revealed that the database under-represented prescriptions dispensed for the aboriginal population in the area.[71]

Structured data on processes

Many researchers have devised their own data collection instruments to ensure that relevant data pertinent to the processes of the service and the evaluation are obtained.[5,17,21–23,46,72–82] Researchers decide for themselves on the appropriate variables, the level of detail required and the feasibility of data collection. Information collected in this way commonly relates to the processes of service delivery, such as frequency of uptake of services, numbers or characteristics of events, and/or contextual variables. Data were collected on enrolments and timing of the delivery of different aspects of a community pharmacy-based interactive patient health education programme.[77,78] The impact of using pharmacy window space for health promotion about emergency hormonal contraception included the collection of data on the number of enquiries during the campaign, uptake of leaflets and the number of prescriptions for emergency hormonal contraception that were dispensed when compared with a control phase.[83] Community pharmacists have also been asked to maintain logbooks to record details of health promotion activities,[57,73] and to document structured information on oral health queries and advice given.[46] To evaluate a community pharmacy-based telephone drug information service, data were recorded on the number and type of queries.[22] Patients have also been requested to maintain diaries to record particular events and activities.[14,84] Maintaining records in sufficient detail can be a time-consuming and demanding task. Researchers must be assured of the feasibility of data collection procedures in the context of the delivery of the services, for example, reliability and completeness of data at busy times, validity and adherence to study protocols.

Work sampling techniques have been used to obtain data on activities of pharmacists.[17,80,82,85–89] Pagers emitting an audible signal at random intervals prompt participants to record their activities at that time. The number of signals per hour varies between studies. Researchers should ensure that the frequency is acceptable to the participants, while providing sufficient data. The applications, advantages and limitations of work measurement techniques, including sampling methods and validation in pharmacy research, have also been addressed.[88,90] The findings of studies employing work sampling have been reviewed.[91]

Triangulation

There are many examples in the literature of evaluation studies in which researchers have employed a range of methods to obtain information on different aspects of a programme or data from the perspectives of different population groups.[1,20,38,56,77,78,90,92] Combining methods and comparing the data also enables the researchers to validate their findings. To determine the impact of installing consultation areas in community pharmacies, pharmacists recorded customers' health-related queries in logbooks. To validate the data, observation by a researcher of pharmacists' response times and the nature of questions, and structured questionnaires to clients in a subset of pharmacies, were also undertaken.[57]

Measures

The measures selected for an evaluation will depend on the objectives of the service or intervention and its anticipated outcomes. Existing structured measures (identified from the literature) and/or those devised by researchers specifically for their study may be employed. In some cases, evaluation of existing or new services has been conducted by comparison with accepted standards or guidelines derived from the literature, professional bodies or other sources.

An advantage of incorporating existing structured measures is that some testing of their reliability and validity will have already been undertaken. In addition, incorporating measures that have been applied by others enables comparisons between studies. Limitations include difficulties of finding a suitable measure, and the fact that the original validation may have been restricted to certain population groups. Among the most commonly employed existing structured measures in health services research are those devised to assess aspects of health status (e.g. self-perceived health, functional ability, social functioning, pain) or health-related quality of life.

Many structured measures or scales comprise a series of items, the responses to which are combined (often summed) to produce an overall score. The De Tullio score was used to assess patients' inhaler technique to compare outcomes following verbal and computer counselling. A score out of 11 was allocated according to the number of correct manoeuvres (e.g. shaking the inhaler, holding upright, exhaling normally).[93] An established measure was also used to test pharmacists' knowledge of inhaler devices before and after a training programme. Scores were obtained against a checklist specific for each device (e.g. drug contained, age for which suitable, use of the device).[94] Patients' dexterity in managing their medicines was assessed by their ability to perform five tests (e.g. opening child resistant containers). They were allowed one minute for each task and could obtain a score between zero and five.[95]

To compare clients' experiences of counselling for prescription and over-the-counter medicines in two types of pharmacy, respondents reported their experiences of receiving different types of information (e.g. how to take the medication, what it is for, precautions to take when using it) on a five-point Likert scale spanning one (none of the time) to five (all of the time). The general frequency of counselling score for each type of information was then computed by summing the responses. Cronbach's alpha, which is commonly used to examine internal consistency of a measure, was employed by these researchers.[30]

If no suitable measure exists, researchers may opt to devise their own. In an evaluation of the impact of carers' attitudes on the safety of medication procedures in UK residential homes, the researchers discuss how they constructed a scale which comprised a series of statements, some of which were drawn from statements of good practice contained within national guidelines and established codes of practice. Responses of staff were compared with the types of medication administration systems in operation at the homes.[96]

The measurement of attitudes requires the identification of issues that influence a person's viewpoint and the development of a series of items (to which respondents are commonly asked to indicate their level of agreement) which cover the different viewpoints and strengths of opinion, and which discriminate among individuals with different attitudes (see Chapter 2). To assess attitudes of pharmacists to audit, researchers adopted a questionnaire that had previously been developed and used with general medical practitioners.[97]

Evaluation has also been undertaken by comparing practice with accepted standards, guidelines or policy recommendations, which thus provide a criterion for reference.[31,34,46,98–104] For example, patient medication records held by pharmacies in Scotland were evaluated against a checklist derived from the requirements specified in a health service circular[98]; advice given by pharmacists in response to oral health queries was assessed against existing guidelines,[46] and treatment of tuberculosis was evaluated by documenting the extent of adherence to protocols for its treatment.[99] To assess the impact of guidelines a before-and-after study was conducted prior to, immediately after and 10 months following, the introduction of treatment guidelines for antibiotic use.[102]

Physiological measures

Physiological measures have formed part of studies to assess the feasibility of clinical activities in community pharmacy settings. These have included blood glucose monitoring,[23] therapeutic drug monitoring services based in community pharmacies,[105–107] or a role for pharmacists in early identification of (or prediction of potential) adverse drug reactions.[108] Measures included a range of biochemical and haematological parameters and plasma drug concentrations. Physiological parameters have also been employed as outcome measures in evaluating the impact of pharmaceutical interventions. Evaluation of a pharmacist-run anticoagulant clinic included an assessment of the extent to which patients' INRs (international normalised ratios) were maintained within the range specified by their clinician.[31] The evaluation of a pharmaceutical care model for the management of non-insulin-dependent diabetes included measurement of fasting plasma glucose, glycated haemoglobin concentrations and other measures, such as blood pressure, creatinine and cholesterol.[109] In some cases, physiological parameters were combined with other measures, such as symptoms,[110] health status,[109] hospitalisation and need for emergency care.[111,112]

Measurement of health status

Rather than relying on physiological parameters, researchers may wish to include measures that reflect the impact of a disease or drug therapy on an individual's ability to perform various activities of daily life, their general well-being or wider aspects of their health status or health-related quality of life. In any study, a number of measures may be used in combination. There are many instruments available for the measurement of health status and health-related quality of life. These include generic health status measures (e.g. SF36, SF12, HSQ12), disease-specific measures (e.g. GHQ for anxiety and depression, Arthritis Impact Measurement Scale, McGill pain questionnaire), measures of functional ability and self-perceived health. The development and application of both generic health status and disease-specific measures have been comprehensively reviewed by Bowling.[113,114] New measures are continually being developed, and many existing measures are being validated, revised and/or updated for use among different population groups. If suitable instruments exist it is advisable to use these rather than attempt to develop another. The application of these measures in pharmacy practice research has been reviewed by Pickard *et al*.[115]

In developing a health status or health-related quality of life measure, the researcher must identify those components of health status and quality of life important to the population being researched. However, although they may be common features, all individuals will identify a unique range of concerns, priorities, hopes and expectations in life. For any individual, these may change with time. The validity of an instrument is dependent upon the researchers identifying the 'domains' that are important determinants of the quality of life of a population, which then provide a basis for the development of an instrument that is a reliable and accurate reflection of these. The development and validation of measures requires extensive fieldwork. Established instruments cannot be assumed to be transferable across different population groups. The SF36 was investigated among different cultural groups that make up the population of New Zealand. For some of these cultural groups, the analysis of data revealed a similar factor structure to that found in other populations; however, researchers questioned the validity of the instrument (in that the physical and mental health components were not clearly differentiated) when applied to others.[116]

Interventions intended for individuals with specific health problems or using particular drugs require the selection of measures relevant to the expected outcomes. It is important that the measures selected are sufficiently sensitive to ensure that differences are identified. For this reason, disease-specific measures that focus on particular aspects of health status relevant to people with particular conditions will be more likely to detect improvements or deterioration over time or with different therapies. To assess the impact of a diabetes management programme, differences between the intervention and control groups were detected on a number of variables. However, a generic health status measure derived from the SF36 was used to compare intervention and control groups and revealed no significant differences between the two groups in any of the domains of the instrument.[109] Researchers assessing non-prescription drug use among elderly patients combined established measures with their own. Two aspects of psychological state were assessed: cognitive impairment (Jacob's cognitive screen) and the geriatric depression scale. Health status was ascertained through self-reports. The number of health problems was counted in terms of the number of 'body systems' affected (e.g. heart, breathing, stomach).[117] To assess the mental state of patients following an initiative to rationalise prescribing, a rating scale developed by a local psychiatrist was adopted. This included 21 symptoms: for example, hallucinations, delusion and memory. Each symptom was rated as 0 (absent), 1 (slight), 2 (mild), 3 (moderate), 4 (severe).[63] An evaluation of domiciliary pharmacy visits included measurement of cognitive ability using the abbreviated mental test.[95]

In some studies, assessments have been undertaken by a professional or other carer rather than the individual. In an evaluation of pharmacists' interventions in an elderly care facility, a clinical assessment including mood, alertness, sleeping patterns, constipation, confusion, dizziness, frequency of falls and incontinence was performed by the matron.[118] A clinical evaluation of community pharmacists' interventions included an assessment of the likely impact on patients' everyday activities and the degree of patient discomfort as estimated by a clinical expert panel.[119] Some measures are designed for use by carers on behalf of their care-recipient. The responses obtained cannot be assumed to provide similar results to those that would be obtained from the individuals themselves.

Pain

A range of instruments has been developed in health services research for the measurement of pain.[114] Assessment of pain and/or pain relief has been incorporated into the evaluation of a number of pharmacy interventions. In an evaluation of patient-controlled analgesia, postoperative pain was recorded on a scale of 1–10. Pain scores were measured on a verbal rating scale from 'no pain' to 'unbearable pain' and a 10-cm visual analogue scale. A pain score of four or less as a target level of pain control after 24 hours was agreed with the responsible clinician.[120] In a study of patients with rheumatoid arthritis receiving non-steroidal anti-inflammatory drugs, the McGill pain questionnaire was used to measure pain relief. Patients rated their expectations of pain relief, their satisfaction with pain control and their average and worst pain over the previous month.[121] A poor outcome of therapy was designated by four distinct measures: a pain relief score on the visual-analogue scale, a deliberate change in therapy by patients without consulting their general medical practitioner, the presence of potential adverse drugs reactions, and/or dissatisfaction with therapy.[121]

The evaluation of a programme to educate postoperative patients on the use of patient-controlled analgesia included measures of pain as well as the number of successful and unsuccessful attempts to obtain analgesia and the incidence of nausea and vomiting. Pain was assessed at rest and on movement by asking patients to breathe deeply and touch the opposite side of the bed with a hand. Pain was measured as 0 (no pain at rest or on movement), 1 (no pain at rest, slight pain on movement), 2 (intermittent pain at rest, moderate on movement), 3 (continuous pain at rest, severe on movement). The authors report that this scale has been reported in the literature to correlate with visual analogue scales of pain.[28] Q methodology has also been employed in the measurement of pain. From an analysis of accounts of pain from different sources, researchers derived a pool of statements which through sorting and analytical procedures were reduced to a final Q set which reflected the experiences, patterns and perspectives found in the narratives.[122]

Self-perceived health

Self-perceived health is a component of many health status measures. A question on self-perceived health has been incorporated into a number of studies investigating aspects of pharmaceutical care, either as part of an established measure or as a separate item. A typical question is: 'how would you describe your health – excellent, very good, good, fair or poor?' The question employs subjective quantifiers (see Chapter 2) in which individuals employ their own terms of reference and perceptions in assessing their health status. However, self-perceived health is viewed as an important component of health status, and some validity is conferred by its correlation with morbidity.

Measuring satisfaction and acceptability

Consumer satisfaction with services has become an important indicator of their quality. The British Government includes assessment of consumer satisfaction as part of its regular review of health service reforms.[123] In the evaluation of pharmacy services, the views of clients are commonly sought. In some cases (e.g. a study in which different levels of information were provided in community pharmacies[124]), consumer satisfaction may be a principal outcome measure.

The measurement of satisfaction with health services presents a number of difficulties. Satisfaction will depend on consumers' perceived needs and expectations. For instance, they may take for granted that clinical care will be good and their satisfaction may depend on inter-personal skills of staff, the length of a consultation or the degree of privacy. Professionals and consumers may differ in their views regard-ing the goals of care. In assessing the quality of advice, pharmacists may focus on the content and delivery, while consumers are concerned about the cost of products or the time they have to wait. Dissatisfaction with a single aspect of care can also have a big impact on an overall rating. In reporting overall satisfaction, an individual may be pre-occupied with a single aspect of a service (possibly deemed unimportant by health pro-fessionals), which has a major effect on their rating. Thus, overall ratings of satisfaction may be of limited value to health professionals who wish to provide consumer sensitive services. In addition to difficulties of identifying the relevant issues and ensuring that questions used are a valid reflection of the satisfaction 'construct', the reproducibility of responses has also been questioned. For example, in an investigation of predictors of satisfaction, in which satisfaction was operationalised with the global question: 'Overall, how satisfied are you with the care you received for this problem – excellent, very good, good, fair or poor?', the authors reported that proportion of people responding 'excellent' changed as time-lapsed.[125]

A feature of many of studies in which satisfaction with pharmacy studies is measured is the extent to which favourable responses are obtained. In the vast majority of cases, pharmacy researchers report high levels of satisfaction. (In one study of non-prescription advice in the pharmacy, all clients reported being satisfied.[26]) However, in relation to health promotion services in community pharmacies, the validity of the positive findings of many studies and presumptions often made regard-ing the acceptability of services to consumers have been questioned.[24] There are many possible explanations for the reported favourable responses. It is a common view that the high levels of satisfaction with pharmacy services that are reported in many studies are a reflection of low expectations of clients. The true picture may be distorted by publi-cation bias, in which researchers may be more likely to submit positive findings and/or editors more likely to accept them.

The predominance of positive findings may also be a feature of methodology. Responders may include a higher proportion of people who valued a service than the non-responders. People who do respond may be less inclined to share negative than positive views, especially (as is sometimes the case with pilot projects) if they believe they might be identifiable.

In most cases the respondents are restricted to individuals who participated in the programme. This is often justifiable in that the objective of the evaluation is to obtain views of participants on the value of the programme and their experiences of it. However, individuals who opt to participate in the first place are often self-selecting and their comments may not be applicable to a wider population; thus, the findings may provide useful insights into the attractions and problems of a service for those who use it, but limited data on why others do not. The favourable findings of these studies may also, of course, be a reflection of the genuine positive experiences of service users.

The views and experiences of health professionals, especially pharmacists and medical practitioners, are common components in the evaluation of services.[2–5,11–13,16,21,23,29,34,38,39,126–129] Acceptability to health professionals is considered an important prerequisite for the success of service developments, in terms of both feasibility of operation of a programme in a health-care setting and its perceived value. In the evaluation of collaborative meetings between pharmacists and general practitioners (GPs), participants were asked to comment on both 'operational matters' (e.g. frequency, preparation time for meetings and duration) and to give their views on the value of the meetings.[2]

Questions regarding the usefulness of initiatives are often included.[2–4,11,12,128] That the initiative is perceived as useful may be important for its success, although it will not necessarily translate into a measure of utility in a practice setting. Also, as with surveys of satisfaction among pharmacy clients, responses may reflect expectations of participants and be influenced by other methodological factors.

In the evaluation of prescribing interventions by pharmacists, measures often include prescribers' reports of the acceptability of recommendations. However, researchers have found that reported acceptability of a recommendation does not always result in its implementation.[127] In one study, GPs were asked if they would alter their prescribing as a result of verbal presentations by pharmacists. Researchers subsequently noted that, although some changes in prescribing in line with recommendations were made, this did not extend to all participating GPs or all drugs.[12]

Costs

Economic evaluation has been defined as the comparison between costs and outcomes of all alternatives available.[130] Methods employed by health economists for the economic evaluation of health care programmes include cost-minimisation, cost-effectiveness, cost–benefit and cost–utility analyses. The principles and processes of these procedures are detailed and discussed by Drummond et al.[131] There are examples of the application of these methods in the pharmacy literature.

Cost-minimisation analysis involves the comparison of the costs of different alternatives for which the outcomes are assumed to be identical. A cost-minimisation study was undertaken to compare the costs of glyceryl trinitrate tablets and sprays. The researcher included differences in acquisition prices, prescription costs, wastage in both sprays and tablets and the willingness of the consumer to pay for the advantages conferred by a change in formulation. The results were employed to argue that improvements in drug delivery systems could be accompanied by cost savings.[130]

Cost-effectiveness, cost–benefit and cost–utility analyses, in addition to an assessment of costs, also require a comparison of the outcomes. In cost-effectiveness analysis, the outcomes of the alternative options are measured in the same units (e.g. reduction in blood pressure, hours of pain relief), so for each alternative costs per unit of effectiveness are established. A cost-effectiveness analysis was undertaken to compare oral and intravenous ganciclovir in the maintenance treatment of newly diagnosed cytomegalovirus retinitis in patients with AIDS. Disease progression was a main outcome measure.[132]

The cost-effectiveness of a pharmaceutical intervention in assisting people to stop smoking included the costs of the training programme, the costs of nicotine replacement product purchases and counselling costs. To assess training costs researchers devised an 'opportunity costs' questionnaire for completion by participating pharmacists. This provided data on the costs of attending the workshop, alternative activity foregone, lost income, and means and time of travel. Information on costs to the pharmacy was also collected. Data were gathered in participating and control pharmacies on individuals who had quit smoking after nine months. The researchers then calculated an average 'cost per quitter'. They concluded that the cost-effectiveness ratio was £300 (approximately 500 euros) per additional quitter who had received intensive support and that the programme demonstrated value for money.[133]

Cost–benefit analysis involves the comparison of a range of outcomes or benefits of a programme. In addition to decisions regarding what costs to include, and costs to whom (e.g. the health authority which wishes to contain its expenditure, knock-on effects for community practitioners, the patients themselves and their relatives, friends or other carers), the researcher also has to make a decision regarding identification and measurement of benefits. These are then assigned a monetary value. A comparison of the total prescribing costs of several antimicrobial regimens included an assessment of the costs of the drug itself, preparation and administration costs (calculated from staff time), consumables and waste. Costs of clinical monitoring, laboratory tests, toxicity and patient outcomes were excluded.[46] In a prospective, observational cost analysis of patient-controlled analgesia, the costings included equipment, staff time, disposables and drug use, from a hospital perspective. The authors point out that no social or economic outcome measure to reflect overall benefits was included.[51] An evaluation of a model of pharmaceutical care in community pharmacy included costs to the health sector, pharmacy services and patients.[134]

In applying the economic theory of consumer surplus to estimate the benefits of dispensing doctors and prescribing pharmacists, researchers included benefits to patients (e.g. prescription charges, time and travel costs), and benefits to society (e.g. GPs' time and pharmacists' dispensing fees). They also discussed side-effects, detection of prescribing errors and professional counselling.[135] In a study of costs and benefits of an intervention to rationalise prescribing in long-stay psychiatric wards, data on costs of all drugs before and after the intervention were compared using hospital pharmacy computer data. The researchers also included a measure of mental health status, although this was not incorporated into the cost–benefit analysis.[63]

Many initiatives by pharmacists to influence prescribing include an assessment of their impact on costs, whether or not this is their primary aim. Prescribing data are often routinely collected and provide a suitable database. The total number of items prescribed and costs per item for selected therapeutic drug groups were used in the evaluation of medical practice formularies.[136] Similarly, the introduction of a laxative prescribing policy was assessed by comparing expenditure on laxatives before and after the study period and then a year later to establish whether or not the reduction in spending had been sustained.[62]

The costs of implementation of an intervention may also be included in the analysis.[61,65] Meetings between pharmacists and general medical practitioners were evaluated by examining costs of the scheme (e.g. the facilitator, secretarial support, payments to pharmacists and medical practitioners, costs of training, travel and miscellaneous overheads), as well as subsequent trends in costs of prescribed medicines.[61] To compare costs and potential savings at ward level of different dosing schedules, researchers included costs of nursing time (in preparation and administration of drug doses), which was based on salary plus employer costs, material costs (e.g. syringes, needles, medicine cups) and dose frequencies of the different dosage forms. A formula was derived to establish theoretical annual cost savings of changing to medication with an alternative dose frequency.[137] In an analysis of costs of patient-controlled analgesia, researchers included the costs of the equipment, side-effect treatment, additional analgesia, staff time, equipment disposables and drugs used.[120]

To compare the total prescribing costs of several antimicrobial regimens, costs were broken down into the cost of the compound itself and 'hidden' costs which included consumables, waste disposal, preparation and administration costs. Timed measurements were evaluated based on hourly rates of pay for the members of staff concerned. The researchers reported that they did not include costs relating to clinical monitoring, laboratory tests, toxicity and patient outcomes.[138] These might, of course, be important factors to decision-makers when choosing between alternative treatment options. In a study of growth in prescribing costs, prescribing cost data were used to investigate relative changes in different therapeutic categories.[139]

Sensitivity analysis is sometimes employed to ensure that conclusions of economic analyses are robust. Economists recognise that, in any evaluation, assumptions are made regarding costs and valuations of different variables. Sensitivity analysis involves repeated analyses in which assumed values are replaced with the highest and lowest that might be obtained for each variable. An assessment of the sensitivity of the conclusions of the study to changes in the assumed values for each variable can then be made. A number of researchers have evaluated the cost implications of the use of patients' own drugs during their hospital stay or at discharge.[76,140,141] The differing conclusions of these studies (identified by the authors[76]), may reflect differences between settings and/or in the operation of the scheme, the effect of decisions regarding which costs to include and/or procedures for their valuation and assessment. Thus comparison of study findings may not be justified.

A preliminary economic analysis of nurse prescribing assessed changes in frequency and costs of prescribing with a range of 'scenarios' which were identified and described by the authors as representing alternative patterns of care that could have occurred in the absence of nurse prescribing. A comparison of costs based on the eight scenarios enabled a sensitivity analysis to assess the robustness of the researchers' conclusions.[14]

Prescription interventions

Prescription interventions by pharmacists have been evaluated in descriptive studies (documenting the frequency and type of intervention) and in terms of the potential or anticipated value of the intervention to patients.

Definitions and classification of prescription interventions

Researchers in New Zealand defined an intervention as: 'any action taken to clarify or change a prescription to optimise the patient's drug therapy and/or minimise the risk of harmful effects'.[142] In a study of monitoring of discharge prescriptions by ward pharmacists an intervention was defined as 'a recommendation, a query or a problem which had occurred with the discharge prescription and which required contact with the prescribing doctor or nursing staff or referral to the medical notes'.[75] Clinical pharmacy interventions have also been distinguished as reactive (those for which dispensing could not occur without further consultation) and proactive (those for which the pharmacist could have proceeded with dispensing without further consultation). These researchers also defined an overall clinical intervention rate: number of interventions/number of prescription items, which was found to be 1.5 per cent, with a ratio of reactive to proactive of 4:1.[119]

Classification of prescription interventions has generally been according to reasons for the intervention (e.g. prescribing omission, prescribing error, drug interaction and drug therapy monitoring problem[142]), the action taken by the pharmacist and/or the outcomes (or expected outcomes). Categorisations based on actions taken by pharmacists in a community pharmacy setting have included: prescription dispensed as written, prescription clarified and dispensed, prescription changed and dispensed, prescription not dispensed, patient educated/counselled, and other.[142] In the evaluation of a repeat medication clinic run by a clinical pharmacist, interventions were classified as: review of medication, change of medication, change of formulation, modification of dose, continuation of medication, archive, monitor, add new drug, and discontinue medication.[143] Pharmacists' recommendations for changes to drug therapy (stop the drug, change the drug, change the dose or change the preparation) formed a basis for the assessment of a programme for the review of repeat prescriptions.[11] Researchers evaluating the impact of pharmaceutical care activities in a mental health unit classified interventions according to actions which were linked to expected outcomes: problem identified, problem resolved, problem prevented, improved drug therapy, improved drug supply and monitoring.[144]

In a study documenting pharmacists' involvement in drug therapy decisions, interventions were classified into four levels: annotative (e.g. clarification of prescription), corrective (e.g. to effect a change), consultative (e.g. pharmacist consulted regarding a prescribing decision) and proactive (e.g. pharmacist raises issue). A fifth (other) category was also included.[145]

Drug-related problems in a study of interventions by community pharmacists were defined as 'circumstances of drug therapy that may interfere with a desired therapeutic objective'.[146] This definition was intended to include problems identified by pharmacy personnel as well as those presented by the patient.

Evaluation of prescription interventions

In the evaluation of prescription interventions, one of two approaches has commonly been employed. The use of rating scales on which health professionals score each intervention for its likely or potential clinical significance is an approach that has been adopted by many researchers to evaluate interventions in terms of their contribution to patient care.[17,119,127,143,144,147–151] Most of the scoring systems provide an opportunity for positive and negative judgements concerning the impact of the intervention. Assessments have been undertaken by clinical pharmacists, clinicians and teams of health professionals. In an evaluation of service provision by community pharmacists to community hospitals, ratings of interventions by expert panels were compared with those of a peer group.[151]

A six-point scoring system was employed for the assessment of interventions by ward pharmacists:

1   intervention detrimental to patient's well-being
2   intervention of no significance to patient care
3   intervention significant, but does not lead to improvement in patient care
4   intervention significant and results in an improvement in the standard of care
5   intervention very significant and prevents a major organ failure or adverse reaction of similar importance
6   intervention potentially life-saving.

The system was validated by comparing the scores assigned by one pharmacist and three doctors on a sample of interventions.[148] The clinical significance of interventions has also been rated by other researchers as: information only, fine tuning of therapy, important to act, life threatening, intervention deemed invalid, intervention deemed detrimental to patient.[143] In an evaluation of the impact of medication review by community pharmacists, a 'clinical panel' was established to assess clinical significance of a subset of cases. Members independently evaluated changes on a scale which was developed in earlier research[152,153] spanning:

0–1 no effect to negative effect
1   minor significance, any improved standard of care
2   significant, improves standard of care or optimises therapy
3   very significant, prevents major toxicity and/or end organ damage
4   potentially life saving.[153]

Attempts have been made to assess the significance of interventions on wider aspects of a patient's 'quality of life' rather than a narrower interpretation of 'clinical significance'. Assessors were asked to estimate both the extent of interference with a patient's everyday activities and the degree of discomfort had the intervention not occurred. These estimates were recorded on a from 0 to 6 scale (spanning normal everyday activity to no normal activity). This approach did present some difficulties, and the authors acknowledged the poor agreement between assessors as demonstrated by *Kappa* statistics.[119]

In developing a rating scale, a decision has to be made regarding the number of intervals (see Chapter 2). Too few intervals will compromise the discriminatory power of the scale in that the assessors will be forced to place cases which they perceive as dissimilar in the same category. A scale with too many intervals will be unreliable in that assessors will have difficulty in selecting the appropriate position for any given case. Researchers also have to decide on either an odd or even number of intervals. In scales spanning positive and negative judgements, an odd number provides a central, non-committal position. Anchoring of visual analogue scales by providing a description at either end often improves the reliability of results by ensuring similar interpretations by the assessors regarding the attribute that is being assessed. If all points of the scale are anchored by a description,[143,148] the scale represents a categorical (nominal or ordinal) measure rather than a linear visual analogue scale.

Researchers have also assessed prescription interventions according to whether or not they met with the approval of, or were accepted by, prescribers.[118,145,150] In a study of prescription interventions in residential homes, outcomes were categorised as: advice accepted, advice partially accepted, advice withdrawn on discussion, advice rejected, doctor to review patient, no discussion took place.[127] In some studies these measures were extended to take into account whether or not the recommended courses of action were subsequently implemented and/or maintained.[38,127,154,155] Authors have reported that not all recommendations on which prescribers agreed to act were ultimately implemented.[127,154] The reasons for the discrepancies were unclear, they may be many and varied; however, these findings raise the question as to whether verbal acceptance is a valid indicator of the prescriber's views. In an evaluation of interventions by a community pharmacist, researchers adapted the 'number needed to treat' (NNT) concept. The number of prescriptions that needed to be reviewed to result in one intervention that led to actual, or potential, clinical improvement was calculated.[150]

In the evaluation of a model of pharmaceutical care in Australia, operational definitions of patients' problems were provided under eight categories: need for additional therapy, unnecessary drug, wrong or inappropriate drug, wrong or inappropriate doses, adverse drug reactions, compliance, drugs out-of-date and lifestyle issues.[134]

Appropriateness of prescribing

In assessing the appropriateness of prescribing, many researchers have based their assessment on the extent to which practice concurs with the views of 'experts' or accepted recommendations or guidelines. Thus, criteria for the appropriateness of prescribing in a nursing home setting were agreed by an expert panel and then applied to residents' drug profiles.[156] In a study of the level of inappropriate prescribing for patients aged 65 or over, the main outcome measure was the prevalence of prescribing 20 medications that, according to criteria developed by a panel of experts in geriatric medicine and pharmacology, should be avoided in elderly people.[157]

Hanlon et al.[158,159] have developed a medication appropriateness index (MAI) for assessing prescribing. This MAI score is based on ten items: indication, effectiveness, dosage, correct directions, practical directions, drug–drug interactions, drug–disease interactions, duplication, duration and expense. Inter-rater reliability was assessed by comparing the ratings by two clinical pharmacists of 65 medications. The association between MAI score and specific outcomes (hospitalisation, unscheduled ambulatory or emergency care and blood pressure control) has been investigated.[111] Researchers have also compared elderly people's and clinicians' ratings of MAI criteria.[160]

In a study of interventions in an elderly care facility, drug-related problems were classified in terms of appropriateness of prescribing: use of drugs in the absence of clear diagnosis, presence of common side-effects from two or more drugs on medication profile (additive side-effects), concurrent use of drugs that may produce an adverse drug reaction (interaction), use of two or more drugs with same pharmacological profiles for a problem usually treated with a single agent (duplicate therapy), exceeding the recommended dose, and use of six or more drugs on a medication profile (polypharmacy).[118]

The appropriateness of prescriptions for extemporaneous products has been assessed in terms of therapeutic appropriateness: that is, whether the product was a recommended treatment for the stated diagnosis according to the medical literature.[64]

Initiatives to influence prescribing

There are many examples of initiatives by pharmacists to influence prescribing behaviour. Cost implications, acceptability to practitioners (see above) and changes in prescribing habits are the factors most often included in the evaluation.

Prescribing practices, as apparent in routinely collected prescribing data, have been used as a measure of the impact of many initiatives.[5,12,39,65,66,68,69,139,161,162] This information enables a comparison of costs before and after an intervention, as well as providing data on prescribing patterns of individual target drugs or products.

Health authority prescribing data were used to measure the effects of an academic representative, who adopted behaviours typical of commercial representatives, on prescribing behaviour. A 'prescribing index' was devised which was defined as the ratio of the cost of prescribing of the target drug to the costs of prescribing competitor drugs plus the target drug. This prescribing index was seen as an indicator of propensity to prescribe the target drug, its value ranging from 0 to 1 (in which 1 represented 100% prescribing of the target drug).[69] In another study, a controlled trial in which intensive pharmacist support was provided to eight general practice surgeries, the changes in prescribing expenditure between the eight trial and control surgeries were compared using prescribing costs data. These differences were then assessed against the costs of employing the pharmacists to provide the support.[163]

In some studies, DDDs (defined daily doses) have been used as a measure of prescribing of individual drugs.[39,65,68] DDDs were devised and defined by the World Health Organization to facilitate comparisons of drug use in different countries or settings. The volume of each drug supplied is converted into standardised units, based on an average adult maintenance dose for the particular drug when used for its major indication.[164]

Ward pharmacy services and discharge from secondary care

In addition to evaluation of clinical pharmacy interventions and prescription monitoring, researchers have also evaluated ward pharmacy activities in terms of the processes and delivery of services.[17,80,82,85,86] The measures frequently employed include time spent by pharmacists and/or other members of staff on various ward pharmacy-related activities. Work sampling methods have been used by a number of researchers in these studies,[17,80,82,85,86] with a range of predetermined categories being devised for the documentation of activities. The impact on pharmacy staff and others has also been assessed. The effects of automated dispensing systems on the extent of medication-related and non-medication-related activities of nurses and health unit co-ordinators before and after implementation were monitored.[82] In addition to time spent on different tasks, researchers have investigated the frequency and processes of identification and resolution of prescription-related problems, and the processes of supply of stock and non-stock items to the wards. In a study to compare hand-written and computer-generated charts, medication administration errors were categorised according to ASHP (American Society of Health-system Pharmacists) definitions: omissions, wrong time, unauthorised drug, improper dose, wrong dosage form, wrong administration technique, deteriorated drug, and other.[44]

A number of researchers have evaluated aspects of hospital discharge processes and outcomes, including pharmacists' roles.[21,72,75,165,166] The impact of decentralisation of pharmacy services on the processes of obtaining the discharge medication was assessed by investigating changes in the timing of steps in the process: the writing of the prescription, its arrival in pharmacy, availability of medication for the patient. This enabled the identification of the stages of the process affected by the change.[72] The views of community health professionals on the transfer of discharge information have also been sought.[3,4]

The impact of issuing letters at discharge has been measured in terms of the prescribing discrepancies arising following hospital discharge. For this the 'number needed to treat' (NNT) measure was adopted. (The NNT for an intervention indicates the average number of cases receiving the intervention in order to achieve an attributable outcome in one case.[167]) In this study, the researchers calculated the number of patients that needed to be discharged with a letter in order to prevent one unintentional discrepancy that would be expected to lead to an adverse effect. A consensus panel was convened to enable separate calculations for the 'number of unintentional discrepancies' and the 'number of unintentional discrepancies deemed clinically significant'.[165]

Evaluation of advice-giving

There have been many descriptive studies investigating the nature and quality of advice-giving in community pharmacies. The methods of data collection and findings of those undertaken in the UK have been reviewed.[168] Most of these studies have employed 'process' measures, gathering data on the circumstances and characteristics of advice-giving. Although these measures do not in themselves provide information on ultimate outcomes, they may be expected to be associated with optimal outcomes and/or features important to clients.

An assessment of non-prescription advice in community pharmacies included a measure of pharmacist availability (whether physically present in the pharmacy), accessibility (i.e. capable of being reached, there being no physical barrier in the pharmacy to reduce the chance of reaching the pharmacist or gaining his or her attention), and approachability (a trait of the pharmacist, perceived or actual, as being easy to meet and converse with, willing to help, and responsive). These factors were seen as important measures in demonstrating whether consumers who wanted advice on non-prescription medicines had difficulty in receiving it.[169] To evaluate the impact of consultation areas in community pharmacies, measures included place of consultation in the pharmacy, pharmacists' response times, numbers and nature of questions.[57] A study assessing the impact of the position of the pharmacist (in dispensary, on shop floor, etc.) on advice-giving compared the proportion of clients purchasing non-prescription medicines who were advised, the source of advice and the initiator of the encounter, with the siting of the pharmacist.[45]

In assessing the quality of advice, researchers have focused on both the content (e.g. questions asked and advice given) and features of communication between the pharmacist and client. Studies by the Consumers' Association, UK[50,51] and other researchers[46] measured the quality of advice by comparing the content with established guidelines or the views of 'experts'. Assessment of the delivery of advice has included analysis of the numbers and types of questions (e.g. open, closed, leading), the extent to which the pharmacist responds to clients' questions, and the clarity of explanations given.[26,48,170,171]

Researchers have attempted to evaluate pharmacy advice-giving in terms of outcomes. This presents difficulties in demonstrating that the subsequent actions of clients are attributable to this advice. In an evaluation of pharmacists' non-prescription medicine advice, patients were followed-up and points assigned for 11 parameters of appropriate use:

- use with interacting non-prescription drug
- use with interacting prescription drug
- inappropriate product for the symptoms
- frequency of use
- dose used
- use with food or water
- use with alcohol
- driving if dizzy or drowsy
- duration of use intended
- interaction with medical condition
- consultation with a doctor.

Knowledge was assessed regarding precautions, side-effects and contraindications.[36]

The extent to which clients could recall advice has also been measured. Advice was broken down into separate items, an item being defined as 'a phrase which standing alone could be meaningful'.[26,172] Items correctly reported were classed as 'recalled', items not reported or misreported were considered 'forgotten'.[26] In addition, items were coded as either essential or secondary on the basis of views in the literature regarding what information is essential to customers.[172] The accuracy and extent of customers' recall was reported, along with its association with other factors, such as the number of drugs and the extent to which customers were active or passive in their discussions with pharmacists.[172]

Health promotion

The potential for community pharmacists to contribute to health promotion has long been acknowledged. The ultimate goal of health promotion activity is to encourage individuals to adopt healthier lifestyles that will have a positive impact on their health status. Influences on lifestyle and factors leading to changes in behaviour are complex. Thus, evaluating the role of pharmacists in terms of these outcomes is difficult.

In evaluating health promotion initiatives, researchers commonly focus on processes of delivery of programmes, gathering data on the provision and uptake of services, and the views of pharmacists and clients regarding their acceptability and perceived value.[10,18,19,24,35,73,78,83,173]

In the evaluation of smoking cessation programmes based at community pharmacies, success has been measured in terms of the proportion of participants who reported themselves to be smokers or non-smokers immediately after completing the programme and then between 3 and 12 months later,[29,174] the cost-effectiveness of the programme based on individuals who quit[133] and in the advice-giving of pharmacists following participation in a training programme.[55]

Comparison of immunisation rates between a group receiving a letter from a community pharmacy advising on immunisation and a control group provides an example of a randomised controlled trial to evaluate pharmacists' impact regarding a specific disease-prevention intervention. The outcome measures were the proportion in each group who were vaccinated and the likelihood of an unvaccinated patient being vaccinated after receipt of the letter.[175]

Educational initiatives

For many education programmes, the evaluation has been based on the views of participants. Researchers have gathered information on perceived relevance, improvements in knowledge and/or skills base, expected changes in practice, comments on individual components of the course and overall value and acceptability.[6,8,10,176–178] In some cases these data have been combined with other measures, such as an independent assessment of the knowledge and/or skills base.[9,35,92,179]

In the evaluation of educational initiatives, difficulty arises in establishing the relationship between reported or perceived benefits of a course, such as an improved knowledge and/or skill base, and resultant changes in a practice setting. For example, an assertion skills course was assessed by a questionnaire administered before and after attendance. The questionnaire included a range of situations in hospital pharmacy, where appropriate assertive responses may lead to positive outcomes. For each situation respondents were asked how they felt and what they would say and do. This evaluation would show how, as a result of the course, participants were able to identify the assertiveness option and their intentions regarding their actions. However, the evaluation does not provide an indication of whether or not these behaviours would be adopted in practice.[180]

Similarly, in the evaluation of a training programme on asthma management, researchers reported improvement, at least in the short-term, in the knowledge-base of participants. While they concluded that such training could potentially enhance pharmacists' input into the management of asthma, the evaluation did not provide data on the extent to which these benefits resulted in changes in practice.[94] In an evaluation of guidelines to promote appropriate advice in community pharmacies, pharmacists' knowledge before and after dissemination of the guidelines was assessed by questions based on the content of the guidelines. To provide some data on application in a practice setting, pharmacists were also requested to maintain records regarding their use or non-use of the guidelines.[81]

This issue was also addressed in a study of the effects of a training programme on advice-giving relating to smoking cessation. A covert participant researcher (researcher posing as a client) requested advice in pharmacies where the pharmacist had or had not taken part in the training. The advice given by the two groups was compared.[55] A training programme for pharmacists, and its subsequent implementation in community pharmacy, was assessed in terms of its cost-effectiveness.[133] An initial evaluation after nine months was followed by two further annual evaluations to assess longer term change.[181]

Patient knowledge

Patients' knowledge of their medication has been used as an outcome measure in many studies.[31,95,182–185] Researchers are generally aware of the tenuous relationship between knowledge and medicine-taking behaviour. Measures of knowledge are sometimes combined with other aspects of medicine-taking such as compliance or adherence, the ability to read labels and manage packaging, perceived effects of medicines and/or physiological and clinical measures.[31,182–185]

In measuring knowledge, researchers commonly focus on the name and purposes of medicines. Other questions may include the dose, frequency, duration and side-effects for each prescribed or purchased drug.[95,182,185,186] The accuracy of responses has been compared with information on the label or other written information. Researchers evaluating a pharmacist-developed anticoagulant clinic also assessed patients' knowledge regarding limits imposed on lifestyle; the information collected was believed to be required for good compliance.[31] Recalling the correct dosage was deemed the important information in a study among clients at village pharmacies in Burkina Faso, West Africa.[186]

Measures of compliance/adherence

Many studies have included measures of compliance with, or adherence to, prescribed medication regimens. A variety of methods have been employed, all of which present their own problems of reliability and validity.

Tablet counting has been used by many researchers.[95,182–184,187,188] The number of doses remaining in a container is compared with the number that would be expected if the drug had been taken according to instructions.

To assess the effects of computer-generated reminder charts, a compliance score for each medicine was calculated: number of tablets taken/correct number × 100, leading to a mean compliance score for each patient.[183] As people commonly do not take medicines precisely as instructed, researchers have to decide the extent of deviation from dose directions to be permitted before an individual is designated as non-compliant. In this study, a score of at least 85% was accepted as indicating compliance.[183] A similar approach was used to assess the effects of a self-medication programme prior to hospital discharge.[184] Compliance data from electronic monitoring devices, from which data on times of opening the medication containers would be obtained, and pill counts were combined in a study in which pharmacists made recommendations regarding therapy for people with diabetes.[188]

Researchers using these methods are aware of the problems they present in terms of reliability, for example, that people may transfer tablets between containers, the date on which the container was put to use might be unclear, number of doses removed from the container might not correspond to those taken, outer containers may be removed, and that no information on timing of doses is available. Researchers are also aware that patients may not wish to appear non-compliant. Some authors report that patients were not told that in the course of research their tablets would be counted.[182,183]

Because of the difficulties that measurement of compliance presents, many researchers combine tablet counts with other methods, often self-reports.[95,183,184,187,189] Scores have also been calculated from self-reports[95]: % compliance = total number of doses prescribed minus the number of doses omitted / total number prescribed × 100.

In a study of health beliefs and compliance of South African out-patients with antihypertensive medication, compliance was measured in terms of the number of scheduled appointments that were kept, and also in a question whereby respondents were asked to report the number of days in the previous week when no medicine had been taken. Authors also adapted questions from the health belief model to include a measure of the patient's knowledge of their medication, the patient's health beliefs regarding their medication and the patient's assessment of the importance of regular intake of medicines. The most commonly reported reason for non-compliance was inability to pay the clinic fees; other patients questioned the importance for health of repeated use of medicines as scheduled.[189]

Compliance in a study of patients discharged from hospital was based on self-reports: 'How often do you forget to take your medicines – daily, weekly, monthly, never?' A patient admitting to daily or weekly omission was classed as non-compliant, irrespective of the level, and as an alternative measure actual doses remaining were examined after identifying the prescription history post-discharge. A patient was classified as non-compliant on either or both criteria.[190] A study of compliance with anti-malarial prophylaxis among tourists following their return home was measured by self-reports in a questionnaire at the end of the four-week period during which travellers are advised to continue their medication.[191]

In measuring compliance with advice from village pharmacies in Burkina Faso, researchers assessed both 'buying' compliance, if clients bought the products as advised, and 'drug-taking' compliance, derived from the number of pills remaining in the household.[186] In an evaluation of pharmacists' advice to elderly patients taking multiple medications, compliance was described as 'the concurrence of daily dose claimed to be taken by the patient [reported during a domiciliary visit] with the dose stated in the GP's records'. The authors reported that this measure of compliance was compromised by the frequent lack of a specific dose being recorded by the doctor.[185] In one study, clients who had received advice in the pharmacy were considered to have adhered to it if, when followed up by telephone, they reported using the product in both the quantity and the frequency stated by the manufacturer.[26]

The assessment of compliance using prescription refill data (the extent to which patients obtain repeat prescriptions when due) has been used to assess long-term adherence to anti-retroviral therapy, in which adherent patients were those meeting at least 80% of required doses.[192] A review of studies employing 'refill' compliance found that studies assessing the validity of these measures found significant association between refill and other compliance measures, concluding that 'refill' compliance could be a useful source of compliance information when direct measurement was not possible. They also found no correlation between compliance and population characteristics, inconsistent association with the total number of drugs prescribed, and better compliance for drugs with fewer daily doses.[193]

Grymonpre *et al.*[187] compared medication adherence calculated from pill counts, self-reported adherence (number taken per day compared with labelling directions) and prescription claims data (refill frequency). They reported statistically significantly lower adherence scores using pill counts than the other methods. The accuracy of measures of compliance has been discussed by Gregoire *et al.*[194] who compared non-compliance to antihypertensive medication using pill counts and pharmacy records. They concluded that pharmacy records could be effective in identifying non-compliance, although they presented some limitations.

To evaluate a therapeutic drug monitoring programme in community pharmacy, compliance was estimated from computer-based patient medication records from the previous year: % compliance = number of dose units dispensed / required number of dose units (predicted from dose regimen). In this study, compliance between 80 and 120% was considered normal.[107] Again, the reliability of this measure may be unclear.

Adherence in terms of administration by caregivers was incorporated in the evaluation of a pharmaceutical advisory service. The proportion of medicines administered in accordance with prescribers' wishes was documented.[110] Compliance/adherence, however it is measured, is not necessarily an indicator of clinical outcome or health status. In this study, compliance with prescribers' instructions was combined with the number of patients who were no longer constipated and/or free of other possible drug-induced problems.[110] The evaluation of a pharmacist-run anticoagulant clinic included a comparison of patients' INRs (international normalised ratios) with the INR range specified for them by their clinician. By agreement with the haematologist, patients within 0.5 of their specified range were deemed compliant.[31]

A conceptual shift from compliance (in which patients are expected to follow instructions) to adherence (in which it is acknowledged that people take an active role in decisions regarding the use of their prescribed medicines) has impacted on the way in which this variable is measured. Researchers are now often interested in the decision-making processes of individuals regarding the use of their medicines. Acknowledging that people may not be comfortable admitting to non-compliance, and to improve the validity of self-reports, researchers have described asking questions 'in a non-threatening way'.[95] prefacing their questions with reassurances that people do not always remember to take their tablets,[195] and/or acknowledging that people may alter doses or take an active role in regulating the use of medicines according to their perceived needs.[196–198]

A review of studies assessing medication compliance identified many shortcomings in the methods employed.[199] However, this is a complex topic. What is important is that researchers are aware of complexities of achieving reliable and valid assessments and the implications of whatever approaches and methods are selected.

Conclusion

Pharmacy services are many and varied, and new initiatives are essential to ensure the provision of consumer-sensitive services relevant to the needs of the populations they serve. In the evaluation of initiatives from the perspectives of different population groups, researchers have drawn upon a wide range of methodologies. The range of outcomes and potential outcomes of health programmes can also be extensive. It is important that the major consequences and implications of new services are identified, so that relevant and sensitive measures can be incorporated. Although many of these outcomes may be readily quantifiable, for others measurement is problematic. The selection, adaptation and development of suitable measures against which to assess their actual and potential contribution to health care will remain an important task of pharmacy practice researchers.

References

1. Watson P. Community pharmacists and mental health: an evaluation of two pharmaceutical care programmes. *Pharm J* 1997; 258: 419–22.
2. Pilling M, Geoghegan M, Wolfson D J, Holden J D. The St Helens and Knowsley prescribing initiative: a model for pharmacist-led meetings with GPs. *Pharm J* 1998; 260: 100–2.
3. Cook H. Transfer of information between hospital and community pharmacy – a feasibility study. *Pharm J* 1995; 254: 736–7.
4. Eadon H. Use of pharmacy discharge information for transplant patients. *Pharm J* 1994; 253: 314–16.

5. Bentley E M, Mackie I C, Fuller S. Pharmacists and the 'smile for sugar-free medicines' campaign. *Pharm J* 1993; 251: 606–7.

6. Mottram D R, Rowe P H. Evaluation of the impact of recent changes in post-graduate continuing education for pharmacists in England. *Int J Pharm Pract* 1996; 4: 123–8.

7. Whittlesea C M C, Walker R. An adverse drug reaction reporting scheme for community pharmacists. *Int J Pharm Pract* 1996; 4: 228–34.

8. Savela E, Lilja J, Enlund H. Continuing education by teleconference to remote areas. *J Soc Admin Pharm* 1996; 13: 159–66.

9. Savela E, Hannula A M. Different forms of in-company training and their suitability for pharmacies. *J Soc Admin Pharm* 1991; 8: 76–80.

10. Sinclair H, Bond C, Lennox A S, *et al*. An evaluation of a training workshop for pharmacists based on the Stages of Change model of smoking cessation. *Health Educ J* 1997; 56: 296–312.

11. Ghalamkari H H, Rees J E, Saltrese-Taylor A. Evaluation of a pilot health promotion project in pharmacies: 3. Clients' further opinions and actions taken after receiving health promotion advice. *Pharm J* 1997; 258: 909–13.

12. Roddick E, Maclean R, McKean C, *et al*. Communication with general practitioners. *Pharm J* 1993; 251: 816–19.

13. Baigent B. Evaluation of clinical pharmacy in a mental health unit. *Pharm J* 1993; 250: 150–3.

14. Ferguson B, Luker K, Smith K, *et al*. Preliminary findings from an economic analysis of nurse prescribing. *Int J Pharm Pract* 1998; 6: 127–32.

15. Smith F J. Referral of clients by community pharmacists: views of general medical practitioners. *Int J Pharm Pract* 1996; 4: 30–5.

16. Steward M, Gibson S. Evaluation of the Farillon vaccine delivery service to GP practices. *Pharm J* 1994; 253 :650–1.

17. Eadon H J, Batty R, Beech E F. Implementation of a patient-orientated pharmacy service. *Int J Pharm Pract* 1996; 4: 214–20.

18. Ghalamkari H H, Rees J E, Saltrese-Taylor A. Evaluation of a pilot health promotion project in pharmacies: 2. Clients' initial views on pharmacists' advice. *Pharm J* 1997; 258: 314–17.

19. Ghalamkari HH, Rees JE, Saltrese-Taylor A. Evaluation of a pilot health promotion project in pharmacies: (3) Clients' further opinions and actions taken after receiving health promotion advice. *Pharm J* 1997; 258: 909–13.

20. Lindsay G H, Hesketh E A, Harden R M. Community pharmacy-based interactive patient education: 3. patient acceptability. *Pharm J* 1994; 252: 578–9.

21. Cromarty E, Downie G, Wilkinson S, Cromarty J A. Communication regarding the discharge medicines of elderly patients: a controlled trial. *Pharm J* 1998; 260: 62–4.

22. Muhammed T, Ghalamkari H, Millar G, Hirst J. A community drug information service. *Pharm J* 1998; 260: 278–80.

23. King M J, Halloran S P, Kwong P Y P. Blood glucose measurement in the community pharmacy. *Pharm J* 1993; 250: 808–10.

24. Anderson C. Health promotion by community pharmacists: consumers' views. *Int J Pharm Pract* 1998; 6: 1–12.

25. Ashcroft D M, Clark C M, Gorman S P. Shared care: a study of patients' experiences with erythropoietin. *Int J Pharm Pract* 1998; 6: 145–9.

26. Evans S W, John D N, Bloor M J, Luscombe D K. Use of non-prescription advice offered to the public by pharmacists. *Int J Pharm Pract* 1997; 5: 16–25.
27. Livingstone C R, Pugh A L G, Winn S, Williamson V K. Developing community pharmacy services wanted by local people: information and advice about prescription medicines. *Int J Pharm Pract* 1996; 4: 94–102.
28. Berwick S J, Lanningan N A, Ratcliff A. Effect of patient education in postoperative patients using patient-controlled analgesia. *Int J Pharm Pract* 1994; 3: 53–5.
29. Isacson D, Bingefors C, Ribohn M. Quit smoking in the pharmacy – an evaluation of a smoking cessation scheme in Sweden. *J Soc Admin Pharm* 1998; 15: 164–73.
30. Krass I. A comparison of clients' experiences of counselling for prescriptions and over-the-counter medications in two types of pharmacies: validation of a research instrument. *J Soc Admin Pharm* 1996; 13: 206–14.
31. Radley A S, Hall J. The establishment and evaluation of a pharmacist-developed anticoagulant clinic. *Pharm J* 1994; 252: 91–2.
32. Timmins A. The contribution of the intensive care pharmacist in the United Kingdom. *Pharm J* 2000; 265: 341–4.
33. Servizio di Informazione e di Educazione Sanitaria, Farmacie Comunali Italiane. What information for the patient? Large scale pilot study on experimental package inserts giving information on prescribed and over-the-counter drugs. *BMJ* 1990; 301: 1261–5.
34. Norman F, Scrimshaw A. Do residential homes benefit from registration with a community pharmacy? *Pharm J* 1994; 252: 97–9.
35. Anderson C, Alexander A. Wiltshire pharmacy health promotion training initiative: a telephone survey. *Int J Pharm Pract* 1997; 5: 185–91.
36. Rantucci M J, Segal H J. Over-the-counter medication: outcome and effectiveness of patient counselling. *J Soc Admin Pharm* 1986; 3: 81–91.
37. Dowell J S, Snadden D, Dunbar J A. Rapid prescribing change: how do patients respond? *Soc Sci Med* 1996; 43: 1543–9.
38. Goldstein R, Hulme H, Willits J. Reviewing repeat prescribing – general practitioners and community pharmacists working together. *Int J Pharm Pract* 1998; 6: 60–6.
39. Damsgaard J J, Folke P E, Launso L, Schaefer K. Effects of local interventions towards prescribing of psychotropic drugs. *J Soc Admin Pharm* 1992; 9: 179–84.
40. Franzen S, Lilja J, Hamilton D, Larsson S. How do Finnish women evaluate verbal pharmacy over-the-counter information? *J Soc Admin Pharm* 1996; 3: 99–108.
41. Rickles N M, Wertheimer A I, McGhan W F. The selective attention model for patient evaluation of pharmaceutical services (SAMPEPS). *J Soc Admin Pharm* 1998; 15: 174–89.
42. Hoog S. Positive and negative incidents perceived by self-care pharmacy customers. *J Soc Admin Pharm* 1994; 11:86–96.
43. Indritz MES, Artz MB. Value added to health by pharmacists. *Soc Sci Med* 1999; 48: 647–60.
44. Cavell G F, Hughes D K. Does computerised prescribing improve the accuracy of drug administration? *Pharm J* 1997; 259: 782–4.

45. Stevenson M, Taylor J. The effect of a front-shop pharmacist on non-prescription medication consultations. *J Soc Admin Pharm* 1995; 12: 154–8.

46. Sowter J R, Raynor D K. The management of oral health problems in community pharmacies. *Pharm J* 1997; 259: 308–10.

47. Ferraz M B, Pereira R B, Paiva J G A, *et al*. Availability of over-the-counter drugs for arthritis in Sao Paulo, Brazil. *Soc Sci Med* 1996; 42: 1129–31.

48. Smith F J. Community pharmacists and health promotion: a study of consultations between pharmacists and clients. *Health Promotion Int* 1992; 7: 249–55.

49. Anderson C W, Alexander A M. Response to dysmenorrhoea: an assessment of knowledge and skills. *Pharm J* 1992; 249: R2.

50. Consumers' Association. Advice across a chemist's counter. *Which?* 1985; August: 351–4.

51. Consumers' Association. Pharmacists: how reliable are they? *Which? Way to Health* 1991; December: 191–4.

52. Krska J, Greenwood R, Howitt E P. Audit of advice provided in response to symptoms. *Pharm J* 1994; 252: 93–6.

53. Smith F J, Salkind M R, Jolly B C. Community pharmacy: a method of assessing quality of care. *Soc Sci Med* 1990; 31: 603–7.

54. Lamsam G D, Kropff M A. Community pharmacists' assessments and recommendations for treatment in four case scenarios. *Ann Pharmacother* 1998; 32: 409–16.

55. Anderson C. A controlled study of the effect of a health promotion training scheme on pharmacists' advice about smoking cessation. *J Soc Admin Pharm* 1995; 12: 115–24.

56. Brendstrup E, Launso L. Evaluation of a non-drug intervention programme for younger seniors. *J Soc Admin Pharm* 1993; 10: 23–35.

57. Harper R, Harding G, Savage I, *et al*. Consultation areas in community pharmacies: an evaluation. *Pharm J* 1998; 261: 947–50.

58. Konradsen F, Amerasinghe PH, Perera D, *et al*. A village treatment centre for malaria: community response in Sri Lanka. *Soc Sci Med* 2000; 50: 879–89.

59. Davis S, Coulson R A, Wood S M. Adverse reaction reporting by hospital pharmacists: the first year. *Pharm J* 1999; 262: 366–7.

60. Lee A, Bateman D N, Edwards C, *et al*. Reporting of adverse drug reactions by hospital pharmacists: pilot scheme. *BMJ* 1997; 315: 519.

61. Geoghegan M, Pilling M, Holden J, Wolfson D. A controlled evaluation of the effect of community pharmacists on general practitioner prescribing. *Pharm J* 1998; 261: 864–6.

62. Patel K. A policy for rationalising laxatives use and expenditure. *Pharm J* 1993; 250: 185–6.

63. Cloete B G, Gomez C, Lyon R, Male B M. Costs and benefits of multidisciplinary medication review in a long-stay psychiatric ward. *Pharm J* 1992; 249: 102–3.

64. Kettis-Lindblad A, Isacson D, Eriksson C. Assessment of appropriateness of extemporaneous preparations prescribed in Swedish primary care. *Int J Pharm Pract* 1996; 4: 117–22.

65. Ekedahl A, Petersson B-A, Eklund P, *et al*. Prescribing patterns and drug costs:

effects of formulary recommendations and community pharmacists' information campaigns. *Int J Pharm Pract* 1994; 2: 194–8.

66. Th van de Poel G, Bruijnzeels M A, van der Does E, Lubsen J. A way of achieving more rational drug prescribing? *Int J Pharm Pract* 1991; 1: 45–8.

67. Anderson S. Measuring the performance of hospital pharmaceutical services: the Swedish experience. *J Soc Admin Pharm* 1993; 10: 92–8.

68. Braybrook S, Walker R. Influencing prescribing in primary care: a comparison of two different prescribing feedback methods. *J Clin Pharm Ther* 1996; 21: 247–54.

69. Newton-Syms F A O, Dawson P H, Cooke J, *et al.* The influence of a representative on prescribing by general practitioners. *Br J Clin Pharmacol* 1992; 33: 69–73.

70. Roughead E E, Gilbert A L, Primrose J G. Improving drug use: a case study of events which led to changes in use of flucloxacillin in Australia. *Soc Sci Med* 1999; 48: 845–53.

71. Kozyrskyj A L, Mustard C A. Validation of an electronic population-based prescription data-base. *Ann Pharmacother* 1998; 32: 1153.

72. Taheney K, Tyrrell A, Cairns C, Bunn R. Influence of patient focussed care on managing medicines for discharge. *Pharm J* 1999; 262: 368–71.

73. Ghalamkari H H, Rees J E, Saltrese-Taylor A, Ramsden M. Evaluation of a pilot health promotion project in pharmacies: 1. Quantifying the pharmacist's health promotion role. *Pharm J* 1997; 258: 138–43.

74. Choo G C C, Cook H. A community and hospital pharmacy discharge liaison service by fax. *Pharm J* 1997; 259: 659–61.

75. Elfellah M S, Jappy B M. Outcomes following discharge prescription monitoring by the ward pharmacist. *Pharm J* 1996; 257: 156–7.

76. Miles S A, Bourns I M. Resource implications of using patients' own drugs at discharge from hospital. *Pharm J* 1995; 254: 405–7.

77. Lindsay G H, Hesketh E A, Harden R M. Community pharmacy-based interactive patient education: 1. implementation, 2. pharmacist opinion. *Pharm J* 1994; 252: 541–4.

78. Hesketh A, Lindsay G, Harden R. Interactive health promotion in the community pharmacy. *Health Educ J* 1995; 54: 294–303.

79. Rogers P J, Fletcher G, Rees JE. Clinical interventions by community pharmacists using prescription medication records. *Int J Pharm Pract* 1994; 3: 6–13.

80. Beech E F, Barber N D. Ward pharmacy services: is a once daily visit less efficient than a twice daily visit? *Int J Pharm Pract* 1995; 3: 124–7.

81. Bond C M, Grimshaw J, Taylor R, Winfield A J. The evaluation of clinical guidelines to ensure appropriate 'over-the-counter' advice in community pharmacies: a preliminary study. *J Soc Admin Pharm* 1998; 15: 33–9.

82. Guerrero R M, Nickman N A, Jorgenson J A. Work activities before and after implementation of an automated dispensing system. *Am J Health Syst Pharm* 1996; 53: 548–54.

83. Sharma S, Anderson C. The impact of using pharmacy window space for health promotion about emergency contraception. *Health Educ J* 1998; 57: 42–50.

84. Cantrill J A, Vaezi L, Nicolson M, Noyce P R. A study to explore the feasibility

of using a health diary to monitor therapeutic outcomes from over-the-counter medicines. *J Soc Admin Pharm* 1995; 12: 190–8.

85. Beech E F, Barber N D. The development of a self-reporting multidimensional work sampling measure to study ward pharmacy services in the UK. *J Soc Admin Pharm* 1993; 10: 157–62.

86. Deshmukh A A, Eggleton A G, Monteath A J. Evaluation of ward pharmacy activity and effects of a change in non-stock ward supply. *Int J Pharm Pract* 1995; 3: 236–40.

87. Rutter P M, Hunt A J, Darracott R, Jones I F. A subjective study of how community pharmacists in Great Britain spend their time. *J Soc Admin Pharm* 1998; 15: 252–61.

88. Rutter P M, Hunt A J, Darracott R, Jones IF. Validation of a subjective evaluation study using work sampling. *J Soc Admin Pharm* 1999; 16: 174–85.

89. Emmerton L, Becket G, Gillbanks L. The application of electronic work sampling technology in New Zealand community pharmacy. *J Soc Admin Pharm* 1998; 15: 191–200.

90. Rutter P M, Brown D, Jones I F. Pharmacy research: the place of work measurement. *Int J Pharm Pract* 1998; 6: 46–58.

91. Savage I. The changing face of pharmacy practice – evidence from 20 years of work sampling studies. *Int J Pharm Pract* 1999; 7: 209–19.

92. Rees J A, Collett J H, Mylrea S, Crowther I. Subject-centred learning outcomes of structured work-based learning in a community pharmacy training programme. *Int J Pharm Pract* 1996; 4: 171–4.

93. Stapleton L J, Liddell H, Daly M J. Inhaler technique – a pilot study comparing verbal and computer counselling. *Pharm J* 1996; 256: 866–8.

94. Wilcock M, White M. Asthma training and the community pharmacist. *Pharm J* 1998; 260: 315–17.

95. Begley S, Livingstone C, Hodges N, Williamson V. Impact of domiciliary pharmacy visits on medication management in an elderly population. *Int J Pharm Pract* 1997; 5: 111–21.

96. Rivers P H. The impact of carers' attitudes on the safety of medication procedures in UK residential homes for the elderly. *J Soc Admin Pharm* 1995; 12: 132–43.

97. Bond C M, Williams A, Taylor R J, *et al.* An introduction to audit in Grampian: a basic course for pharmacists. *Pharm J* 1993; 250: 645–7.

98. Noble S C, MacDonald A. Monitoring of patient mediation records in two Scottish health board areas. *Pharm J* 1992; 249: 406–8.

99. Maponga C C, Nazerali H, Mungwindiri C, Wingwiri M. Cost implications of the tuberculosis/HIV co-epidemic and drug treatment of tuberculosis in Zimbabwe. *J Soc Admin Pharm* 1996; 13: 20–9.

100. Hughes C M, Turner K, Fitzpatrick C, *et al.* The use of a prescribing audit tool to assess the impact of a practice pharmacist in general practice. *Pharm J* 1999; 262: 27–30.

101. Sheridan J, Strang J, Lovell S. National and local guidance on services for drug misusers: do they influence practice? Results of a survey on community pharmacists in south-east England. *Int J Pharm Pract* 1999; 7: 100–6.

102. McCaig D J, Hind C A, Downie G, Wilkinson S. Antibiotic use in elderly hospital inpatients before and after the introduction of treatment guidelines. *Int J Pharm Pract* 1999; 7: 18–28.

103. Marriott J F. BNF recommendations on substitution: are they followed in practice? *Pharm J* 1999; 263: 289–92.

104. Laumann J M, Bjornson D C. Treatment of medicaid patients with asthma: comparison with treatment guidelines using disease-based drug utilisation review methodology. *Ann Pharmacother* 1998; 32: 1290–4.

105. Hawksworth G M, Chrystyn H. Therapeutic drug and biochemical monitoring in a community pharmacy: Part 1. *Int J Pharm Pract* 1995; 3: 133–8.

106. Hawksworth G M, Chrystyn H. Therapeutic drug and biochemical monitoring in a community pharmacy: Part 2. *Int J Pharm Pract* 1995; 3: 139–44.

107. Maguire T A, McElnay J C. Therapeutic drug monitoring in community pharmacy – a feasibility study. *Int J Pharm Pract* 1993; 2: 168–71.

108. Broderick W M, Purves I N, Edwards C. The use of biochemical screening in general practice – a role for pharmacists. *Pharm J* 1992; 249: 618–20.

109. Jaber L A, Halapy H, Fernet M, *et al.* Evaluation of a pharmaceutical care model on diabetes management. *Ann Pharmacother* 1996; 30: 238–43.

110. Deshmukh A A, Sommerville H. A pharmaceutical advisory service in a private nursing home: provision and outcome. *Int J Pharm Pract* 1996; 4: 88–93.

111. Schmader K E, Hanlon J T, Landsman P B, *et al.* Inappropriate prescribing and health outcomes in elderly veteran outpatients. *Ann Pharmacother* 1997; 31: 529–33.

112. Coast-Senior E A, Kronor B A, Kelley C L. Management of patients with type 2 diabetes by pharmacists in primary care clinics. *Ann Pharmacother* 1998; 32: 636–41.

113. Bowling A. *Measuring Health: a Review of Quality of Life Measurement Scales.* Buckingham: Open University Press, 1991.

114. Bowling A. *Measuring Disease: a Review of Disease-specific Quality of Life Measurement Scales.* Buckingham: Open University Press, 1995.

115. Pickard A S, Johnson J A, Farris K B. The impact of pharmacist interventions on health-related quality of life. *Ann Pharmacother* 1999; 33: 1167–72.

116. Scott K M, Sarfati D, Tobias M I, Haslett S J. A challenge to the cross-cultural validity of the SF-36 health survey: factor structure in Maori. Pacific and New Zealand European ethnic groups. *Soc Sci Med* 2000; 51: 1655–64.

117. Mount J K. Non-prescription drug use among high risk elderly patients. *J Soc Admin Pharm* 1991; 8: 25–34.

118. Bellingham M, Wiseman I C. Pharmacist intervention in an elderly care facility. *Int J Pharm Pract* 1996; 4: 25–9.

119. Caleo S, Benrimoj S, Collins D, *et al.* Clinical evaluation of community pharmacists' interventions. *Int J Pharm Pract* 1996; 4: 221–7.

120. Hopkinson P, Hutton J. Cost analysis of patient-controlled analgesia. *Pharm J* 1998; 260: 244–6.

121. Read R W, Krska J. Targeted medication review: patients in the community with chronic pain. *Int J Pharm Pract* 1998; 6: 216–22.

122. Aldrich S, Eccleston C. Making sense of everyday pain. *Soc Sci Med* 2000; 50: 1631–41.

123. Government White Paper. A first class service: quality in the new NHS. London: Department of Health, 1998.

124. Whitehead P, Atkin P, Krass I, Benrimoj S I. Patient drug information and consumer choice of pharmacy. *Int J Pharm Pract* 199; 7: 71–9.

125. Jackson J L, Chamberlain J, Kroenke K. Predictors of patient satisfaction. *Soc Sci Med* 2001; 52: 609–20.

126. Morrison A, Elliott L, Cowan L, *et al*. The Glasgow pharmacy summer protection campaign. *Pharm J* 1997; 258: 641–2.

127. Rees J K, Livingstone D J, Livingstone C R, Clarke C D. A community clinical pharmacy service for elderly people in residential homes. *Pharm J* 1995; 255: 54–6.

128. Wood K M, Mucklow J C, Boath E M. Influencing prescribing in primary care: a collaboration between clinical pharmacology and clinical pharmacy. *Int J Pharm Pract* 1997; 5: 1–5.

129. Langham J M, Boggs K S. The effect of a ward-based pharmacy technician service. *Pharm J* 2000; 264: 961–63.

130. Malek M. Glyceryl trinitrate sprays in the treatment of angina: a cost minimization study. *Pharm J* 1996; 257: 690–1.

131. Drummond M F, O'Brien B, Stoddart G L, Torrance G W. *Methods for the Economic Evaluation of Health Care Programmes*, 2nd edn. Oxford: Oxford University Press, 1997.

132. Rachlis A, Smaill F, Walker V, *et al*. Incremental cost-effectiveness analysis of intravenous ganciclovir versus oral ganciclovir in the maintenance treatment of newly diagnosed cytomegalovirus retinitis in patients with AIDS. *Pharmacoeconomics* 1999; 16: 71–84.

133. Sinclair H, Silcock J, Bond C M, *et al*. The cost-effectiveness of intense pharmaceutical intervention in assisting people to stop smoking. *Int J Pharm Pract* 1999; 7: 107–12.

134. March G, Gilbert A, Roughead E, Quintrell N. Developing and evaluating a model for pharmaceutical care in Australian community pharmacies. *Int J Pharm Pract* 1999; 7: 220–9.

135. Ryan M, Bond C. Using the economic theory of consumer surplus to estimate the benefits of dispensing doctors and prescribing pharmacists. *J Soc Admin Pharm* 1996; 13: 178–87.

136. Tordoff J M, Wright D. Analysis of the impact of community pharmacists providing formulary development advice to GPs. *Pharm J* 1999; 262: 166–8.

137. Wallenius K, Tuovinen K, Naaranlahti T, Enlund H. Savings at ward level through simplification of dose schedules. *Int J Pharm Pract* 1996; 4:55–8.

138. Smyth E T M, Barr J G, Hogg G M. Potential savings achieved through sequential, intravenous to non-parenteral, antimicrobial therapy. *Pharm J* 1998; 261: 170–2.

139. Avery A J, Rodgers S, Heron T, *et al*. A prescription for improvement? An observational study to identify how general practices vary in their growth in prescribing costs. *BMJ* 2000; 321: 276–81.

140. Semple J S, Morgan J E, Garner S T, *et al*. The effect of self-administration and reuse of patients' own drugs on a hospital pharmacy. *Pharm J* 1995; 255: 124–6.

141. Bowden J E. Reissuing patients' medicines – a step to seamless care. *Pharm J* 1993; 251: 356–7.

142. Hulls V, Emmerton L. Prescription interventions in New Zealand community pharmacy. *J Soc Admin Pharm* 1996; 13: 198–205.

143. Burtonwood A M, Hinchliffe A L, Tinkler G G. A prescription for quality: a role for the clinical pharmacist in general practice. *Pharm J* 1998; 261: 678–80.

144. Kettle J, Downie G, Palin A, Chesson R. Pharmaceutical care activities within a mental health team. *Pharm J* 1996; 256: 814–16.

145. Wood J, Bell D. Evaluating pharmacists' involvement in drug therapy decisions. *Pharm J* 1997; 259: 342–5.

146. Westerlund T, Almarsdottir A B, Melander A. Drug-related problems and pharmacy interventions in community practice. *Int J Pharm Pract* 1999; 7: 40–50.

147. Kinky D E, Erush S C, Laskin M S, Gibson G A. Economic impact of a drug information service. *Ann Pharmacother* 1999; 33: 11–16.

148. Eadon H. Assessing the quality of ward pharmacists' interventions. *Int J Pharm Pract* 1992; 1: 145–7.

149. Warholak T, Rupp M T, Salazar T A, Foster S. Effect of patient information on the quality of pharmacists' drug use decisions. *J Am Pharm Assoc* 2000; 40: 500–8.

150. Granas A, Bates I. The effect of pharmaceutical review of repeat prescriptions in general practice. *Int J Pharm Pract* 1999; 7: 264–75.

151. Woolfrey S, Asghar M N, Gray S, Gray A. Can community pharmacists provide a clinical pharmacy service to community hospitals? *Pharm J* 2000; 264: 109–11.

152. Western Australian Clinical Pharmacists Group. Recording clinical interventions: is there a better way. *Aust J Hosp Pharm* 1991; 21: 158–62. Cited in Krass I, Smith C. Impact of medication regimen reviews performed by community pharmacists for ambulatory patients through liaison with general medical practitioners. *Int J Pharm Pract* 2000; 8: 111–20.

153. Krass I, Smith C. Impact of medication regimen reviews performed by community pharmacists for ambulatory patients through liaison with general medical practitioners. *Int J Pharm Pract* 2000; 8: 111–20.

154. Corbett J. Provision of prescribing advice for nursing and residential home patients. *Pharm J* 1997; 259: 422–4.

155. Schmidt I K, Claesson C B, Westerholm B, Nilsson L G. Physician and staff assessments of drug interventions and outcomes in Swedish nursing homes. *Ann Pharmacother* 1998; 32: 27–32.

156. Lunn J, Chan K, Donoghue J, *et al*. A study of the appropriateness of prescribing in nursing homes. *Int J Pharm Pract* 1997; 5: 6–10.

157. Aparasu R R, Fliginger S E. Inappropriate medication prescribing for the elderly by office-based physicians. *Ann Pharmacother* 1997; 31: 823–9.

158. Hanlon J T, Scmader K E, Samsa G P, *et al*. A method for assessing drug therapy appropriateness. *J Clin Epidemiol* 1992; 45: 1045–51.

159. Fitzgerald L S, Hanlon J T, Shelton P S, *et al*. Reliability of a modified medication appropriateness index in ambulatory older persons. *Ann Pharmacother* 1997; 31: 543–8.

160. Volume C I, Burback L M, Farris K B. Reassessing the MAI: elderly people's

opinions about medication appropriateness. *Int J Pharm Pract* 1999; 7: 129–37.

161. Strang J, Sheridan J. Effect of Government recommendations on methadone prescribing in south-east England: a comparison of 1995 and 1997 surveys. *BMJ* 1998; 317: 1489–90.

162. Bangen M, Grave K. Introduction of a standard prescription form for drug prescribing to farmed fish in Norway. *J Soc Admin Pharm* 1995; 12: 159–62.

163. Rodgers S, Avery AJ, Meecham D, *et al*. Controlled trial of pharmacist intervention in general practice: the effect on prescribing costs. *Br J Gen Pract* 1999; 49: 717–20.

164. Serradell J, Bjornson D C, Hartzema A G. Drug utilization study methodologies: national and international perspectives. In: Hartzema A G, Porta M S, Tilson H H, eds. *Pharmacoepidemilogy: An Introduction*. Cincinnati: Harvey Whitney Books Co., 1988.

165. Duggan C, Feldman R, Hough J, Bates I. Reducing adverse prescribing discrepancies following hospital discharge. *Int J Pharm Pract* 1998; 6: 77–82.

166. Sexton J, Brown A. Problems with medicines following hospital discharge: not always the patient's fault. *J Soc Admin Pharm* 1999; 16: 199–207.

167. Bandolier: evidence-based health care. Number needed to treat. *Bandolier* 1999; 6(1): supplement i-iv.

168. Tully M P, Hassell K, Noyce P R. Advice-giving in community pharmacies in the UK. *J Health Serv Res Policy* 1997; 2: 38–50.

169. Taylor J, Greer M. NPM consultations: an analysis of pharmacist availability, accessibility and approachability. *J Soc Admin Pharm* 1993; 10: 101–8.

170. Morrow N, Hargie O, Donnelly H, Woodman C. 'Why do you ask?' A study of questioning behaviour in community pharmacist–client consultations. *Int J Pharm Pract* 1993; 2: 90–4.

171. Pilnick A. 'Why didn't you just say that?' Dealing with issues of asymmetry, knowledge and competence in the pharmacist/client encounter. *Sociol Health Illness* 1998; 20: 29–51.

172. Wilson M, Robinson E J, Blenkinsopp A, Panton R. Customers' recall of information given in community pharmacies. *Int J Pharm Pract* 1992; 1: 152–9.

173. Anderson C. Health promotion by community pharmacists: consumers' views. *Int J Pharm Pract* 1998;6:2–12.

174. Bower A, Eaton K. Evaluation of the effectiveness of a community pharmacy based smoking cessation programme. *Pharm J* 1999; 262: 514–15.

175. Grabenstein J D, Hartzema A G, Guess H A, Johnston W P. Community pharmacists as immunisation advocates: a pharmacoepidemiological experiment. *Int J Pharm Pract* 1993; 2: 5–10.

176. Totten C, Morrow N. Developing a training programme for pharmacists in coronary heart disease prevention. *Health Educ J* 1990; 49: 117–20.

177. Morrow N C, Benson M A. A self-instructional management course for pre-registration trainees. *Pharm J* 1993; 251: 288–90.

178. Sykes D, Westwood P. Training community pharmacists to advise GPs on prescribing. *Pharm J* 1997; 258: 417–19.

179. Collett J H, Rees J A, Crowther I, Mylrea S. A model for the development of work-based learning and its assessment. *Pharm J* 1995; 254: 556–8.

180. Batty R, Barber N, Moclair A, Shackle D. Assertion skills for clinical pharmacists. *Pharm J* 1993; 251: 353–5.
181. Sinclair H K, Bond C M, Lennox A S. The long-term learning effect of training in stage of change for smoking cessation: a three year follow-up of community pharmacy staff's knowledge and attitudes. *Int J Pharm Pract* 1999; 7: 1–11.
182. Binyon D. Pharmaceutical care: its impact on patient care and the hospital–community interface. *Pharm J* 1994; 253: 344–9.
183. Raynor D K, Booth T G, Blenkinsopp A. Effects of computer-generated reminder charts on patients' compliance with drug regimens. *BMJ* 1993; 306: 1158–61.
184. Lowe C J, Raynor D K, Courtney E A, *et al*. Effects of a self-medication programme on knowledge of drugs and compliance with treatment in elderly patients. *BMJ* 1995; 310: 1229–31.
185. Fairbrother J, Mottram D R, Williamson P M. The doctor–pharmacist interface: a preliminary evaluation of domiciliary visits by a community pharmacist. *J Soc Admin Pharm* 1993; 10: 85–91.
186. Krause G, Benzler J, Heinmuller R, *et al*. Performance of village pharmacies and patient compliance after implementation of an essential drug programme in rural Burkina Faso. *Health Policy Plann* 1998; 13: 159–66.
187. Grymonpre R E, Didur C D, Montgomery P R, Sitar D S. Pill count, self-report and pharmacy claims data to measure medication adherence in the elderly. *Ann Pharmacother* 1998; 32: 749–54.
188. Matsuyama J R, Mason B J, Jue S G. Pharmacists' interventions using an electronic medication-event monitoring device's adherence data versus pill counts. *Ann Pharmacother* 1993; 27: 851–5.
189. Kruger H S, Gerber J J. Health beliefs and compliance of Black South African outpatients with antihypertensive medication. *J Soc Admin Pharm* 1998; 15: 201–9.
190. Shaw H, Mackie C A, Sharki I. Evaluation of effect of pharmacy discharge planning on medication problems experienced by discharged acute admission mental health patients. *Int J Pharm Pract* 2000; 8: 144–53.
191. Abraham C, Clift S, Grabowski P. Cognitive predictors of adherence to malaria prophylaxis regimens on return from a malarious region: a prospective study. *Soc Sci Med* 1999; 48: 1641–54.
192. Ostrop N J, Hallett K A, Gill M J. Long term patient adherence to antiretroviral therapy. *Ann Pharmacother* 2000; 34: 703–9.
193. Steiner J F, Prochazka A V. The assessment of refill compliance using pharmacy records: methods, validity and applications. *J Clin Epidemiol* 1997; 50: 105–16.
194. Gregoire J-P, Guilbert R, Archambault A, Contandriopoulos A-P. Measurements of non-compliance to antihypertensive medication using pill counts and pharmacy records. *J Soc Admin Pharm* 1997; 14: 198–207.
195. Morgan M, Watkins C J. Managing hypertension: beliefs and responses to medication among cultural groups. *Sociol Health Illness* 1988; 10: 561–78.
196. Stimson G V. Obeying doctor's orders: a view from the other side. *Soc Sci Med* 1972; 8: 97–104.

197. Donovan J L, Blake D R. Patient non-compliance: deviance or reasoned decision-making. *Soc Sci Med* 1992; 34: 507–13.
198. Conrad P. The meaning of medicines; another look at compliance. *Soc Sci Med* 1985; 20: 29–37.
199. Nichol M B, Venturini F, Sung J G Y. A critical evaluation of the methodology of the literature on medication compliance. *Ann Pharmacother* 1999; 33: 531–40.

Index